Nutripoints

HEALTHY EATING MADE SIMPLE!

Dr. Roy Vartabedian & KATHY MATTHEWS

FOREWORD BY KENNETH H. COOPER, M.D.

NUTRIPOINTS

CAN WORK FOR YOU TOO!

"The Nutripoints Program seems to be exactly what I need to have a healthy lifestyle. I hate the thought of counting calories, mainly because I never felt I was getting the proper combinations of foods. Nutripoints makes counting so easy, maybe some day products will be labeled with Nutripoints."

Bonnie Moeller

Indianapolis, Indiana

"I have enjoyed your book and keep it with me at all times. I have lost 50 pounds and finally feel I am getting a balanced diet. I teach 6th grade and use your information in class."

Ron Roberson

Inman, South Carolina

"I am hooked on the Nutripoints Program! Thank you for your inspiration to start a healthful, safe and permanent eating plan."

Riva Rosenfeld

North York, Ontario

"I've been on your Nutripoints Program for about three weeks and I'm surprised at the extra energy it has developed; I'm *73. Nutripoints* has become a daily reference work in our home."

James L. Jones

Allen Park, Michigan

"It is fascinating, positive and addictive. So several of us are about to get compulsive about counting Nutripoints. Thank you, and thank you."

Ellen M. Davis, et al.

The Winston School

Dallas, Texas

"I have been on your diet for six weeks and feel great. Before I started I didn't have much energy and felt twice my age. Thanks for saving my life."

Marilyn Hofmeister

Renton, Washington

Neither the Nutripoints concept nor this book is sponsored or affiliated with Nutri/System, Inc., or the Nutri/System® Weight Loss Program.

Designs for Wellness Press
P.O. Box 1671
Carlsbad, CA 92018

ISBN: 0-9641952-3-2.

Fifth Edition: October, 2005

Cover design artist: George Foster, Foster Covers, www.fostercovers.com

A hardcover edition of this book was published in 1990 by Harper & Row Publishers, Inc., ISBN 0-06-106275-9. First printing of paperback edition published in 1991 by *HarperCollins Publishers*, ISBN 0-06-109917-1.

Printed in United States of America

Visit our website: http://www.Nutripoints.com

TO MY GRANDMA, LOUISE VARTABEDIAN

It was my Grandma Louise's energy, positive attitude, and zest for living, combined with her compelling interest in foods that were "poisons" or "wonder foods" that inspired me to undertake nutrition and health science as my life's work. Grandma Louise lived well into her eighties. My wish is that you may benefit from the culmination of my grandmother's inspiration—Nutripoints—and that by following its principles you may enjoy as full and long a life as she did.

CONTENTS

FORWARD

Nutrition in the 21st Century is more sophisticated and more scientific than ever before. No longer do we guess at whether we are getting optimal nutrition; we will measure it accurately.

In 1968 I developed a simple and easy-to-follow point system for exercise called "aerobic" points. It revolutionized our concept of exercise. Now, at last, the same thing has been done for nutrition. A simple and easy-to-follow point system has been developed that has permanently changed the way we look at foods and nutrition.

After painstaking research and development using the Cooper Clinic Nutrition Database at the Aerobics Center, among others, Dr. Roy Vartabedian has formulated the Nutripoint rating system. Nutripoints, based on nutrient density, precisely quantifies the quality of 3,600 common foods by carefully comparing each food, nutrient by nutrient, to RDA standards. In addition, the system adjusts for cholesterol, sodium, total and saturated fat, sugar, caffeine, and alcohol in each food. The result is *one number* that, taking into account all these factors, tells you the bottom-line nutritional value of the food. I believe that Nutripoints will promote a major change in the American diet and will be an enormous help to everyone interested in avoiding "life-style" diseases, particularly heart disease and cancer.

A balanced program for total well-being must make nutrition its cornerstone. Nutripoints simplifies the complexities of nutrition with a point system that helps you compare foods and track your progress. The system has been used with tremendous success at the Cooper Wellness Programs at the Aerobics Center, and I'm convinced that, coupled with an effective exercise program, it can help you achieve a healthier, happier life.

Kenneth H. Cooper, M.D.

ACKNOWLEDGMENTS

I owe a debt of gratitude to Dr. Kenneth Cooper for his assistance in making this book possible. Dr. Cooper's application of a point system to exercise in his landmark book, ***Aerobics***, inspired me to apply this simple, practical concept to nutrition. In addition, his support in allowing me to devote time and energy to this book while directing the Cooper Wellness Programs at the Aerobics Center made the project possible. By introducing me to his literary agent, Herbert M. Katz, he made this book a reality. I am deeply indebted to Herb Katz. In addition to undertaking the standard responsibilities as the agent for ***Nutripoints***, Herb acted as the "godfather" of the book from its inception, becoming its first champion and promoter as well as a thoughtful and discerning reader. His guidance throughout the publishing process has been invaluable.

Bill Shinker of Harper & Row has been a galvanizing force. His marketing vision and energetic commitment to ***Nutripoints*** have from the beginning made my association with his company an exciting experience.

Larry Ashmead, my editor at Harper & Row, has provided the enthusiasm that has kept ***Nutripoints*** on course right from the beginning. His immediate appreciation of the book's concept and his unflagging support have been greatly appreciated.

Margaret Wimberger, Eamon Dolan, and Anne McCoy, of the editorial staff of Harper & Row, have been meticulous readers and have contributed greatly to the ultimate cohesion of the book.

I would also like to thank Karen Mender, Linda Michaels, Brenda Segel, Steve Magnuson, and Martin Weaver, all of Harper & Row, for their support, hard work, and dedication to this book.

My thanks to Mike Smith and Suzan Lewis, founders of Constructive Solutions, for their hard work. Many of the mathematical formulations and computations for ***Nutripoints*** were completed efficiently and accurately through their efforts, contributing to the book's scientific validity.

Kathleen Duran, R.D., now Director of Nutrition at the Cooper Wellness Programs, supplied many of the menus and recipes for ***Nutripoints***, culling them from the recipes she developed in the Programs. She also acted as my nutritional consultant.

Ava Halleran, M.S., Associate Director of the Cooper Wellness Programs, is my able associate who helped keep things running smoothly in the Programs and allowed me to focus on applying the Nutripoints principles with participants.

Susan Hill, my data-processing specialist, performed the Herculean task of plugging 50,000 pieces of information into the computer in order to analyze the more than 3,000 foods found in the original version of *Nutripoints.*

Thanks to my wife Renée, and son, Alex who patiently gave up of their time with me as I worked long hours compiling my research and writing revisions to update the book for the latest version. Renée also assisted with the book editing, ideas and support along the way, and helps me personally get all my *Nutripoints* at home with her excellent food choices, new recipes, and great cooking!

A WORD FROM DR. VARTABEDIAN

When I was growing up, my Grandmother Louise was the "health nut" of the family. She read "Prevention" magazine, all of Adele Davis' books, and often spoke of foods that were "miracle foods" or "poisons". Each morning she took a bottle-full of supplements and made a cereal that contained blackstrap molasses, brewer's yeast, and wheat germ. It smelled *horrible*, and most of our family thought she was a health *fanatic!* Everyone, that was, except me—because she was the most positive, energetic, enthusiastic person I knew, and I wanted to be just like her! Grandma Louise loved life so much that she wanted us to freeze her body after she died so we could bring her back later when a cure was found! She was the one who inspired me to go into the nutrition and health field, and to set a personal goal to live to be at least 100—and to help as many others come along with me as possible.

My questions to Grandma were endless, "Is this food good for you?", "What about this one?" Grandma became so tired of answering my questions that one unforgettable day she said, "Roy, if it's a food, it's good for you!" With that, my individual quest began to find out *which were the best foods for the human body* that could help people live to 100.

I continued learning as much as possible before attending Andrews University in Berrien Springs, Michigan, where in 3 years I earned a Bachelors Degree in the dual majors of Health Science and Business Administration. Prepared for graduate school, I was accepted at Loma Linda University in southern California. There, I powered ahead and in another 3 years completed my Master of Public Health degrees in Health Education and Nutrition, and a Doctorate of Public Health degree in Preventive Care.

Ready to apply my knowledge, my work in the Family Practice Residency at Florida Hospital in Orlando commenced, and I hit a *brick wall!* My job was to teach Family Practice Residents (new doctors) about Patient Education and Preventive Medicine. The only problem was that I was 24 years old and they had little interest in *preventing* illnesses—they were focused on *treating* them!

After 4 years of working with the doctors in the residency program, we had converted about half of them to the philosophy of wellness and teaching patients how to do their part in keeping healthy. How did we do it? By incorporating a mandatory 1-month rotation in my program where we focused on health improvement for the doctors *personally.* Once they tasted the success of personal health change and total wellness, they were ready to motivate others to do the same. It was rewarding to know that we had started a positive ripple that would emanate outward to the thousands of patients these doctors would see during the life of their practices!

It was during my stay at Florida Hospital from 1980 to 1985 when I began working on the first version of *Nutripoints*. The more I educated my patients about all of the things they needed to keep track of in food to stay healthy, the more frustrated they became. They wanted a simpler way to figure it all out. They asked me the same questions I had asked my grandmother years earlier—then I knew how she felt! Thus, *Nutripoints* was born and was in it's infant stages.

From there I had the wonderful opportunity of working with Dr. Kenneth Cooper, the greatest pioneer in Preventive Medicine of our time, to spearhead a new live-in program aimed at helping people jump-start their life to a healthier lifestyle. I refined the *Nutripoints* analysis and expanded the food database while testing aspects of the program with the live-in participants. The early versions were enthusiastically welcomed and this encouraged me to perfect the whole program and write the first version of this book which was published in 1990.

The book was a runaway best-seller and spread to 13 countries in 10 languages. I was excited and overwhelmed at the same time! My idea inspired by my grandmother had reached fruition and was now helping others answer the questions they had about the best foods. Later that year, I left the Cooper Clinic to start my own company aimed at educating the masses about designing their lives for wellness and optimal health.

For the past 15 years and 5 editions later, that's just what I have been doing—and loving every minute of it! As for myself, I am married now to my beautiful and wonderful wife, Renée, who is a chiropractor from Palmer College with a prevention-oriented philosophy of health very similar to mine. She has contributed to the information in this book and has been a guiding force, enthusiastic supporter, and facilitator of the evolution of the *Nutripoints* concept. Our young son, Alex, has the best chance of being healthy and living to be 100 of anyone I know. He reminds me of Grandma Louise so much with his happy demeanor, high energy, enthusiasm and love for life. We hope he follows in our footsteps to help others achieve optimal health when he, "grows up into a big man", as he says!

I hope to see you someday at a seminar or hear from you in a letter telling me how *Nutripoints* has impacted your life, or ideas you have to make the system work better for you. My ultimate goal is to help you increase the quality of your life, and the quantity of your years!

Roy E. Vartabedian, Dr.P.H.

Nutripoints guidelines and recommendations were developed for the average healthy adult free from disease or major risk factors. Physical variations from individual to individual may necessitate modifications of the book's suggestions. As always, common sense must be used when following a certain program or regime, and extremes must be avoided. Before starting any nutrition or exercise program, you should consult a physician who will supervise your overall program. None of the information presented here should supersede your physician's or dietitian's advice. If you experience any adverse health effects while on the ***Nutripoints*** program, check with your physician or dietitian.

PART I

INTRODUCTION

A WORD FROM KATHY MATTHEWS

The words ***REVOLUTIONARY** and **BREAKTHROUGH*** are so commonplace these days that when something that truly earns these descriptions comes along we're left tongue-tied. ***How do you describe a nutritional system that replaces counting calories, worrying over fats, sugar, and sodium, calculating cholesterol, and figuring out RDAs—a system that does all this, and more, with a single number that tells you all you need to know to maintain a healthy diet?***

Revolutionary, it certainly is.

A breakthrough, unquestionably.

In the same week that I met Dr. Vartabedian, creator of Nutripoints, I received a frantic phone call from a friend. I've known Carol since college and we've been through the diet wars together. About twenty pounds overweight, she had just decided to go on a simple, safe, low-calorie diet—one of those popular diets I'm sure you've heard of. She had also just visited her doctor who, because of her family medical history, had warned her that she must make a serious effort to get plenty of calcium in her diet. He also warned her to avoid cholesterol-rich foods, such as whole milk and other dairy products. He said that the diet she planned to use was a good one but that she should be careful not to skimp on the recommended protein: adequate protein was essential if she wanted to lose weight safely and permanently.

Carol is a motivated and intelligent bank vice president. She is quite sophisticated in her knowledge of nutrition, but her head was spinning. "Kathy," she said on the phone, "this isn't getting easier, it's getting harder. I want to lose weight but I don't want to have to become a professional dietitian. You've written two books on nutrition that were best-sellers. What can I eat?"

I promised to help Carol but I knew that it would be a complicated and relatively tedious task. She needed high-quality protein that was low in fat and cholesterol and probably a lot of green vegetables, some of which would help her obtain her calcium requirement. Would a broiled, skinless breast of chicken be a better choice than a broiled veal chop? And what about the days when Carol had no time to cook; were there any frozen, prepared meals that were really good, nutritionally speaking? Was it really possible to get in a full day's nutrition—all the vitamins and minerals as well as adequate protein and carbohydrates—on a low-fat, low-calorie diet? When you came right down to it, what *were* the best foods to eat? Carol's words rang in my ears and I realized that despite, or perhaps because of, the constant flood of nutritional information, finding your way through the food maze just isn't getting any easier.

Then I met Dr. Vartabedian, a nutritional pioneer who has assimilated a great deal of contradictory data, and who has gone a step beyond anyone in his field. Dr. Vartabedian had already helped nearly a thousand patients grappling with the same problems faced by my friend Carol, and who, like Carol, are intelligent, self-motivated readers of dozens of books and articles that have put them on a nutritional seesaw, trying to balance the benefits and disadvantages inherent in any given food. For example:

- A food is high in calcium but also high in fat (whole dairy products).
- A food is low in fat but high in sodium (crackers, canned soups, pickles).
- A food is high in protein but also high in cholesterol (many types of meat).
- A food is low in cholesterol but high in saturated, or "bad," fat (margarines, palm oil, coconut oil).
- A food is low in calories but not very nutritious (iceberg lettuce, celery, diet drinks).

When I recited the litany of seemingly contradictory nutritional recommendations that confuse us all, Dr. Vartabedian acknowledged the confusion as the inspiration for Nutripoints. The following pages contain Dr. Vartabedian's explanation of the Nutripoint concept and how it works.

"UPDATE OVERLOAD" AND THE CONFUSED CONSUMER

I think it is wonderful that nutritional updates have become fixtures in the news. Unfortunately, in my experience as a nutritionist who has seen thousands of patients over the course of a career, the result of all this information is confusion. If a research finding doesn't help you in the kitchen or at the dining table, where it really counts, it can't do you any good.

When I was a student of nutrition, all my questions about the body and the foods that fuel it were readily answered by my distinguished professors. Nutrition on the molecular level, while complicated, is relatively straightforward. It was only when I began my practice that things became almost intolerably confusing, a confusion reflected in the case histories that follow:

- Mary had read in a women's magazine that if she didn't eat enough protein while trying to diet, she would lose muscle rather than fat and so regain any lost weight very quickly. But how much was enough protein? And didn't protein come mainly from meat and have a lot of fat? How could she find protein that didn't have a lot of calories?

• Roberta ate out at restaurants all the time. She knew the principles of good nutrition (avoid fried foods and creamy sauces, and so on), but what were the best, and most healthful, foods on a typical restaurant menu? Was fresh grilled tuna better or worse than baked flounder? What about a small, very lean baked pork chop compared to a few slices of lean baked ham?

• James had suffered two heart attacks and was on a low-cholesterol diet, but he frequently had to eat at restaurants and just didn't know which foods, particularly meats, were low in cholesterol. He used to think that shrimp was OK, but now he wasn't sure. Everything he read about "good" and "bad" cholesterol confused him even more.

• Ted called himself a "businessman/athlete." He jogged every morning and was in training for a local triathlon competition. He knew he needed to eat well, but he resorted to fast food all the time because he didn't like to cook. Was he getting enough of the right types of foods? Was a Celentano Chicken Primavera entree that he could cook quickly in the microwave a good nutritional choice? How would it compare with, say, a Mrs. Paul's Light and Natural Flounder Fillet?

• Barbara had three kids who were very picky eaters. She knew that it was important for them to get proper nutrition in their growing years, but their eating habits were so erratic she had no confidence that she was having any success. If they loved peanut butter and jelly sandwiches, was that better or worse than a tuna sandwich? She avoided buying breakfast cereals with a lot of sugar, but aside from that, was one brand really better than another in terms of nutrition?

• Lori and her husband had retired and faced many of the nutritional problems of the elderly: they had diminished appetites and had to carefully watch cholesterol and fat intake. Because they were eating less, they had to be particularly careful to get adequate nutrition. Lori wanted to know if those substitute foods such as Egg Beaters and Molly McButter were really OK to use. And would a vitamin pill take care of them on those days when they skipped a meal?

• Phil found himself eating at fast-food restaurants at least five times a week because they were quick and convenient. But what type of nutrition was he getting from this kind of food? Was a McDonald's Quarter Pounder better or worse than a Jack in the Box Beef Fajita Pita? What were *the best* fast foods in terms of nutritional value?

These people came to me, as an expert, with their very real and pressing questions, and I found it difficult to answer them. Most of us know what foods are "good" for us; no one would argue that a carrot or an orange is not "good." And we also feel fairly comfortable pinpointing "bad" foods; fried pork rinds and fudge sauce would be picked out of any list of suspects by just about anyone. But what about all those foods in between "good" and "bad"? How do you judge them? There was no gradient scale that could measure whether an apple was better than an orange or a fried pork rind worse than a strip of fried bacon. *Were* there any dairy foods that were low in fat and high in calcium? *Were* high-fiber breakfast cereals, particularly oat bran, really good nutritional choices? *Were* some "good" vegetables better than other "good" vegetables?

These questions frustrated me as well as my patients. I realized that it was very easy to tell people what *not* to eat, but much harder to tell them what they *should* eat. Indeed, there was an entire spectrum of food values from very good to very bad, but there was no way to measure anything between those extremes. No one believed you could compare apples and oranges, and no one had tried.

There was another factor involved. Suzanne put her finger on it for me when she came to see me about getting sufficient calcium in her pregnancy diet, while avoiding too many unnecessary calories (a very common concern).

"Dr. Vartabedian," she complained, "I'm really interested in nutrition and good food. And of course"—she gestured toward her growing waistline—"never more so than now. But lately I've noticed that every time I think about food I feel anxious. Is it good for me? Good for the baby? Is it really nutritious? Does it have too much fat? Do embryos need to restrict their cholesterol intake?

"Sometimes I'm jealous of my mother, who never worried about palm oil in her crackers, and just ate what she wanted and tried not to eat too much. I read recently that stress increases your cholesterol level. If that's true, it made me wonder if we aren't all taking one step forward and two steps back: we are so worried about how to eat right that even when we *do* eat the right things, our cholesterol levels are going up anyhow from anxiety."

Suzanne's feelings about food and eating had, over a period of years, gone from blithe unconcern, except for calories, to anxiety: diet anxiety. She knew a lot about food, but she didn't know enough to put it all together.

Suzanne was an inspiration to me. Her words rang in my ears long after her healthy baby was born and I'd moved to a fascinating job at Dr. Kenneth Cooper's Aerobics Center in Dallas. The center offers the most comprehensive, state-of-the-art wellness programs available in the world, and it gave me the opportunity to work with one of the most advanced nutritional data bases available. I knew that there must be a solution to Suzanne's dilemma—diet anxiety—and I set about to find it.

Over the course of years, working with hundreds of patients, I finally refined a system that I believe answers *all* of today's perplexing nutritional questions. It's a system that not only tells you which foods are good and which are bad but also establishes a gradient scale that measures all foods. Not only does it rate all foods, it provides a simple system that gives you an optimally balanced diet, one that allows you the luxury of choice.

Nutripoints is my answer to all the patients whose questions I had so painstakingly researched. Nutripoints is the tool that will allow them, and anyone else interested in good nutrition, to find an optimum diet.

We should not be confused about food. Above all, we should not be anxious about what we eat. My hope is that Nutripoints will be a giant step toward returning us to safe, pleasurable, healthful eating.

THE NUTRIPOINTS REVOLUTION

The Nutripoints program is something very different from anything you've come across. It is an actual nutritional advance and a quantum leap in our ability to know that we are eating healthful meals. It will provide you with an entirely new approach to eating. Here are the four revolutionary features of the Nutripoint program that make it so effective and appealing:

1. Nutripoints is the only nutritional information you'll ever need.

Nutripoints assures you that you will meet or exceed all the major nutritional guidelines—including those of the American Heart Association, the American Cancer Society, the National Cancer Institute, and the American Dietetic Association—regarding daily intakes of every major nutrient, including protein, carbohydrates, fiber, vitamins, and minerals, while at the same time staying well below the allowable levels of fat, cholesterol, sugar, and sodium.

Have you ever stood in the supermarket trying to figure out what grams of fat mean in terms of calories? Have you ever wondered what it means when a packaged food provides 100 percent of your daily requirement of one vitamin and 0 percent of everything else? Have you been on diets that you later learned were damaging to your health, even though they might be effective? Do you get confused about whether 1-percent or 2-percent milk is better for you in terms of fat content? And do you know which cheeses are lowest in cholesterol?

Before Nutripoints, you would have had to do twenty-six mathematical calculations on each food you eat to have only the *basis* for the information Nutripoints gives in one number.

Now you can forget about calories, grams of fat, and milligrams of sodium—and even forget about reading labels. And you don't have to abandon hope when you go to a fast-food restaurant. Nutripoints weighs *all* the bad factors in a food against *all* the good factors, and comes up with a simple number that tells you everything you need to know to provide the human machine with the best possible fuel.

Say you're choosing among juices. Here is a small sample of the Nutripoint ratings for juices:

Juice	***Nutripoints***
Unsweetened grapefruit juice	11.0
Minute Maid frozen orange juice	10.0
Dole pineapple juice	5.0
Ocean Spray Cranapple juice	1.5
Lucky Leaf apple juice	1.0

A quick glance at this chart tells you that canned pineapple juice is only half as good as orange juice. And some brands of apple juice are only one-fifth as good as some brands of orange juice. The Nutripoint charts make it easy to choose a juice that you and your family like, as well as a juice that provides good nutrition. You don't even have to know the scientific basis for the Nutripoint score, namely, that those with a higher number contain more vitamin C and less sugar than the juices with a lower score.

Now let's say you're choosing a cereal. Here are the numbers for just a few:

Cereal	*Nutripoints*
Whole Wheat Total	64.5
Kellogg's Product 19	56.0
Nabisco 100% Bran Cereal	31.0
Quaker Oat Squares	17.0
Kellogg's Special K	14.0
Kellogg's Fruit Loops	13.0
Post Cocoa Pebbles	7.5
Quaker 100% Natural cereal	1.0

The general trend with cereals is that the more sugar and processing that come into play and the original whole food, if any, is adulterated, the lower the level of nutrition. Consequently, cereals scoring high on the scale contain more bran or whole grain as well as less sugar (and possibly more added vitamins) than the others. Once again, if you're concerned with good nutrition, you need only look for the high numbers to find the best choices.

Whether you're choosing between broccoli or Brussels sprouts, snapper or salmon, cheddar or goat cheese, or even Mars Bars or Milky Ways and Chicken McNuggets or Big Macs, *Nutripoints* is your good-food bible.

2. Nutripoints is the first positive approach to nutrition that eliminates rigid adhesion to menus and meal plans, because the balance is "built in."

Any diet in the past has had to rely on various meal plans that sometimes got pretty complicated. That's because there was no other way to ensure that people would get the right balance of foods. You can't just eat low-calorie foods and be well nourished: you need to eat from a broad spectrum of foods. The best diets were well constructed: someone figured out how much fat, protein, complex carbohydrates, and so forth were in each food and in each meal and made sure that these amounts were adequate. But you had to follow a very specific daily menu plan or a complicated system of "substitutions" in order to maintain a nutritional balance. Nutripoints makes that rigid approach history because it provides *a comprehensive system* that allows you to create your own meal plans. By following the recommendations concerning numbers of servings from the six Nutrigroups, you'll be guaranteed an optimum diet—one of your own choosing.

Though you'll find menus for those who need and/or want them, the Nutripoint program is totally flexible. Once you're familiar with Nutripoints, you need only focus on the foods you like and the foods that are readily available to you to create meals that give you the best possible nutritional value. You won't be shopping for fish to broil on a day that you're really in a mood for pasta. I've even provided some lists of the best nutritional values, in terms of your food budget, which will help you achieve an optimum diet on limited funds.

Once you're familiar with Nutripoints, you'll find it will become an instinctive way of eating. Best of all, you'll find that simply by choosing your foods from the top of the Nutripoint charts, and getting the recommended servings from every Nutrigroup, you'll be getting at least 100 percent of the RDA (Recommended Daily Allowance) for every vitamin and mineral, as well as the optimum amount of fiber, protein, carbohydrates, and fat. You'll also be limiting your total fat, saturated fat, cholesterol, sugar, sodium, caffeine, and alcohol intake.

Hundreds of Nutripoint converts agree that it's the best remedy for diet anxiety.

3. Nutripoints not only lets you know what's bad, it separates the best from the merely good.

Most foods have some bad things in them as well as some good. But how much bad and how much good? How do you evaluate this difference? Dairy foods seem to be particularly confusing today because of a very real concern about calcium. People know they need to get adequate calcium, but the foods that are very high in calcium, such as milk and cheese, are also very high in fat. Nutripoints eliminates the confusion. The higher the Nutripoint score, the lower in fat *and* the higher in calcium is the rated food. *Evaluating the critical differences in foods is what Nutripoints is all about.*

Here's an illustration of how processing lowers the Nutripoint score of a particular food.

4. Nutripoints allows for recovery from "being bad."

We've become so chained to the "calories per day" or "fat per day" notion of nutrition that it's a relief to substitute the Nutripoints concept, which deals with *real* nutrition in the real world. The fact is, in terms of nutrition, a day is a very short time frame. For example, your body stores vitamin A for weeks. With the Nutripoints program you no longer have to think about a twenty-four-hour make-it-or-break-it eating pattern: you can spread things out over the course of a few days. Although, for the sake of convenience, you'll still be aiming for a daily total of at least 100 points, you can be flexible enough to go over or under on any given day and make up for the lack within another day or two.

Because Nutripoints gives you a way of *measuring* the values of the foods you eat, it gives you an opportunity to get back on track if you fall behind.

Nutripoints is such a simple "numbers game" with negative and positive numbers that if you have a really bad day in which you eat the wrong foods—a day with a negative total of Nutripoints—you can still wind up with an excellent nutritional week.

This expansion of the basic diet time frame removes one of the most persistent and discouraging psychological barriers to effective dieting—the old "I've blown it today, so I might as well forget it" rationale.

FUTURE FOODS

You're probably aware that the foods you eat are very different from those eaten by your grandparents. What determines how "food styles" change? Agricultural trends, food storage, and distribution methods all have some effect, but a big determinant is simple fashion. It's no longer fashionable, for example, for a woman or man to display wealth with girth. It made cultural sense, once upon a time, to achieve status with the evidence of rich and lavish meals. The lean and hungry peasant would look with longing at the tubby lord. Today that trend is fully reversed: for years now people have believed that you can never be too thin or too rich.

In addition to fashion, there are practical reasons for a constantly changing and diverse national diet. A farmer, faced with a day of work from sunrise to sunset, is going to have nutritional needs that differ substantially from those of a stockbroker or a bank teller. The latter simply don't need the greater amounts of fuel required by a body that's doing hard labor.

The great nutritional challenge we face today can be simply stated. Our optimum diet has two principles that seem diametrically opposed: we need to get high levels of nutrients (to keep our bodies functioning well while helping them to fight the effects of disease, aging, and pollution), and we need to achieve this in fewer and fewer calories (to avoid excess weight that affects our appearance and our health).

These needs force us to scrutinize our foods in a new way. If we want to achieve optimum health and longevity we have to think about *nutrients per calorie.*

Nutrients per calorie is the basic cost/benefit analysis we have to keep in mind when we choose foods. It's analogous to our efforts to get the most value per dollar when buying a product. Because we are usually limiting our calorie intake, every calorie has to count in terms of overall nutritional value. Here's an example: there is ample vitamin C in half an avocado, but it will "cost" 160 calories, while a cup of grapefruit juice has nine times the vitamin C of the avocado at a "cost" of only 95 calories.

This concept of nutrients per calorie explains why junk foods are *junk:* they provide virtually no nutrition and a lot of calories. Take, for example, a typical fast-food lunch: a Big Mac with a large order of fries and a Coke. This meal gives you only 25 to 40 percent of major nutrients at a cost of 1,064 calories. For many people that's the *total* number of calories they should have in a day, and they wouldn't have gotten *half* their necessary nutrients. With Nutripoints, you can get over 100 percent of any RDA, along with optimum amounts of fiber, protein, and complex carbohydrates, with *the same* number of calories. You must remember, also, that it costs vitamins and minerals to burn up calories. If you're not getting adequate nutrients along with the calories you're burning up, the body's stores of vitamins and minerals must be called upon to make up for the lack in the food itself. This is the not uncommon predicament that can lead to clinical or subclinical deficiencies and less-than-optimal function of various body processes.

A high nutrient-per-calorie ratio is the basic principle of every healthful diet. *Nutripoints* rates every food on the basis of this critical nutrient-per-calorie ratio. Moreover, because *Nutripoints* rates just about every conceivable food, it allows you to create your own diet, one that suits your tastes and your lifestyle.

NUTRIPOINT NUMBERS

Nutripoints is a very simple way of dealing with something very complex. It is a number system for rating foods. The Nutripoint program has 4 important principles:

Nutripoint Values

Each food has a given Nutripoint value. It is amazingly simple: the higher the Nutripoint score of a given food, the higher it is in "good" components (including all the important vitamins and minerals, and fiber and protein), and the lower it is in "bad" components (including calories, cholesterol, total fat, saturated fat, sodium, sugar, caffeine, and alcohol). Just about every food imaginable, including basic foods, processed foods, fast foods, and even "health" foods, have been evaluated and assigned a number.

Some foods fall in a "not recommended" level and some foods are so low in Nutripoints that they have negative Nutripoint values—such as Mars Bars at −3.5 Nutripoints. Nutripoint values are provided for *all* types of foods, even poor nutritional choices. This is the way in which Nutripoints differs from typical diets. *All foods are evaluated in terms of Nutripoints.* This allows you to compare the bad with the good as well as the good with the best.

A glance at the Nutripoints for various foods is an eye-opener. For instance, we all know the old adage about an apple a day, but did you know that cantaloupe is a far better choice? In the fruit Nutrigroup, although both are "good" for you, one-quarter cantaloupe has 29 Nutripoints whereas an apple has only 4.5. The cantaloupe has fewer calories (50 versus 80) and more iron, fifty times the vitamin A, ten times the vitamin C, more folacin, thiamine, and riboflavin, and more of virtually every other nutrient than the apple. Spinach (75 Nutripoints) is a much better vegetable than plain iceberg lettuce (18 Nutripoints), even though both are low in calories.

Many people are surprised to learn that some cuts of lean beef are better choices than some types of fish. For example, lean round steak (4 Nutripoints) is a better choice than baked flounder (3.5 Nutripoints). Many people wouldn't guess that three ounces of lean, baked ham (5 Nutripoints) is a better choice than a three-ounce, lean, broiled hamburger (3 Nutripoints). Broccoli (38.5 Nutripoints) is a terrific nutritional value compared to a baked potato (8.5 Nutripoints).

As I mentioned, there are negative Nutripoints, and there's also a cut-off point below which foods are not recommended. The numbers are interesting just as a basis of comparison between foods, but you also need them to figure out your daily Nutripoint scores.

Nutripoint Quotas

The numbers assigned to foods have to be put into a workable context: what do they really add up to? You can't just eat a few servings of spinach a day and get a lot of Nutripoints and consider yourself well nourished. There has to be a balance of different types of foods over a period of time.

The Nutripoint program recommends that you get at least 100 Nutripoints per day, which will give you approximately 100 percent of the RDAs. Not only will you get the necessary amounts of eighteen important nutrients, you will at the same time limit the calories, sugar, cholesterol, total fat, saturated fat, sodium, caffeine, and alcohol in your diet—in one easy step helping to prevent and help control heart disease, hypertension, diabetes, obesity, osteoporosis, cancer, and other lifestyle diseases.

Here's how Patrick, a salesman, rated on a typical day before he began the Nutripoint program:

Patrick's Diet

Food	*Nutripoints*
Breakfast	
2 fried eggs	– 25.0
3 strips fried bacon	– 1.0
1 cup coffee	– 3.5
1 Danish	– 2.5
Lunch	– 2.0
McDonald's Big Mac	
French fries	– 2.0
Coke	– 6.0
Dinner	0.0
3 pieces fried chicken	
½ cup mashed potatoes	2.0
with gravy	0.0
Salad	33.0
with dressing	– 2.5
Total:	**– 9.5**

You can readily see that –9.5 Nutripoints is a very poor score for a day if the goal is at least 100 points. It means that Patrick is probably eating far too much fat, sodium, and calories, and is not getting nearly enough fiber and nutrients. A daily diet with a Nutripoint total in this range could spell the beginning of future health problems, as well as minor immediate symptoms. Patrick probably would complain of headaches, general sluggishness, digestive problems, inability to concentrate, and afternoon fatigue.

Of course, 100 Nutripoints is just a basic goal: you may fall below it on some days and exceed it by a wide margin on others. The following chart shows you how to assess a daily Nutripoint score:

Daily Nutripoint Scores

25 — Very poor

50 — Poor

75 — Fair

100 — Good

150 — Excellent

200+ — Superior

Nutripoint Balance

In order for the Nutripoint program to work, your diet must be balanced. You can't eat a cup of turnip greens (79 Nutripoints), some asparagus (44 Nutripoints), some raw radishes (29 Nutripoints), and some cucumber (20 Nutripoints) for a total of 172 Nutripoints, and call it a day. You have to choose from various food groups to be sure that you cover all the nutritional bases.

There are six basic Nutrigroups. To achieve a Nutripoint balance, you must achieve a Nutripoint goal for each group, and *you must do it within the recommended number of servings.* The serving quota is a limiting device: you want to score the highest possible number of Nutripoints, but you can't do it by simply eating enormous quantities of foods.

By following the Nutripoint program of Nutrigroups, you are assured you will meet or surpass recommendations of the American Heart Association, the American Cancer Society, the National Cancer Institute, and the American Dietetic Association.

The following is a simple breakdown of the food group system:

Daily Nutripoint Recommendations

Servings	*Nutrigroup*	*Nutripoints*
4	Vegetables	55
3	Fruits	15
2	Grains	10
1	Legumes	5
2	Milk/dairy	10
1	Meat/poultry/fish	5
	Total:	**100**

What does the chart mean to you on a daily basis? You are going to be making sure that you get four vegetable servings daily. Many vegetables are very high in Nutripoints, and I think you'll find it quite easy to get 55 points per day. For example, you might have a tossed salad (33 Nutripoints) at lunch, broccoli (38.5 Nutripoints) and a baked potato (8.5 Nutripoints) at dinner, and a glass of V8 juice (24.5 Nutripoints) as a snack. This would give you four vegetable servings for a total of 105.5 Nutripoints—well above the 55 Nutripoints you're supposed to get from the vegetable group.

Of course, now and again you might have a day in which you don't do very well. Maybe you'll have a chef's salad (−1.5 Nutripoints), some French fries (1 Nutripoint), some cooked zucchini (15 Nutripoints) and some Fritos (Fritos are in the vegetable group because their principal ingredient is corn), worth −1.5 Nutripoints. Your total score on that day would be 13 Nutripoints from four servings in the vegetable Nutrigroup. You can boost your score with excellent choices from the other groups, and you can boost your long-term score with Nutripoint recovery.

Nutripoint Recovery

What does it really mean if you get more or fewer than 100 Nutripoints daily? It's an opportunity to see your nutritional status in terms of more than just one day.

Most diets are limited to a one-day pattern that, for many dieters, means walking a nutritional tightrope—if you break down and have some barbecued

The following is a breakdown of how some of the nutrients worked out for Patrick's good and bad days:

	Bad Day	***Good Day***	***Ideal***
Calories	3,087	1,049	1,000–2,000
% fat calories	57	15	20–30
% carb. calories	23	50	50–70
Tsp. sugar	10	3	0
Grams fiber	7	29	25–35
Mg. sodium	4,845	2,565	fewer than 3,000
Mg. caffeine	223	0	fewer than 200

While both Patrick's sample days provided virtually all the essential nutrients (except fiber on the bad day), on the good day he achieved this with one-third the calories while limiting all negative factors, such as fat, sugar, and sodium. This illustrates the concept of "nutrition per calorie": what makes Patrick's bad day so bad is that he got bad nutritional value per calorie. No one can afford to do that today.

I want to emphasize that Nutripoints does not encourage or even allow for regular diet lapses. It just doesn't make nutritional sense to try to eat well most of the time but, say, twice a week, have a small binge. The Nutripoints program assumes that you're serious about good nutrition. It simply recognizes that there will be occasions when you'll eat something that isn't of good nutritional value. There's no sense in pretending this doesn't happen, and so Nutripoints takes it into consideration and figures it into the system.

People have found the recovery feature of Nutripoints very reassuring. Many studies have shown that "restrained eaters," who are severely limited in the type or amount of food they can eat, will eventually binge or relapse. Nutripoints provides powerful psychological motivation because it allows you to make up for lapses. It's also far more realistic to assume that people will have good and bad days: Nutripoints gives you a framework that takes real life into consideration.

The extraordinary benefit of Nutripoints is that if you've adopted the nutritional goals of the Nutripoint program you will probably be better nourished than you've ever been in your life, even if you have a bad day.

NUTRIPOINTS IN THE REAL WORLD

It's one thing to come up with the best all-round system for evaluating foods, but the best and most sophisticated charts in the world won't help people if they don't, or can't, use them. Nutripoints' track record for changing people's lives is convincing evidence that it's a system that's easy to live with no matter what your lifestyle.

The story of Joni, a Nutripoint convert who came to the program reluctantly, follows. I want to tell you about Joni because, while some patients have experienced more dramatic changes in their overall health profile, Joni illustrates two key elements of the Nutripoint program:

1. It's incredibly easy to live with.

2. It's valuable even for people who think that their diet is already nutritionally sound.

Joni is a 42-year-old manager of a corporate health plan for a large national company based in New York. Her job gives her reason and opportunity to keep up with the latest medical advances and theories, but she's also personally interested. When it came time for her company to make an arrangement with a corporate health center to do complete physicals on its employees, Joni became a "guinea pig" so that she could get a good understanding of the services offered by the center.

Though Joni hadn't had a complete physical in a few years, she had no complaints that she considered serious, or even worthy of mention. She often had a headache in the afternoon, and she was usually exhausted after work but thought that these symptoms had more to do with her demanding schedule than anything else. Although she counseled employees to get regular exercise, Joni herself was sedentary except for an occasional tennis game in the summer. She knew that she should lose about ten or fifteen pounds, but she thought her diet was pretty good except for regular business lunches when she found it impossible to eat lightly. All in all, Joni thought she was healthy, and she didn't expect any surprises from her physical.

When the printout from the health center arrived, Joni was shocked. Her cholesterol level was 228, her blood pressure was slightly elevated, her fifteen pounds of overweight was confirmed, and her treadmill time, which measured her aerobic endurance level, was terrible. Worse, her family history of osteoporosis indicated that she'd have to dramatically increase her calcium intake but, because of her high cholesterol level and her overweight, be especially careful to avoid fat. She also had a family history of breast cancer, and the latest evidence showed that a reduction in her fat intake would be imperative if she wanted to improve her chances of avoiding this disease.

Because of her work in the health field, Joni had heard about the Cooper Aerobics Center and she enrolled in our four-day Aerobics Wellness Weekend. When she arrived, she told me that the results of her physical had really overwhelmed her; it was the first time she'd felt really "mortal," as she put it. She was also confused. Though she knew what her dietary goals should be, she didn't know how to achieve them. She hated the idea of a typical diet because she really didn't believe she'd be able to stick with one. She felt she needed a "crash course" on nutrition to get her on track. Joni was very frank when she told me that she didn't expect to change her life; she just wanted to pick my brains to learn what she should be eating, and then go about things her own way. She warned me not to expect her to stay with any eating program once she was back on her home turf.

I began by giving Joni a brief explanation of the Nutripoints program. She was fascinated by the numbers and eager to see how they'd apply to her own life. I asked Joni to chart a typical day's eating. She felt she was on solid ground here. She was convinced that her diet was excellent. The following record is what she came up with:

Breakfast	*Nutripoints*
1 oat bran muffin (no butter)	3.0
Coffee	– 3.5
Cream	– 1.5
Snack	
1 container blueberry yogurt	1.0
Lunch	
Pasta primavera	3.0
Bread	2.5
Butter	– 4.0
1 glass wine	–13.0
Salad	33.5
Italian dressing	– 2.5
Dinner	
Weight Watchers frozen sweet and sour chicken	1.5
Yoplait frozen peach yogurt	– 2.0
2 glasses wine	– 26.0
Total:	**– 8.0**

Joni said that on some days she ate much more than usual, and on others less, but that this was a fairly typical meal pattern. She thought it was pretty good—after all, she didn't eat much meat or any eggs, and she tried to avoid sweets. The fact is, Joni's total daily Nutripoint score was –8! Even if you forget about the wine she drank, which dramatically lowered her score, you're left with a score of 31. This is a dismal score, particularly when you consider that Joni thought of herself as someone well versed in nutrition.

It's shocking when you become familiar with Nutripoints and when your sense of what constitutes good nutrition changes, but Joni's diet was typical of someone who knows a fair amount about nutrition in the 1990s. She knew to avoid certain fats and sweets, but she had no notion about the *positive* elements missing in her diet. She was also eating a lot of *hidden* fats and sweets. Joni was really short-changing herself, and her body was beginning to show the symptoms.

Because Joni was so resistant to a "diet," I decided to ease her into the Nutripoint program. I told her we'd stick with her typical eating pattern but that we'd *upgrade* it with Nutripoints. The following table shows Joni's typical day on Nutripoints:

Breakfast	***Nutripoints***
Kellogg's corn flakes	18.0
Skim milk	9.5
¼ cantaloupe	29.0
Decaffeinated coffee	−0.5
with skim milk	2.5
Snack	
Plain, nonfat yogurt	9.0
Frozen strawberries	8.0
Lunch	
Lentil soup	8.0
Pasta with marinara sauce	1.0
Bread (no butter)	3.0
Tossed salad	33.0
"Lite" Italian dressing	−0.5
Fresh fruit salad	13.0
Dinner	
Celentano frozen Chicken Primavera	6.0
Green Giant frozen broccoli, cauliflower, carrots	33.0
Frozfruit Chunky Strawberry	1.0
Total:	**173.0**

Joni couldn't believe that she was eating nearly the exact same things she'd been eating before, and yet improving her diet by about 175 percent. A few simple tricks improved her Nutripoint score dramatically. For example, she found that it was no trouble to toss some frozen berries in a cup of nonfat yogurt in the morning before she left for work. The berries helped keep the yogurt cold and by the time she was ready for her snack, they were defrosted. She says the "fruit added" yogurt now tastes sickeningly sweet to her. After three days at the center eating similar meals that I had devised for her on the basis of her own preferences, Joni was a convert.

After two months on Nutripoints, Joni called me to tell me the results of her latest physical. She'd gone back to the corporate health center to get an update, and she was delighted with the news: her cholesterol level was 186, down 18 percent; her weight was down twelve pounds; and her blood pressure was completely normal.

Joni was quick to tell me that she didn't stick religiously to the program. Every now and again she slipped, but not because she wanted to. It was always because she found herself in a situation—usually a social one, such as a dinner party—in which it was nearly impossible to stick with her new patterns. For example, her worst day included a dinner party at the home of a business associate. She had a glass of red wine (−14 Nutripoints), a crabmeat appetizer with hollandaise sauce (−3.5 Nutripoints), chicken Kiev (0 Nutripoints), a salad with blue cheese dressing (19 Nutripoints), and carrot cake with cream cheese frosting (−2.5 Nutripoints). Even though Joni tried to only sample some of the dishes she thought were the worst Nutripoint values, she still found herself with a score of −4.5 Nutripoints for that meal. As she said, "The cook spent an enormous amount of time and trouble to plunge me into negative Nutripoints!" On the day of that dinner, Joni's Nutripoints came to 53. But she was only more resolved to make up for the loss and go for the top of the list for the rest of the week.

WHY NUTRIPOINTS COULD BE *YOUR* NUTRITIONAL BREAKTHROUGH

One morning, not too long ago, the phone rang in my office. It was Richard, a computer analyst who had visited the Aerobics Center two months previously with his wife. Richard had made the visit for his wife's sake, but he had no real interest in participating. As Richard was extremely overweight, but also reluctant to try any kind of diet, I was surprised to hear from him. By the time he left the Aerobics Center I believed that he had a psychological problem that was preventing him from making an effort.

"Dr. Vartabedian," Richard said, "I have a confession to make. When I got home from the Aerobics Center, I was upset. I guess I really believed that if I paid the money to be there, it would *have* to help me. Yes, I was there for my wife's sake, but I also wondered if the visit could really help me too. I almost had a chip on my shoulder about it.

"I guess because I didn't have any success, I'm ashamed to say that I made fun of the food charts my wife was using. She was making real progress and I guess I just couldn't take it. Well, a week after I got home I found myself standing at the refrigerator eating raw chocolate-chip cookie dough, right out of the roll, by the spoonful. By the time I had finished half the roll, I felt awful—dizzy and light-headed. I went to lie down, and as I was stretched out on the couch I thought, really thought, about what I had done. I was so disgusted with myself I wasn't sure which was making me sicker, the cookie dough or my own behavior. I decided to give Nutripoints a try. I knew I couldn't change overnight, but I remembered enough about what you'd said about Nutripoints to know that I could do it at my own pace. And I wanted to thank you because as of today I've lost twenty-one pounds. I also wanted to tell you that it's the only thing that's ever worked for me. The only reason that it's worked is because it's really easy. I have a long way to go, but for the first time in my life I know I'm going to make it."

I'm telling Richard's story because he illustrates what I think is the most important feature of Nutripoints: it's easy. Although many people want to improve their lives, without major motivation it's just too hard. I believe that's because diet and exercise programs are just too difficult. They're not fun: they're grim and they make you feel like a penitent. They demand major changes, that you give up patterns and habits acquired over a lifetime. Most people never experience the pleasure of a body enjoying optimum nutrition, or anything near it.

If you want to improve your nutrition but are discouraged by difficult diets with complicated menus, the Nutripoint program will change your life. One of my goals in developing Nutripoints was to find something that *everyone*—even people who would never follow a typical diet—would find accessible.

Here are the features that I think will make the difference for you. First, you'll find that it's the simplest and most positive approach to nutrition you've ever encountered. If you like, you can ease into it: just use the charts to improve the quality of everything you eat. Focus on the positive, and you'll soon find yourself avoiding the negative. I've seen many people ease into the system this way with great success. Maria is an example. She came to our thirteen-day Aerobics Program for Total Well-Being at the Aerobics Center with her husband, who was showing early signs of heart disease. She was there only to offer moral support; she exercised regularly and, though she would have liked to lose a few pounds, she didn't want to diet. As she now says., "Once I realized that I could lose a bit of weight and dramatically improve the quality of my diet simply by doing some informed comparisons of foods and eliminating a few foods that tipped the balance the wrong way, I couldn't *help* but do it. My nutritional status was not great. I was eating bad stuff, and I guess without realizing it I was on a gradual decline. You just don't stop and see what you're doing to yourself day to day.

"I never would have thought about making a change without Nutripoints. It never occurred to me before Nutripoints just why typical reducing or health-oriented diets turned me off. They all seemed to be complicated or offer a gimmick that I couldn't really believe in. But Nutripoints is not really a diet; it's *a tool* based on real science that allows you to go as far as you want to improve your nutrition. My husband has certainly changed his life and dramatically improved his health—his cholesterol is already down 46 points—but I always felt convinced that would happen if he made major changes in his diet. The real surprise is me. I never would have believed that I'd jump on the Nutripoints bandwagon and, given the fact that I didn't think I needed any improvement, I'm amazed at the changes I see in me and my husband. I've lost those few extra pounds, and the general improvement in the way both my husband and I feel is really wonderful. We've got more energy, we're more calm. We feel just great."

There's a second, bonus benefit to Nutripoints: you won't have to wait years to enjoy its effects. The following are the average changes experienced by participants in the thirteen-day Aerobics Program for Total Well-Being:

Weight	8 lbs., or 4% decrease
Cholesterol	14% decrease
Cholesterol/HDL ratio*	16% decrease
Glucose	10% decrease
Triglycerides	40% decrease
Treadmill time (fitness level)	19% increase
Blood pressure	6% decrease

These participants are working on exercise and stress reduction in addition to nutrition. But if you undertake the Nutripoints program with any measure of seriousness, and you work on stress reduction and exercise too, there's no reason why you can't experience similar improvements. From a short-term point of view, you'll probably experience freedom from digestive problems, sluggishness, inability to concentrate, frequent headaches, and irritability. And in mid-afternoon, when many people start to fade, you'll find that you have the energy and stamina to keep going.

*Cholesterol levels can be measured in two ways: total cholesterol measures all types found in the blood whereas high-density cholesterol (HDL) refers to good, protective cholesterol only. The higher the HDL is in relation to total cholesterol, the better. Therefore the lower the ratio (cholesterol/HDL), the better.

PART II

THE SCIENCE OF OPTIMAL NUTRITION

SCARED SMART

FOR A MOMENT, FORGET PILLS, FORGET EXERCISE, FORGET RELAXATION techniques. The fact is, the single most important step you can take today to improve your overall sense of well-being and your long-term health is to improve your nutrition. Exercise works the body; food *makes* the body. There are trillions of cells in your body, and each one is made up of, and nourished by, the food you eat. You simply can't function at your best, as we'll see, if you don't eat the best foods. Of course, exercise, stress-reduction techniques, and all sensible efforts at better health make sense, but if you don't improve your nutrition, your other efforts will be virtually pointless.

Does it really matter that you keep your fat, cholesterol, and sodium levels down? That you make a point of getting all the vitamins and minerals your body needs? I'm so used to dealing with the educated demands of my clients at the Aerobics Center that I sometimes forget that anyone today needs convincing.

The people who come to me for help with their diets are highly motivated. In many cases, *motivated* is a euphemism for *terrified*. Some of my patients are actually staring death in the face. They've suffered a heart attack, maybe two. I think of these people as "scared smart." They have decided *they* want to live, and they're prepared to do anything it takes to make that possible. The Nutripoint program is an enormous relief to them. It's an eating program that can help them to literally save their own lives. In addition, it is easy to incorporate into their lifestyles, and it allows them to devise their own eating program: many of these people believed that they would have to live on a terribly restricted, boring diet for the rest of their lives.

I hope that most of the rest of us—the lucky ones who haven't been forced to change their diets through personal illness—have moved out of the Dark Ages of nutrition, where we believed we could eat whatever we wanted and trust to luck or good genes to get us through. It just doesn't work that way. It really is up to you.

Cholesterol was the red flag that alerted millions of Americans to the fact that diet really does matter—that what we're eating every day is going to make a difference in how we feel both today and tomorrow. But cholesterol is only part of the story. Today, largely because of their diets, over 50 percent of Americans are at risk for heart disease, diabetes, hypertension, and cancer. The American Cancer Society announced that they expected 1.4 million Americans to hear a cancer diagnosis in 2005. In addition to more than one million new cancer cases, the society projected over half a million cancer deaths for 2005. Direct cancer-related medical costs for 2004 were $16.4 billion. Thirty-five percent of cancers—only one of the leading causes of death—are diet related. Former U.S. Surgeon General Koop recently said 85% of the diseases we are dying from in the U.S. today are contributed to or directly caused by our lifestyles.

It's no news that the American diet can be dangerous to your health. As early as 1977 George McGovern headed a congressional committee that investigated the long-term effects of what Americans eat. The McGovern committee studied the relationship between the average diet and the nation's major killers—heart disease, cancers of the colon and breast, stroke, high blood pressure, obesity, diabetes, arteriosclerosis, and cirrhosis of the liver. They estimated that if Americans modified their rich diets, there would be an 80-percent drop in the number of obese people, a 25-percent drop in deaths from heart disease, a 50-percent drop in deaths from diabetes, and a 1-percent annual increase in longevity.

It seems that every day there's a new study that demonstrates the dangers of fats and cholesterol, and the importance of fiber and various nutrients, such as calcium, in the diet. A recent study reported in the *New York Times* confirmed yet again the dangers for women of a high-calorie, high-fat diet. This study, which was the largest survey done to date, overwhelmingly demonstrated that women who ate the most fats, saturated fats, and animal protein had a three times greater chance of getting breast cancer than those whose intake of these substances was lowest. Moreover, it showed that a high-calorie diet made women almost twice as likely to develop breast cancer.

A diet high in fat, cholesterol, and calories has been definitively linked to the major lifestyle diseases. The answer couldn't be more obvious: if you want to avoid the major killing and debilitating diseases, improve your diet.

BEYOND CALORIES

How *do* you improve your diet? Well, you try to cut fat and cholesterol, and probably calories. But how do you actually go about doing this? The first thing you do is to discard your old notions about how to judge foods. If you're like most people, the calorie is the only food measure that you're really familiar with. It's time to forget calories and move on to Nutripoints.

To understand just how revolutionary Nutripoints are, you need only take a look at what has existed in the past to help people choose among foods.

We are all calorie nuts. We have some notion from high school that we have to have variety (something about choosing from various food groups, or using a food pyramid), but counting calories has been the most common system for comparing foods. Most people who pay attention to what they eat are trying to lose weight. They look for foods that are low in calories. But we now know that calories are just one measure of the value of various foods. A diet extremely low in calories can also be a diet that is nutritionally unsound—even absolutely dangerous, as we've seen from some fad diets. A diet extremely low in calories is not necessarily a diet that will promote permanent weight loss.

RDAs (Recommended Dietary Allowances) provide some measure of food value. These figures were arrived at by the Food and Nutrition Board, a committee of the National Academy of Sciences–National Research Council. RDAs are sup-posed to be the "levels of intake of essential nutrients considered, in the judgment of the Food and Nutrition Board on the basis of available scientific knowledge, to be adequate to meet the known nutritional needs of practically all healthy persons."

RDAs are assigned to all foods, but unprocessed foods don't provide the handy labels that would help you determine whether a white or a sweet potato is a better choice in terms of your nutritional needs. RDAs are concerned with vitamins and minerals, but ignore critical analyses of the fat, carbohydrate, and protein contents of foods. So, while a useful beginning, it's difficult to translate RDAs into a healthful diet.

In 1973 the FDA (Food and Drug Administration) adopted its basic nutritional labeling regulations. Making use of RDAs, this was a step forward in helping people determine the nutritive value of foods. Three kinds of foods must be labeled: those that make any kind of nutritional claim, such as "high in fiber," those that are fortified with nutrients, and those that are specifically intended for children under age four. Manufacturers of other types of foods are free to voluntarily include nutritional labeling. Foods that are so labeled list the percentage of the RDA of each nutrient the food contains. Nutritional labeling is very useful in comparing the relative nutritional value of two similar foods.

While nutritional labeling is an advance for consumers, it's of limited value. Although in 1975 it was believed that roughly 85 percent of all manufacturers would be using nutritional labeling soon, by 1985 less than half of packaged foods were labeled. In 2005 most all packages are now labeled, but many labels are almost deceptive. For example, a manufacturer must list ingredients in descending order of amounts, but sugar can be listed in various forms, such as sugar, dextrose, corn syrup, honey, molasses, and so on. If you're not sophisticated about reading labels, you can wind up buying a product that has far more sugar than a cursory glance would reveal.

Another major drawback of nutritional labeling is that it tends to highlight the vitamin/mineral content of foods while downplaying the importance of fat, carbohydrates, protein, and fiber. These major nutrients are usually listed as amounts (for example, a frozen dinner might have 8 grams of fat) rather than as percentages. If a percentage is listed, it is given as a percent of the daily requirement, which is useless. The percentage you want to see is the percent of total calories in the food. This makes it more difficult for the consumer to tell how nutritious the food really is.

While labels might list the amounts of certain nutrients, this information still doesn't tell you what you need to know: how much is good? If you know the amount of fat, protein, fiber, or complex carbohydrates in a certain food, can you tell if it's a good choice in terms of the ideal, or in terms of what you've already eaten today? Most people just don't know if a food with 10 percent complex carbohydrates is a good choice. Finally, it is enormously time consuming to stand in a supermarket and compare labels to check varying percentages of nutrients.

Nutritional labeling is great as far as it goes, but it doesn't offer any help with the foods we should be eating the most of: whole, unprocessed foods. You can check a label to see if Count Chocula cereal has more sugar than Fruity Pebbles, but there are no handy labels to help you determine whether an apple versus a banana, or a pork chop versus a veal chop, is a better choice in terms of your nutritional needs.

The fact is, nutritional labeling and RDAs are a useful beginning, but for most people they are simply raw data in a form too complicated to be of much use. It's good to know that a product contains 15 percent of your daily requirement of protein, but where do you go from there? Is that an acceptable amount? Is it a good contribution to your daily protein intake? And how does it compare to other, similar products?

It's almost as if food labeling is only an intriguing set of puzzle pieces that the average consumer is unable to put together in any useful way. (Now that the FDA has passed a rule that allows companies to make health claims in their food labels, consumers can even be misled: a soup high in fiber can claim that the fiber in the soup helps reduce the risk of cancer, without mentioning that its high sodium content contributes to hypertension.)

Unfortunately, and despite the enormous interest in nutrition today, the experts can't be of much help in determining which foods offer better nutritional value. They know that a bran muffin is better than a Twinkie...probably...unless, come to think of it, the bran muffin is commercially manufactured with palm oil and contains a lot of cholesterol.

No doctor or nutritionist can tell you which foods are best to eat because, up to now, they haven't had the "software." While the government has charts that list all of the nutrient values in thousands of foods, most people (including doctors and nutritionists) are overwhelmed in trying to translate this vast sea of data into any useful information. It's just too complicated. The best anyone could do up to now is to point out that some foods are better than others. Some foods low in cholesterol are high in sugar or salt. Some foods low in calories have virtually no nutritive value. Some foods that are high in protein are surprisingly high in fat.

Nutripoints has made use of the most up-to-date information available on foods today. It has looked at nutritional labeling, RDAs, calorie and cholesterol counts, and so on, as *raw data,* which is what it really is as far as the consumer is concerned, and gone one step beyond by providing the first accurate, practical nutritional guidebook.

PUTTING THE NUTRIENTS BACK IN NUTRITION

- Anemia, from lack of iron in the diet, is the most common nutritional-deficiency disease in the country today. Symptoms include immune disorders, fatigue, learning problems in children, muscle weakness, among many others.

- Only 22 percent of Americans past the age of one meet the top recommended dietary allowances of vitamin B_6. According to the USDA, only 8 percent of women consume 100 percent of the dietary allowances of B_6. Such deficiencies have been linked to everything from asthma and PMS, to diabetes, cardiovascular disease, and cancer.

- Only 42 percent of the population consumes the recommended daily allowance of calcium. The people who need it most consume the least: 80 percent of teenage and middle-aged women consume less than half of the recommended daily allowance. Most people have heard about osteoporosis and calcium deficiency, but lack of sufficient calcium in the diet can also contribute to gum disease, high blood pressure, and even colon cancer.

These are a few facts that illustrate how many of the people in the "best-nourished nation in the world" are suffering from the first stages of malnutrition. How could this have happened? In large part it's due to our obsession with dieting, which translates into a never-ending desire to lose weight. In fact, losing weight has become such a primary focus for so many of us that we forget that *diet* refers to a system for nourishing the body rather than a means to lose weight. When was the last time a friend told you he or she was on a "diet" geared to improve consumption of all the major nutrients in order to feel better and prevent disease?

In fact, many diets today take into consideration the negative elements in American eating patterns and help you avoid excess fats, cholesterol, and sodium—although very few help you avoid all three (some now even *promote* eating them). And most diets make you feel like you're the worst kid in second grade: the basic theme is, "don't, don't, don't; no, no, no!" Don't eat this; don't eat that; don't even think about eating all of these things!

Nutripoints goes beyond this negative approach and moves the entire idea of diet into another, positive realm. Most diets set you up for failure; there is no way you can "fail" with Nutripoints. That's because the emphasis is not on avoiding certain foods, or on eating specific foods. Rather, the emphasis is on *choice.* The Nutripoint program assumes that you are intelligent and that you are ready to improve your diet. It provides you with the information—the type of information you've never had before—that will enable you to make intelligent choices.

Most of us think of nutrition in terms of losing weight. We think if we eat foods that are low in calories, and avoid junk food, we're doing well. In fact, there is another popular "point system" today that does just that. Unfortunately, this focus on calories and weight loss has obscured the importance of adequate nutrition. The fact is, most of us are not very well nourished. We eat too much fat, too much protein, too much sugar, and we don't get enough fiber, complex carbohydrates, and certain critical nutrients in our diets.

While Americans have reduced their fat intake 12 percent since 1977, and slightly increased their complex carbohydrate intake, the improvement hasn't been enough. While we're eating 80 percent more yogurt than we were in 1983, and 43 percent more wholesome snacks (including fruits and nuts), our consumption of salty tortilla, taco, and nacho chips rose by 60 percent. We're eating less bacon, but more frankfurters and breakfast sausage. We all claim we're eating fewer sweets, but consumption of "gourmet" chocolate-chip cookies has passed seventy-five million pounds annually. Who's eating all this stuff?

I witnessed a typical example of how some of our misguided notions about foods have more to do with trends than with accurate information on how foods affect our bodies. I was in the supermarket watching a young man who was filling his cart. He carefully chose a bottled water, a "lite" frozen entree, a large bottle of diet soft drink, and then a huge bag of M&M's!

While most Americans are at least aware of the shortcomings in their diets, or at least aware enough to insist that they're doing better (despite the facts that contradict them), they're still vulnerable to disease from too much fat and too little fiber.

The more surprising results of recent USDA and FDA surveys are that our diets are shortchanging us of vital vitamins and minerals. As the two top officials of the U.S. Department of Agriculture's Human Nutrition Information Service reported, "50 percent or more [of the 38,000 people surveyed] had intakes below the RDA for vitamin A, iron, calcium, magnesium, and vitamin B_6; over 30 percent of the individuals failed to meet the 70-percent RDA levels for these nutrients. Zinc and folacin are also known to be short in many diets." The report concluded that "U.S. diets do not show up well...when either the RDA or the [USDA's] Daily Food Guide is used as a standard." So while most of us feel fairly complacent about the nutrients we're getting from our diets, the facts tell a very different story.

The very steps we take to reduce fat (such as cutting out red meat and many dairy products) are further reducing our intake of these important nutrients.

Does it really matter if your intake of, say, iron, is low? Most of us tend to think that a deficiency of any given nutrient is only a remote possibility. We figure that our iron intake must be OK if we don't have anemia. What most people don't appreciate is the subtle interplay of nutrients in our bodies: it doesn't take a diagnosed deficiency to make you feel tired, or make it hard for you to shake a cold. Indeed, lack of sufficient iron in your diet will begin to sap your energy and lower your physical and mental productivity long before it turns into a full-blown deficiency.

The story of Bill Walton, the basketball star, illustrates the need for adequate nutrients. When Walton was under contract with the San Diego Clippers, he had a terrible run of luck. Walton kept breaking bones, and past breaks were troubling him. His left foot had been broken twice, and didn't seem to be healing. When x-rayed, it showed evidence of osteoporosis. If he did have osteoporosis, it would explain why he'd broken so many bones: several fingers and toes, a leg, a wrist, a cheekbone, and his nose, in addition to the two breaks in his foot. But Walton drank what should have been enough milk to provide the calcium the body needs to prevent osteoporosis.

Tests on Walton's blood became an indictment of his diet: while his calcium level was high, his levels of trace elements were alarming. He had an absolute zero level of manganese, and his copper and zinc levels were one-third normal.

Walton's nutritional mistake was not his vegetarian diet, as so many people suspected, but his *unbalanced* diet. He ate mainly brown rice and vegetables supplemented with milk and, occasionally, fish. While too many people today would consider this an ideal diet—low in fat and cholesterol and high in fiber—it was destroying his body and his career. He wasn't getting the critical balance of nutrients his body needed.

When Walton supplemented his diet with the minerals he was missing, he soon recovered, his foot healed, and within six weeks he was back playing basketball.

I was fascinated by Walton's story because it's such a powerful illustration of the necessity of getting *all* the nutrients, even trace elements, if we want to perform properly. It also demonstrates how the lack of one or two nutrients can cripple the entire system. In Walton's case, calcium was unable to do its work of strengthening bones because it didn't have the minerals copper and manganese essential to the task.

Walton's diet was unusual, and his demands on his body accelerated the problems that most of us wouldn't experience so dramatically, but it's not uncommon for the average American to consume a diet that is just as unvaried and nutritionally unsound. Many people, in an effort to lose weight, go on popular diets that put their health at risk.

Many popular reducing diets are unsound, and sometimes we make them even worse by adapting them to our own desires without the requisite knowledge. Inventing our own diets, where we simply cut out foods we believe to be fattening, is another trouble area. In many cases, we wind up eating a shockingly inadequate diet that repeats one or two "low-calorie" meals virtually every day.

As I mentioned before, even people who eat a relatively good diet will unknowingly cut out essential vitamins and minerals when they reduce fat and cholesterol in their diets. Most people simply don't know how to substitute a "good" food for a "bad" one. They're not aware that the right diet can be a simple matter of intelligent substitution.

I think that the goal of *optimum nutrition* will replace concern with the calorie as we learn more about the critical role these nutrients play in ensuring our well-being.

As Paul Saltman, trace element researcher at the University of California, San Diego, says, "There is every reason to believe that millions would have more energy, and would perform at higher levels physically and mentally, if our diet were richer in certain minerals and trace metals." Nutripoints is the best method available today to help you achieve that goal.

THE ADVANTAGE OF NATURAL NUTRITION

"Why can't I just take a vitamin pill?" How many thousands of times have I heard this question? It's not surprising that people are confused on the issue of vitamin supplements. The vitamin supplement manufacturers spend veritable fortunes convincing us that a pill is just as good, if not better, a source of nutrition as food. And who wouldn't *want* to believe them? You don't have to shop frequently for pills. They don't take up much room. You don't have to wash or chop or stir-fry or sauté them. But the fact is, vitamin pills have virtually no real role in achieving natural nutrition.

Did you know, for example, that most of those reports you hear about that demonstrate that vitamin A or vitamin C can cure or mitigate the effects of this or that disease *do not rely on pills, but rather on food, as a source of the vitamin?* Many people hear about research that promises to help their arthritis, PMS, or whatever, and begin to dose themselves on whatever vitamin or mineral was cited as the cure. But frequently, pills had nothing to do with the reported results.

This is just one misconception about vitamins. As I'll demonstrate, there are other, even more compelling reasons for relying on *natural nutrition,* or fuel from food.

One of the cornerstones of Nutripoints is that *pills are not a substitute for food.* Let's take a look at some of the drawbacks of vitamin supplementation.

Even the best vitamins are incomplete.

Despite what you may read or hear, vitamin supplementation is not an exact science. It's a relatively new scientific frontier: by 1913, only two vitamins had been recognized. Moreover, because we're interested in the effects of vitamins on humans, and because humans often cannot be the subjects of experiments for obvious reasons, we're limited in how much we *can* learn about the effects of vitamins on human health.

But we do know a great deal from animal experimentation. For example, guinea pigs eating a totally synthetic diet which contains all the known nutrients needed to sustain their lives will not thrive. Why? Because we're not aware of all the essential nutrients—for guinea pigs or for ourselves. Dr. Jean Mayer, one of the most highly respected authorities on nutrition, has said that "if the history of the development of our science is a dependable guide, there may be nutrients performing significant duties for us that we have not yet identified. In particular, there may be minerals functioning heroically to our benefit and all unknown to us." A vitamin pill contains the *known* micronutrients, and that's the best we can do. But no one can claim that it's complete.

Vitamin D_2, or irradiated ergosterol, for example, can be produced by irradiating yeast with ultraviolet light. Because this is a "natural" process, irradiated ergosterol can be called a "natural" vitamin. Milk and many other food products, as well as vitamin supplements, contain irradiated ergosterol. But this substance, vitamin D_2, is not the same as the D vitamin produced in the body when ultraviolet light strikes the skin. Moreover, vitamin D_2 does not supply the complex of D vitamins found in such foods as fish oils, milk fats from animals feeding on fresh greens, and liver. The fact is, the supplements we create, either naturally or otherwise, may not be exactly the same as those created by nature in foods. If the effects of these created supplements in the body are precisely the same, no one can prove it, and there's room for great skepticism on the part of the consumer.

Even the best vitamins are not perfectly balanced; some are dangerously unbalanced.

The vitamins and minerals that occur naturally in food are balanced. Nature dictates how much of a given nutrient will be present. But the contents of a vitamin pill are dictated by companies—companies that are run for profit and that sometimes pander to the public's ignorance about vitamins and how they work in the body.

It's important to remember that nutrients have to work in concert, and to take too much of one or another can be useless or even dangerous. For example, increasing zinc intake by only 3.5 milligrams per day above the RDA of 15 milligrams per day can decrease copper retention as well as interfere with calcium absorption. Large doses of folic acid can mask a vitamin B_{12} deficiency and result in serious and irreversible neurological damage. In pregnant women, large doses of folic acid can cause zinc deficiencies, which could lead to birth defects. Most people are astonished to learn that megadoses of vitamin C impair B_{12} utilization and can raise blood cholesterol.

Vitamins and minerals work in concert with one another, and we ignore this fact to our peril. Calcium, for example, is one of the most abundant minerals in the body. It's found in bone cartilage, teeth, and blood and nerve cells. We're all wary of calcium deficiencies today because of the threat of osteoporosis. But calcium supplements *can* do more harm than good. Calcium is used by the body in conjunction with magnesium. One of these minerals taken alone will have a totally different effect. For example, magnesium oxide is effective in the relief of constipation. If you take it with calcium, it will have no effect on your bowels. Too many calcium supplements, taken over a long period of time, can result in a disorder called hypercalcemia, which can eventually lead to rheumatoid arthritis. Calcium, taken in its natural form in dairy products and vegetables, eliminates the risk of such an overdose. It is the only guarantee that the body is getting the calcium it needs in concert with magnesium, and in the balance necessary for optimum functioning.

Some popular vitamin formulations completely ignore the concept of balance and can actually put you in danger. One popular brand contains a potentially toxic amount of vitamin A, minerals in insignificant amounts, and eight unrecognized nutrients. It also features a label that lists potency according to the obsolete MDR (Minimum Daily Requirement) standard, instead of the current FDA standard, the RDA (Recommended Dietary Allowance). This vitamin is also among the most expensive available.

The only way to be sure that the nutrients you ingest are properly balanced and readily absorbed by the body is to get them from food.

Vitamins can be toxic.

The body stores excess vitamin A in the liver. The fact that the liver is a storehouse for many excess vitamins is why it is also considered a valuable food (though liver has great drawbacks in nutritional terms). In any case, liver could almost be seen as one of the original megavitamins. And, like commercially produced megavitamins, it can be dangerous. For example, long ago Eskimos learned to avoid eating polar bear liver. They knew it caused death; they didn't know that it did so because of its extremely high content of vitamin A. Polar bear liver contains about one million international units (IU) in three ounces, compared to an RDA of 5,000 IU for men.

In the early sixties, approximately twenty children in New York died from vitamin A overdoses when their mothers doubled the recommended dosage of vitamin supplements. Each child took two capsules daily. This was in addition to the already generous amounts of vitamin A the children were receiving from foods in their diets.

There are also long-term dangers to the use of supplements. For example, some experts worry that consumption of large amounts of iron supplements could cause a buildup of iron in the liver, leading to serious problems in later life.

Although we've talked about the dangers of inadequate calcium intake, there's also a danger in too much calcium. As I mentioned before, due to the threat of osteoporosis, many women have begun to take calcium supplements. But very few of these women are actually aware of how much calcium they are consuming. As more and more foods are supplemented with calcium to cash in on the concern with osteoporosis, people are getting extra calcium in everything from their orange juice to their antacid tablets. This extra calcium is *in addition* to the calcium they're getting naturally in their diets from milk and other sources. Long-term high doses of calcium could have potentially harmful consequences. Moreover, calcium supplements derived from dolomite or bone meal can be contaminated with poisonous metals, such as lead.

Unfortunately, the FDA, with a few exceptions, has no authority to limit the potency of vitamin/mineral supplements. These supplements are considered foods or food additives, not drugs. While the average consumer taking an "insurance" multivitamin will most likely not get into trouble, medically unsupervised megavitamin supplementation is a dangerous game.

Vitamin supplementation can alter your body chemistry.

There's a more subtle problem relative to vitamin/mineral supplementation. While consumers may be aware that high levels of certain nutrients can be dangerous, most are not aware that even low routine doses of vitamins can create problems by conditioning the body to *expect* higher than normal levels of certain vitamins. This is known as *systemic conditioning.* It occurs with water-soluble vitamins, and it can create withdrawal problems when the nutrient is withdrawn. There is a great deal yet to be learned about systemic conditioning in relation to nutrients, but we do know that it can affect offspring as well as the individual taking the nutrient. There have been cases of infants suffering from something called *rebound scurvy,* which causes temporary scurvylike withdrawal symptoms, because their mothers took megadoses of vitamin C while pregnant. You should certainly never take megadoses of any vitamin while pregnant. If you are currently taking megadoses of a water-soluble vitamin (including the Bs and vitamin C), be sure to cut down on your intake gradually to avoid the symptoms of withdrawal. (Megadoses of a fat-soluble vitamin, such as A, D, or E, should be ceased immediately if at toxic levels.)

You should also be aware that vitamin/mineral supplementation can alter the results of various diagnostic tests, particularly blood and urine tests. Large doses of vitamin C can give false readings for blood in stool and sugar in urine. If you take supplements, particularly in high doses, be sure to tell your doctor so that diagnostic tests can be correctly interpreted.

HOW TO TAKE A VITAMIN

Despite what I've just said, I'm not opposed to *intelligent* supplementation. If you perfectly follow Nutripoints, there is really no need for supplements. But in practice I have found that even though we may know what the best foods *are,* often—for whatever reason, we don't *eat* all the best foods we need every day in the real world. So for this reason, I will give some guidelines as to what supplements work, which don't work, and which may even be harmful.

VITAMIN AND MINERAL SUPPLEMENTS: OLD TECHNOLOGY

Until recently, scientists believed that since research studies showed lower cancer, heart disease, and other chronic disease rates in populations who had high blood levels of antioxidants such as vitamins A, C, and E, that supplements containing these nutrients would provide similar results. While studies did show benefit in some instances, one of the startling findings in a major study supplementing beta-carotene (a form of vitamin A) was that beta-carotene in its *isolated form* did not provide the same benefit as it did when it was *eaten in foods,* in fact it could be harmful. The reason, it turns out, is that beta-carotene is only one of many "carotenoids" in the body, so others such as alpha-carotene and lutein are needed as well, and increasing this one carotenoid (which is only 12-percent of all carotenoids in the body), could throw off the body's natural balance. Since most of the studies showing benefits of beta-carotene in the diet were taken from whole foods, not supplements, this all began to make sense.

Thus, supplementing with vitamins and minerals, rather than getting them from whole foods can be tricky because their balance in foods is virtually impossible to duplicate, and they may need to interact with unknown factors in foods to achieve maximum results. Thus, the best vitamin and mineral supplements are balanced with as wide a variety of nutrients, and as close to 100% of the Recommended Daily Values as possible so as to avoid imbalances in the body and simulate the natural amounts in foods as much as possible. (On the other hand, also remember that if you have *a specific* nutrient deficiency/need, *a specific* vitamin, mineral, or other nutrient supplement may be necessary and beneficial.)

NUTRITIONAL BREAKTHROUGH: WHOLE FOOD SUPPLEMENTS

Recently, a new nutritional technology has made it possible to get a "whole food concentrate" in a capsule. The concept is to take a whole food such as a fruit or vegetable, juice it, and isolate it in pill form. Thus, you have the nutrient "essence" of the food, and in a convenient form. Since every food has not only vitamins and minerals, but enzymes, fibers, and many newly discovered "phytochemicals"—or plant micronutrients with a positive effect, you can see how superior this concept is to taking isolated vitamins and minerals. The "natural balance" of complementary nutrients in these supplements enhances the body's absorption for our optimal benefit. Nutrients in whole food-based concentrates are therefore more "bioavailable" to the body, and that's why I believe they are superior and will provide greater protection against cellular oxidation, chronic diseases, and aging.

Several companies have begun producing these superior supplements. In the following table I grade the types and classes of supplements from highest to lowest:

A+ Whole food-based concentrate (WFC) containing a wide variety of high Nutripoint-rated vegetables, fruits, grains, legumes, with a natural spectrum of vitamins and minerals. Provide independent research on product documenting results. Example: Juice Plus+® (NSA®).
A- WFC containing only one or a few high Nutripoint-rated vegetables or fruits, and/or containing added vitamins and minerals in natural quantity and balance. Examples: Super Juice™, Nutrilite® Double-X (Amway®), New Vision® Juice Power™
B Vitamin/mineral supplement (V/MS) containing wide variety of nutrients (at least 15-20) in approximately 100% of Recommended Daily Values. Examples: Advanced Formula Centrum®, One-A-Day® Maximum, Theragran M®, Myadec®, Unicaps®.
C V/MS which is incomplete (i.e.: 5-10 nutrients), imbalanced (i.e. 25% to 3,000+% of RDV's). Examples: One-A-Day® Stressgard, Stresstabs®, GNC® Mega and Ultra Mega.

D V/MS which is incomplete and/or contains unrecognized nutrients (no researched benefits). Example: Buried Treasure Liquid Vitamins .
E V/MS as above which may also contain harmful ingredients such as alcohol, arsenic, aluminum, etc., or harmful levels of nutrients. Example: Geritol® Tonic, Dr. Powers Colloidal Mineral Source.

TIPS FOR TAKING SUPPLEMENTS

- Check the expiration date on your supplements both when you buy to assure initial freshness, and later to make sure the expiration has not past. They will become less effective over time and are best used when fresh. Store them in a cool, dry place.

- Take your supplements with a well-balanced meal. Most nutrients are best absorbed when taken with foods, so that the interactions between nutrients can be facilitated when all are present. This also allows more time for the supplement to be dissolved, and thus better absorbed by the body.

- Spread your daily dosage of supplements over 2 or 3 meals rather than taking them all at once. This will assure balanced absorption and utilization of nutrients and keep blood-nutrient levels high throughout the day. Make sure you have plenty of liquid for the supplement to dissolve, either in the meal, or with a glass of filtered or bottled water.
- Remember that quality in your supplements is important, and usually costs more. Those higher on the grading scale above use higher quality ingredients and have manufacturing processes which are more painstaking to assure nutrient content and quality. On the other hand, there are some ineffective products that cost a lot, too. Use my scale to guide you with the quality and effectiveness part. Then for cost, think about the fact that it's better to spend more on your nutritional intake now (whether for the *best foods* or for *supplements)* than later on medications and treatments, which usually cost more and have side effects or risks as well.

IS OUR FOOD REALLY SAFE?

There is great concern today about the quality of our foods. The various additives and pesticides used to promote the growth and storage life of foods are a troubling fact of life.

I have not taken into consideration additive and pesticide use in my Nutripoint scores for a number of reasons. First, most uses of pesticides and various additives simply don't make enough of a difference in the *nutritive* value of a food. Second, their levels in any given food are simply too difficult to calibrate. Apples, for example, come from so many regions and from so many growers with varying methods of cultivation that it would be impossible to assess each in a book that covers more than 3,600 foods.

While Nutripoints cannot be your guide on how to avoid pesticides and chemicals in your food, I think it's important to be an aware and educated consumer. In 1989 there was a scare concerning the use of the chemical alar on apples. Many people stopped buying apples and apple products. But within a few weeks the *Wall Street Journal*, among others, printed lists of apple juices that had been tested and were found safe in terms of alar content. While some people were complaining about the limited number of juices they could safely give to their children, others knew that there were at least a dozen apple juice brands that were perfectly fine. The lesson is, be aware!

An excellent book that can help you make sense of the dangers of additives and pesticides is *The Goldbecks' Guide to Good Food*, by Nikki and David Goldbeck, published in paperback by New American Library. (This book is also an excellent all-round guide on how to shop for the very best foods.)

ORGANIC VS. NON-ORGANIC

This brings us to the advantages of organic foods. Organic food is produced by farmers who use farming methods that strive for a balance with nature. They focus on soil improvement and rely on biological systems to produce high quality foods and reduce environmental impact. The "organic" label identifies foods grown with practices that:

- Don't use synthetic pesticides, herbicides and soil fumigants.
- Don't use genetic engineering or irradiation in food production.
- Don't use sewage sludge as fertilizer.
- Don't use antibiotics and growth hormones in meat and poultry.
- Use 100-percent organic feed for livestock.
- Improve the quality and fertility of the soil.
- Protect the water quality.
- Reduce soil erosion.
- Rely on biological systems for pest and weed control.
- Reduce the impact of agriculture on the environment.

So you can see it just makes sense to use organic foods when possible. Organic produce clearly contains much lower pesticide levels than produce from conventional growing methods. Studies show that they may also contain more nutrients as well. The *type* of nutrients in food is determined by the genetics of that particular food. The *amount* of these nutrients is determined by many factors including composition of the soil, the amount of sunshine and rain, when it is harvested, and the type of fertilizers used. The absence of pesticides could possibly contribute as well.

A major study published in 2001 compiled data from 41 studies on the nutrient composition of organic vs. non-organically grown foods. Some organically grown foods contained less nutrients and some contained much more—there are variations even among organic growing methods. When all the numbers were averaged, they concluded that organic crops contained significantly more vitamin C, iron, magnesium, and phosphorus and significantly less nitrates and heavy metals than the conventionally grown crops.

When buying organic foods, it's always important to consider others factors as well. For example, if you live in an area where organic foods are not popular and sit on the shelf longer than conventionally grown foods, they could contain much less nutrients—even if they started with more. Today, with consumption of organic food increasing every day, this is less and less of a concern, but make sure there is a quick turnover of the organic foods where you buy them.

How do you know if a food is "organic?" Here is a guideline set up by the USDA in 2002 to help consumers know the exact organic content of the food they buy:

- **100-percent Organic**: All of the product's content is certified organic and may display the USDA Organic seal on the label.
- **Organic**: At least 95-percent of the product's content is certified organic. These products may also display the USDA Organic seal on the label. These products contain some minor ingredients that are not certified organic, such as minerals and vitamins.
- **Made with Organic Ingredients**: At least 70 percent of the product's content is certified organic. Up to three ingredients can be listed on the label with the phrase "made with organic".
- Products containing less than 70-percent organic content may only identify the organic ingredients in the ingredient listing on the label.

Organic foods usually cost more since their farming techniques are more labor-intensive. If your budget makes it difficult for you to afford them, use Nutripoints to help you pick the most nutrient-dense foods overall, so you will be getting the most nutrients your money can buy—literally getting the most nutritional "bang for the buck!"

Another way to do this is to focus your reliance on organic on the most at-risk foods you buy. Foods which are at highest risk for pesticide contamination according to the Environmental Working Group are as follows:

12 Most Contaminated
(buy organic)

- Apples
- Bell Peppers
- Celery
- Cherries
- Grapes (imported)
- Nectarines
- Peaches
- Pears
- Potatoes
- Red Raspberries
- Spinach
- Strawberries

- **12 Least Contaminated:**
- Asparagus
- Avocados
- Bananas
- Broccoli
- Cauliflower
- Corn (sweet)
- Kiwi
- Mangos
- Onions
- Papaya
- Pineapples
- Peas (sweet)

The Environmental Working Group website is a great resource (**www.foodnews.org**) where you can get more details on specific pesticides in various types of produce. There is a handy wallet-sized "Shopper's Guide to Pesticides in Produce" you can download, a "Produce Scanner", and "Report Card for Pesticides in Produce".

From a practical standpoint, how can you minimize the risk you take in eating certain foods? The following are some tips:

- When possible, buy organically grown fruits and vegetables, or those grown under the Integrated Pest Management System, which uses alternative methods of growing and cultivation to keep chemical use at a minimum.

- Try to buy produce that originates in this country. Imported foods may contain residues of pesticides banned here. You'll have to have the cooperation of your greengrocer or supermarket manager to learn the source of produce in your market.

- Wash all fresh fruits and vegetables, and rinse them thoroughly. It's best to use a natural, biodegradable cleanser available at most health food stores. For non-organic produce soaking in water for 5-15 minutes and using a food-grade hydrogen peroxide or bleach is very effective.

- If foods have been waxed, peeling is more effective than washing. Or you can try using a natural, biodegradable fruit and vegetable cleanser available at health food stores.

- Request that your supermarket carry organically grown foods. Write to corporate headquarters and express your concern about pesticide residues.

- Write federal and state government officials about your concerns regarding pesticide use. At the federal level, write the Administrator, Environmental Protection Agency, 401 M Street, SW, Washington, DC 20460; and the Commissioner, Food and Drug Administration, 5600 Fishers Lane, Rockville, MD 20857.

- To avoid risk of salmonella contamination, wash your hands thoroughly before and after handling poultry and eggs. Refrigerate raw and cooked poultry and eggs. Keep raw poultry and eggs away from cooked poultry and eggs. Cook eggs and poultry thoroughly. Wash surfaces that come in contact with raw poultry and eggs with warm, soapy water.

- To avoid parasites, don't eat raw seafood.

IS OUR FOOD REALLY NUTRITIOUS?

Many people today are concerned about the actual nutritional value of foods. In fact, many of my patients have mentioned that they take vitamins, at least in part, because they don't believe that the foods they eat, even supposedly highly nutritious foods, deliver high-quality nutrients. They think this is because of the use of fertilizers, the length of time foods must travel, and the amount of time they spend on the supermarket shelves before we eat them.

Fertilizers used in commercially produced foods are not necessarily a negative in terms of good nutrition. It's interesting that the same people who are opposed to using chemical fertilizers are often devoted to vitamin/mineral supplements, which are, after all, nothing more than chemical fertilizers for the body. That aside, you should not be categorically opposed to fertilizers or chemicals, as some of them actually preserve the nutrients in foods.

What about the idea that foods are lacking in nutrients because they're grown in depleted soils? It has been known for quite some time that soils can be depleted of certain water-soluble nutrients like iodine, and also minerals like selenium. These we know of are usually included in fertilizers to compensate for the nutrients that can become depleted in soils after much use or erosion. The science of farming has advanced to a high degree of efficiency in growing foods per acre of land. Many fear that in doing so, they will deplete the soils to the point where foods do not contain the proper nutrients they should. Although farming techniques strive to use the land in such a way to avoid this fate, and make that fertilizers contain all of the elements we know of that need to be replaced in the soil, the question remains—since some studies show a decline in the nutrient content of some foods over time.

On the positive side, due to the expense of commercial fertilizers and pesticides, and the need to be as efficient as possible, most farmers use some organic fertilizers and techniques (by necessity), even if they are not a "certified organic" type of farm. This recycles some of the natural elements in the soils, and reduces the need for use of commercial products.

In addition, the risk from the effects of soil depletion—although seemingly increased due to high-growth techniques today—could be decreased for the following reason. In the past, our foods were grown more locally and from one specific location or farm. If you ate foods from one or a few local sources and the soil was depleted in certain elements, you would be at high risk. Today, we get our food from hundreds and even thousands of different sources from around the U.S. and even the world. At home we have noticed for example that one week our blueberries are shipped from Michigan, then maybe from Oregon or Maine or Canada the next. So the chances of our foods being low in specific nutrients for certain foods is decreased due to the law of averages.

Beyond pesticides and depleted soil, the question of storage in relation to nutrient content is a valid one. But you might be surprised to learn that the greatest loss occurs in your own kitchen. When the analyses of various foods are done to determine their nutritional content, they're not done on rare, perfectly grown super-foods; they're done on the very same foods you find on supermarket shelves. So when you learn that a raw sweet pepper has 140 milligrams of vitamin C, you can be confident that the sweet peppers you buy in your supermarket have very close to the same amount.

Once food gets to your kitchen, nutrition can be quickly lost through poor storage and processing. Most meats, fish, fruits, and vegetables should be promptly stored in the refrigerator. They should be carefully wrapped, and they should be washed just before eating or cooking them.

PART III

THE NUTRIPOINT BUILDING BLOCKS

THE NUTRIPOINT FORMULA

WHEN I WAS GROWING UP, IT WAS A MEAT AND POTATOES WORLD. Kids were supposed to drink their milk and eat their green vegetables, and parents weren't supposed to eat too many calories. That was just about the extent of common nutritional wisdom. But in my family there was someone who had a different take on the world, particularly the world of food.

My grandma was one of the original "health nuts," at least that's how some people saw her when she arrived at our house with her *Prevention* magazines and her brewer's yeast. But I thought my grandma was someone very special; and, on the face of things, if what she was doing was nutty, at least it worked: she was full of energy and spirit and had one of the most positive approaches to life I've ever seen. She inspired me to believe that there was something to this idea of paying attention to what you ate. As she mixed up her breakfast concoction I would be at her side, asking questions. Is this good for you? Is that good for you? Is this better than that? How much better is this than that? Now I understand why I used to drive her crazy: she really didn't have any way to answer me.

When patients began to ask me the same questions, with a smile I often thought of Grandma. I was in the same position. I knew some foods were bad, and others good, but I didn't know much beyond that. The difference was that Grandma was a grandma and I was *a nutritionist*. That inability to answer nutritional questions, a predicament seemingly handed down from one generation to another, was the original inspiration for Nutripoints.

As I worked with patients and struggled with their questions, I began to think how great it would be if you could reduce nutritional information to simple numbers: just give each food a certain number of points for the good things it had. The major problem faced by my patients was the juggling act they faced with all the nutritional variables. They had to think about cholesterol, sodium, total fat, saturated fat, sugar, complex carbohydrates, vitamins, minerals, fiber, caffeine, and alcohol, in addition to calories. As one patient told me, "I'd have to be a walking computer to figure all this out." I knew what he meant because he'd have to be referring to labels, USDA charts, and RDAs for every food.

In 1981 I worked out a rough formula. I tested it out on a computer using USDA data on 400 foods. It seemed to work, and I was delighted, but put it aside to focus on other things. When I came to the Aerobics Center in Dallas, I revived my old idea and began to use it with patients. I assigned numbers to foods to help people choose the best ones.

The idea of a food having a number attached was a big success; patients loved it. But there was something missing. I needed *a system—some* method of helping people get a variety and a balance of foods as well as the best foods.

In 1985 I started using the basic concepts that evolved into Nutripoints: high nutrient density, low calories, and balance. All of this was done with numbers, and it was wonderfully effective. Many patients at the Aerobics Center had serious health problems—such as coronary heart disease, high cholesterol, high blood pressure, obesity, and diabetes—or were engaging in poor eating habits that were contributing to a major risk for these diseases. While at the center, they had great success with my "numbers" system. There was just one problem with the early versions of Nutripoints. Patients used the numbers when they were at the clinic, but once they got home and tried to find their way without the numbers, they had difficulty sticking with their new, good eating habits.

I knew that if I wanted to help people stick with an optimum eating program, I'd have to come up with a complete system that not only rated the foods but allowed people to achieve variety and balance *within the system.* And, of course, it had to be easy—no more complicated than the simple numbers I was already working with. I could only imagine the problems the person who had never been exposed to a "wellness clinic" must be experiencing.

I began to perfect Nutripoints, working with patients in order to test its effectiveness and confirm its accessibility. It took countless hours with the computer and with data from food manufacturers and fast-food chains to come up with a program that was, first of all, accurate—more accurate than anything currently available—in rating as many foods as possible. It had to make it easy for people to get a completely balanced diet, and to do so by picking their favorite foods, or at least foods they liked, so the system had to be very flexible. Finally, it had to be easy. It had to be something that people could do at home, by themselves, and something they could stick with whether they ate at home, at restaurants, at fast-food restaurants, or at friends' houses. I'm finally satisfied that Nutripoints fulfills all of these goals.

The following pages explain how the Nutripoints formula is set up.

First, I determined the components of each food. How much of each vitamin and mineral, how much fiber, protein, complex carbohydrates, cholesterol, total fat, saturated fat, sugar, caffeine, and alcohol was in each food entry. There were eighteen *essential* elements and eight *excessive* elements in each food, the amount of which needed to be determined.

Where did the information come from? I used various sources. The Cooper Clinic Database provided about half the information initially. The USDA Database was enormously helpful and is updated regularly. I also referred to Pennington and Church's comprehensive *Nutritive Value of Foods,* as well as other nutrition books. The newest source I've added recently is the NutriBase Clinical database, which is extremely comprehensive.

In the case of brand-name foods and fast-foods, the information first came either from the manufacturer's research data or from food labels. I initially wrote to approximately 200 companies and received information from more than three-fourths of them. In the case of fast foods, I wrote to manufacturers and included those foods I received data on. Most of the data is now available online on the company websites—this information is usually the most up-to-date. This is where I currently get most all of the information for new brand-name foods and for updates.

Once I gathered information on all the foods, I needed to analyze it in terms of what nutrients the foods contained, and how the foods compared with how much of those nutrients we need in our diets. For example, a food that has a full day's requirement of vitamin C is better than a food that has 50 percent of a day's requirement of C. The nutrient content needed to be compared with a standard.

I wanted to use a standard for each nutrient that represented the highest level of *essential* nutrients per calorie and the lowest level of *excessive* nutrients per calorie. That way I'd be able to downgrade foods that are high in nutrients but also high in calories, or, say, a food that's very high in a mineral such as calcium but also very high in fat. It was also an attempt to introduce a balance factor that limits credit for a single nutrient. If a food has 50 percent of the RDA for six nutrients, it's a better food than something that has 150 percent of the RDA for only a single nutrient. A food can only get 100 percent credit for an essential (even if it has 200 percent of the RDA for a given factor), but there's no cap on how negatively the excessives can affect a Nutripoint score.

As a standard for the *essential* nutrients, I used the RDA requirements for adults, which are:

Protein (high quality)	45 g
Protein (low quality)	65 g
Vitamin A	5,000 IU
Vitamin C	60 mg
Thiamine (B_1)	1.5 mg
Riboflavin (B_2)	1.7 mg
Niacin (B_3)	20 mg
Calcium	1,000 mg
Iron	18 mg
B_6	2 mg
Folic acid	.4 mg (400 mcg)
B_{12}	6 mcg
Phosphorus	1,000 mg
Magnesium	400 mg
Zinc	15 mg
Pantothenic acid	10 mg

These levels, set by the government, are generally the highest standard for each nutrient based on the National Research Council's recommended daily allowance for various subgroups of the U.S. population. Therefore, these standards should meet, or exceed, the needs of virtually all healthy adults. As to the two kinds of protein, because we're rating each food individually, we quantified the *type* of protein, and the ratings reflect this. High-quality protein is found in animal products, and low-quality protein is found in all other foods. They're so defined because the balance of amino acids is more complete in animal protein. But in practice, you don't need to worry at all about types of protein because the balance of the Nutripoint program takes care of this for you.

Some essentials have no RDA, and therefore the following guidelines were used:

Complex carbohydrates	60 percent of total calories
Dietary fiber	35 g*
Potassium	5,625 mg†

The following standards were used as the upper limit allowable for each of the *excessive* elements in our diet:

Total fat	30 percent of total calories
Saturated fat	10 percent of total calories
Cholesterol	300 mg. per day
Sodium	3,000 mg. per day
Sugar	10 percent of total calories
Caffeine	200 mg. per day
Alcohol	½ ounce of pure alcohol per day

Once I set these standards, the computer converted these figures to a percentage of either the recommended amount (in the case of the essential nutrients), which would be a positive percentage, or the recommended limit (in the case of the excessive nutrients), which would be a negative percentage.

For example, an apple has 6 milligrams of vitamin C. So I would take 6 and divide by the RDA for vitamin C, which is 60. The resulting percentage is 10. So, for vitamin C, one of the eighteen variables, an apple scores 10 percent. The Nutripoint formula does this calculation for each one of the eighteen essentials,which include all the vitamins and minerals as well as fiber, complex carbohydrates, and protein.

Another example: an orange has 66 milligrams of vitamin C, so 66 divided by 60 (the RDA for vitamin C) equals 110 percent. An orange has 110 percent of the RDA for vitamin C. But the formula gives no credit beyond 100 percent for any one of the essentials. (That's done to avoid giving too much credit to a food that is high in only one nutrient. We don't want a food to be at the top of the list if it has an enormous amount of one nutrient, but not much of any other nutrients.) Thus the percentage score for the orange in relation to vitamin C is 100 percent.

***This is the upper limit of the daily recommendation of the National Cancer Institute.**

†Although no RDA for potassium has been set, the National Research Council has set a "recommended safe dietary intake" of several nutrients, including potassium. This level represents the highest level within that range.

A variation of the same procedure is done for the excessives. For example, whole milk has 30 milligrams of cholesterol for an eight-ounce serving. Three hundred is the daily limit of cholesterol, so you determine what percentage of your daily limit is contained in that eight-ounce glass of milk. Three hundred divided by 30 equals 10 percent. Because it's a negative factor, this means it's a negative percentage. So milk gets a 10-percent negative for cholesterol.

All of those percentages, negative and positive, for each food were then added together and divided by the number of positive factors. That percentage was then divided by the total calories in the standard serving of that food. The result is a fraction. The fraction was then multiplied by 100 and rounded to the nearest half or whole number. The resulting figure is the Nutripoint rating for that food.

I considered twenty-six factors for each of the 3,600 foods, which translates into 93,600 info-bits that went into the rankings.

One of the advantages of the Nutripoint formula is that it's flexible. If another nutrient is discovered, or if another negative factor that affects our health is revealed, the formula can be adjusted for this new information, and the numbers re-crunched to come up with new, updated Nutripoint scores for every food. It's a formula that's poised to adapt to the latest nutritional research so that the Nutripoint score for a food will always be the best and most complete evaluation possible.

ANSWERS TO QUESTIONS ABOUT THE NUTRIPOINT FORMULA

While I have just described the basics of how the Nutripoint formula works, I would like to answer the following common questions about it:

Are all the factors weighted equally?

In other words, does a food get as much credit for having 100 percent of the RDA of vitamin C as it does for having 100 percent of the RDA for pantothenic acid? And is having too much fat just as bad as having too much caffeine? It is obvious that some factors should be weighted, and I did so. The following are exceptions to the formula rules:

- *Dietary fiber* is weighted two times positive.

I felt that fiber is of utmost importance in the American diet, so we weighted it more positively to help steer people to foods that are rich in these factors.

Weighting fiber highly also helps to lower the scores of foods that are fortified. This is done because many of them contain a lot of vitamins and minerals, but are low in fiber due to processing.

- *Cholesterol* and *alcohol* are weighted three times negatively.

I felt that cholesterol was an extremely negative factor in today's diet. By weighting it with a triple negative, I ensured that foods high in cholesterol would have lowered Nutripoint scores.

Because alcohol is negative in so many ways, I weighted it particularly negatively. It can be high in calories. It's virtually devoid of nutrients. It drains the body's stores of nutrients, particularly the B vitamins. It's a toxin to the body which the liver must detoxify so you are not poisoned by it. It is also a direct carcinogen to any part of the body which it comes in contact. It can be psychologically harmful, and of course—addictive. For these reasons I wanted to steer people away from alcohol.

Recent studies have shown that red wine contains phytochemicals which may help prevent heart disease, and even provide positive benefits from the alcohol itself. The other side of the story is that these same phytochemicals can be obtained by drinking red grape juice—without the negative effects or risks associated with alcohol consumption. As for the benefits of alcohol in general, every drug which has a positive effect—has a corresponding negative effect on the body. It's like trading off a benefit to one organ of the body to the detriment of another. Are the benefits worth the negatives? In my opinion—no.

What about saturated fat? Doesn't recent research show that it's just as bad, or even worse, than eating cholesterol?

Yes, it does seem that saturated fat, which acts to elevate blood cholesterol, is a particularly negative element in the diet. The Nutripoint formula in effect weights saturated fat doubly negative because both total fat and saturated fat (a part of total fat) are given negative weights separately.

Could the formula for Nutripoints ever change?

Yes. It's possible that we'd find a more accurate way to calculate Nutripoints, especially if there's a research breakthrough on a new nutrient or on an element that's revealed to be particularly harmful to our health. It's important to remember, however, that whatever flaws might exist in the present system, it is consistent in its analysis, and is the best and most up-to-date system we have. Because it does the same things to all foods, and because the foods themselves will not change, it's an extraordinarily reliable guide to food value.

How did you decide what the portion size should be for each food?

The Nutripoint score is *a quality* rating. The serving size correlates with the *calories* in the food. In other words, the quality of the food times the calories equals Nutripoints. In order to make sure the Nutripoint value is correct, I had to be sure that the calories per serving within each group were approximately the same. I also had to be practical about amounts people typically consider to be a serving (although you are allowed to eat the serving size best for you and adjust the corresponding Nutripoints). The following lists show how the calories per serving break down in the various Nutrigroups:

Food Groups

Nutrigroup	*Calories per Serving*
Vegetable	20—60
Fruit	50—100
Grain	100—200
Legume	100—200
Milk/dairy	100–200
Meat/poultry/fish	125—250
Other Groups	50–100
Oil	
Sugar	100–200
Condiment	0—20
Alcohol	100–200

Serving sizes get smaller as the amount of calories and fat goes up. If something has, say, 100 calories, you might have a cup as a serving size, but if it's 200 calories, you might have a half cup.

Were there any surprises in the results of the Nutripoint food ratings?

Yes. For example, I was surprised at how low peanut butter rates. At .5 Nutripoints, it's low down on the legume Nutrigroup list. I thought that because it has no cholesterol and a decent amount of protein it would do better. I was also surprised at the cheeses. The fat and cholesterol in cheese really pulls it down, and many types of cheese are below the recommended level in the milk/dairy Nutrigroup. This makes it obvious that it's important to stick to the low-fat dairy foods. I was surprised at how bad eggs are. While egg whites are fine, a whole cooked egg scores −11.5, a terrible rating! It's really the cholesterol and saturated fat that pulls it down. Lean beef was also a surprise: it's not as bad as many people think. In fact, as you glance down the list you'll find that it's sometimes a better choice than some types of chicken. I'm sure you'll be interested to check your favorite foods in the lists and find how they score. You may be in for some surprises too.

ESSENTIALS AND EXCESSIVES

Now that you know the basics of what went into the Nutripoint formula, you might find it interesting to learn a bit more about the components of foods and how they affect your diet.

I have a somewhat revolutionary proposition to make: let's look at the essentials of our diet in an entirely new light. Instead of breaking things down into "sources of energy" or "percentages of daily requirements," let's be completely practical about what we need to know about food.

In fact, you don't *really* need to know anything but the numbers and Nutrigroups, but you probably have a healthy curiosity about the basic factors that go into figuring the Nutripoint numbers. So let's look at food with a fresh approach.

The factors that have been figured into the Nutripoints formula are all elements in the foods we eat. Some are good for us, but are lacking in our diets; others are good for us, but are consumed in excessive quantities; still others are bad for us, and should be avoided. I've made a practical breakdown of the elements of foods that corresponds only to what you need to know. I've divided them into two groups: *essentials* and *excessives.*

My breakdown of the essential elements in our diet is slightly unconventional. Both fat and cholesterol, for example, are indeed essential to maintain life. But, because they have become problem elements in our diets, I've moved them into the excessives category: no one in this country has to worry about getting enough fat or cholesterol in his or her diet. Calories, too, earn their place on the excessives list, even though we couldn't live without them. My breakdown is as follows:

Essentials	*Excessives*
Complex carbohydrates	Total fat
Protein	Saturated fat
Dietary fiber	Calories
Vitamins*	Cholesterol
Minerals†	Sodium
	Sugar
	Caffeine
	Alcohol

The Essentials

The following are brief descriptions of the role *each* of these elements plays in our diets:

Complex Carbohydrates Carbohydrates, as the name implies, are made up of carbon, hydrogen, and oxygen. Carbohydrates supply energy, in the form of blood sugar, to keep the body functioning. Carbohydrates have always seemed to me a "schizophrenic" food group: on the one hand, complex carbohydrates (those found in cereals, rice, breads, pasta, beans, nuts, and all vegetables) are really good for you. You probably eat too little of them, and one of the aims of Nutripoints is to ensure that you eat more. On the other hand, simple carbohydrates (those found in refined sugars, such as candy, cakes, puddings, soft drinks, sugar-coated cereals, and the like) are terrible for you, and you probably eat too much of them (thus why the low-carb diets work). Nutripoints has made sugar a negative factor in the Nutripoint formula and complex carbohydrates a positive factor so that the numbers reflect what you really need in your diet. In other words, Nutripoints weights fiber as a positive factor, and sugar as a negative factor; the system highlights the *best* carbohydrates for you.

The Nutripoint program emphasizes complex carbohydrates as a primary food. By recommending ten servings of carbohydrates daily (four of vegetables, three of fruits, two of grains, and one of legumes), it recognizes that a diet rich in complex carbohydrates can improve your energy levels and your performance, as well as help you prevent long-term disease. This emphasis on carbohydrates has replaced

*** Vitamins include A, thiamin, B_2, B_3, B_6, B_{12}, C, pantothenic acid, and folacin.**
† Minerals include calcium, iron, magnesium, phosphorus, potassium, and zinc.

the old-fashioned reliance on protein as a "diet" food. Carbohydrates are low in fat, but nonetheless very satisfying. They are rich in vitamins and minerals. They "burn clean" in the body, leaving only carbon dioxide and water to be excreted (as opposed to protein, which leaves nitrogen and sulfur waste). Carbohydrates are also the major source of fuel to the brain, which relies on an optimum level of blood sugar to function properly.

Protein Along with fat and carbohydrates, protein is one of the sources of energy from food. It is essential for life. Every cell in the body contains some protein. Indeed, excluding water, half of the body's weight is protein. It's important that you get sufficient protein in your diet every day to function at an optimum level.

Most of us think of protein as the "safest" food component. We think carbohydrates are bad; we know fat is bad. But protein is something that you should eat a lot of, especially if you're on a diet. Right? Wrong! Most of us eat at least *twice* as much protein as we need. And, unlike a water-soluble vitamin, excess protein is not excreted. It's stored in the body. Because the major sources of protein we consume include meat and dairy products, which are high in fat, our high protein intake is also creating high fat, cholesterol, and calorie intakes. In short, it's making us fat. It's also putting a strain on the liver and kidneys, which are responsible for processing excess protein. Finally, excess protein consumption increases your need for calcium, and can exacerbate problems connected with a low-calcium diet.

The Nutripoints balance assures you that you're getting just the right amount of protein daily. You'll be getting high-quality protein with a balance of all the essential amino acids. But the source of some of your protein will shift: instead of getting most of your protein from meat, you'll be getting more from other sources, such as legumes. I might mention here that I've provided a vegetarian option, a Nutripoints program for those readers who prefer to omit meat entirely from their diets.

Nutri-Tip: Protein

The best approach to giving your diet a better balance in terms of protein is to shift the major source of it from meat and dairy foods to fish, soy products (such as tofu), and dried beans and peas. There are some excellent frozen entrees that rely on tofu as their main source of protein. They're low in calories, without cholesterol, and lower in fat than meat. I highly recommend them. I've also included some delicious main course bean-based recipes, such as bean soups, which I think you'll enjoy.

Fiber Fiber, commonly called "roughage," is a nonnutritive part of food. It has virtually no calories, and is not digested. Fiber is important in giving "bulk" to food, and in helping to move it through the intestines and colon. Lack of sufficient fiber in the diet has been linked to cancers of the colon and rectum, diverticulosis, hemorrhoids, hiatal hernia, varicose veins, and heart disease.

There are two types of fiber present in foods: soluble and insoluble. We've long been aware of insoluble fiber. It was the "rough stuff" we could depend on to promote regularity. It's insoluble because it won't dissolve in hot water. Soluble fiber, which will dissolve in hot water, has an effect on the body's metabolism of fats and sugar. Oat bran has become the most popular soluble fiber—maybe because we can put it into sweet, fatty *muffins* and think we're doing ourselves a nutritional favor. While it's certainly true that certain soluble fibers have a beneficial effect on blood cholesterol, fruits and vegetables, as well as beans, contain soluble fiber that's every bit as beneficial as the fiber found in oat bran.

Following the Nutripoints program will ensure that you're getting enough of both soluble and insoluble fiber. There is no need to take fiber supplements, and they can actually be dangerous if you don't take them with enough water, or if you take them to excess. Moreover, too much fiber, which is more likely to occur if you take supplements, can leach nutrients from your body as it moves food too rapidly through your digestive system. Remember: food, not pills!

In the past, the oat bran craze was superseded by the rice bran craze. Recently it's come full circle to the high-protein low-carb diets of the past. It seems that every few months there's a new nutritional bandwagon you can climb on. It may be megavitamins, or fiber, or tryptophan, or fish oil. As appealing as these trends can be (it's always so tempting to think that you can change and improve your life in one easy step), most of us who have seen these trends come and go recognize that they're often an exaggeration of some very complex research. The oat bran phenomenon started with some research that found that the fiber in certain foods, including beans, carrots, and oat bran, among others, was helpful in controlling cholesterol. Well, carrots and beans are not very sexy, so everyone seized on the oat bran connection. In fact, oat bran is no more effective in controlling cholesterol than a number of other fibrous foods. But who wants to eat some beans or carrots when you can have a huge, rich, sweet, fatty oat bran muffin for breakfast and feel virtuous at the same time? The fact is, if you're serious about good nutrition, the trends are not your best inspiration. So often they turn out to be exaggerated or even wrong.

Nutripoints goes beyond trends in that you'll be eating the very foods that may be discovered in the near future to be beneficial. How can I be sure of this? Because you'll be eating the very best, highest-quality foods. Nutripoints makes optimum nutrition an achievable goal today.

> Nutri-Tip: Fiber
> Beans are an excellent source of fiber, and play too small a role in our diets. To get the most benefit from beans, soak them overnight and then cook them slowly at a low temperature. If you don't soak them and you cook them in boiling water, you'll just toughen them and impede the availability of the fiber and nutrients they're rich in.

Vitamins and Minerals Adequate vitamin and mineral intake is one of the major goals of Nutripoints. The goal of the system is to provide you with *at least* the RDA of every essential vitamin and mineral.

Vitamins are organic substances that are essential to biochemical reactions in our bodies. Vitamins do not give us "energy"; we rely on calories for that. They simply promote the metabolic functions that result in energy. There are thirteen vitamins. Four vitamins are fat-soluble (A, D, E, and K), and nine are water-soluble (C and the eight B-complex vitamins: thiamin, riboflavin, niacin, B_6, folic acid, B_{12}, pantothenic acid, and biotin).

Minerals are inorganic substances that, like vitamins, promote various metabolic functions in the body. The macrominerals, which are needed in relatively large amounts, include calcium, phosphorus, magnesium, potassium, sulfur, sodium, and chlorine. The microminerals, or trace minerals, are needed in tiny amounts. They include iron, zinc, selenium, manganese, molybdenum, copper, iodine, chromium, and fluorine. I haven't included the microminerals in the Nutripoint formula because they're not normally reported in USDA data, and getting information on amounts available in foods is difficult, if not impossible. It's also been shown that foods high in the macronutrients are also high in the micronutrients.

The same is true for the recently discovered and highly beneficial "phytochemicals" in foods (of which there are thousands—and possibly tens of thousands). As we get more information on some of the key ones for every food, we can incorporate them into the formula. But for now—rest assured that most every food highly-rated in Nutripoints is the best based on what we *can identify and measure,* and most likely is also high in these other healthy components in foods that we *can't identify and measure.*

Here's a quick breakdown of every vitamin and mineral considered in the Nutripoint numbers, and some tips on how to guarantee your intake of that particular substance.

Vitamin A I think of vitamin A as the "wrapper" vitamin because it's largely responsible for the health of our wrappers: our skin, hair, and mucous membranes (the linings of our mouths, stomachs, and so on). It's also involved in vision, immunity, and reproduction. Vitamin A is fat-soluble. The most exciting news about vitamin A is that researchers have recently connected a lack of vitamin A with the development of certain cancers. This is important because many of us, particularly children and adolescents, don't get nearly enough vitamin A. At the same time, there is fear among medical experts that some people, hearing of the ability of vitamin A to boost the immune system and prevent cancer, are overdosing on vitamin A. Because vitamin A is fat-soluble, and is therefore stored in the body, toxic amounts can build up and cause jaundice or liver damage. Moreover, vitamin A supplements have not been shown to help fight cancer. Beta-carotene, a precursor to vitamin A, which is found in red and yellow fruits and vegetables, is the cancer fighter, so those foods are your best sources of vitamin A. If you're getting your vitamin A in the form of beta-carotene from foods, you won't have to worry about the dangers of overdosing.

> Nutri-Tip: Vitamin A
>
> One of the best, quickest, and most delicious sources of vitamin A is a sweet potato. It gives you twice the RDA for vitamin A. If you've never tried a baked sweet potato, you're missing something. Just eat it hot from the oven or microwave plain, or with a bit of nonfat yogurt for a great snack or as part of a meal.

Vitamin C Vitamin C (ascorbic acid) is one of the most well known water-soluble vitamins. It's a sort of "glue" vitamin that is important in the manufacture of collagen, which helps hold the body together. Perhaps one of the best-known roles of vitamin C is that of infection fighter.

I've learned that many people, even those who don't take any other type of vitamin, will pop a vitamin C tablet regularly, or when they feel a cold coming on. This obsession is somewhat misguided, as most of us get at least one and a half times the amount of vitamin C we need each day. At least vitamin C, because it is water-soluble, is not one of those vitamins that can readily become dangerous in high levels: the body excretes excess amounts.

> Nutri-Tip: Vitamin C
>
> I think the best vitamin C "supplement" you can take is a sweet red pepper. One-eighth of a red pepper will give you about 95 milligrams of vitamin C, or one and a half times your daily requirement. Red pepper is also very low in calories.

Vitamin B_1 (Thiamin) B_1 is known as the "energy" vitamin because one of its most important roles is in the metabolism of carbohydrates. It's also important in the functioning of nerves. It stimulates growth, helps to maintain good muscle tone, and has been shown to stabilize the appetite. Because thiamin is water-soluble, it's rarely dangerous, even when taken to excess.

> Nutri-Tip: Vitamin B_1
>
> Don't add baking soda to water when you cook vegetables (as some people do to retain bright green colors). This practice depletes thiamin. Also, don't wash enriched white rice before you cook it (you can wash brown and wild rice). Don't boil any kind of rice in a lot of water until done and then drain it. Instead, measure the appropriate amount of rice and the appropriate amount of water (about twice as much water as rice), and then cook the rice until it has absorbed all the water. Throwing out water that rice has boiled in is like throwing out "vitamin soup."

Vitamin B_2 (Riboflavin) Vitamin B_2 is necessary for carbohydrate, fat, and protein metabolism. It boosts the immune system and the formation of red blood cells. It also promotes good vision and helps keep skin, nails, and hair healthy.

> Nutri-Tip: Vitamin B_2
>
> Rely on dairy products! Because so many of the sources of B_2 are foods low in Nutripoints, such as organ meats (which are very high in fats), low-fat or nonfat dairy foods are your best source. Keep up with the Nutripoint food groups and don't neglect your two servings of high-Nutripoint dairy foods daily. Adding some extra nonfat dry milk when you're baking (or to recipes such as meat loaf) can give you a good boost of B_2.

Vitamin B_3 (Niacin) Vitamin B_3 has became a popular vitamin because of the role it plays in reducing cholesterol. In addition to this critical job, niacin is necessary for carbohydrate, fat, and protein metabolism. It helps maintain the health of your skin, tongue, and digestive and nervous systems.

The good news about niacin is that very few people have problems with deficiencies because it is so readily available from so many food sources. Just three ounces of water-packed tuna, for example, supplies about three-quarters of your daily requirement.

For reasons previously discussed concerning vitamins and their dangers, I don't recommend that you try to supplement with niacin to lower your blood cholesterol unless you're doing so under the direction of a physician. There are serious side effects connected with megadoses of niacin.

> Nutri-Tip: Vitamin B_3
> The highest level of the RDA for niacin (for males 19 to 22 years of age) is 19 milligrams. As three ounces of tuna canned in water has 14 milligrams you can see why it is not hard to come by niacin in food. So, my suggestion on niacin is to avoid supplements. Prolonged use of megadoses can result in skin rashes, irritation of peptic ulcers, irregular heartbeat, jaundice, and promotion of gout, among other symptoms.

Vitamin B_6 Vitamin B_6 is a water-soluble vitamin that has many roles in the biochemical life of the body. It's necessary for fat, carbohydrate, and protein metabolism. It's important in the production of red blood cells and of antibodies. It helps to regulate blood glucose levels. Because vitamin B_6 is critical to so many functions, its lack is signaled by a wide variety of symptoms and has been connected to everything from asthma, PMS, and carpal tunnel syndrome, to diabetes, cancer, and cardiovascular disease.

So many people are so deficient in vitamin B_6 that the government has named it a "problem nutrient." In a recent study only 22 percent of Americans past the age of one met their recommended dietary allowances of vitamin B_6. Because B_6 plays such an important role in so many biochemical activities in our bodies, it's important to get an adequate amount. But please don't rely on supplements. While B_6 is water-soluble, and excess amounts are largely flushed from the body, high doses (upward of 200 milligrams a day) can result in nervousness, insomnia, frequent urination, irritability, and bed wetting in children.

> Nutri-Tip: Vitamin B_6
> One banana will give you over a third of your daily requirement of vitamin B_6.

Vitamin B_{12} Vitamin B_{12} is a water-soluble vitamin that is responsible for the formation of blood cells, as well as the metabolism of carbohydrates, fats, and proteins. It's important for cell replication and helps maintain a healthy nervous system.

Because B_{12} is found in so many foods, it's rare to suffer a deficiency. The people most likely to suffer a B_{12} deficiency are strict vegetarians, and even they are not very likely to suffer a deficiency if they vary their diet.

> Nutri-Tip: Vitamin B12
> Stores of B_{12} can last in the body up to fifteen years. As you need only 3 micrograms daily, you really don't need to worry about a deficiency, and you can easily see why supplements of B_{12} would be superfluous for healthy people.

Pantothenic Acid Pantothenic acid is essential for healthy skin, body growth, and the production of antibodies. It's also necessary for the conversion of fats and carbohydrates into energy. Because pantothenic acid is so readily available in foods, there's little danger of deficiency.

> Nutri-Tip: Pantothenic Acid
> Because you need such small amounts, and because it's so readily available, you'll have no trouble getting adequate pantothenic acid.

Folacin Folacin aids in the metabolism of proteins, and is necessary for the growth and division of cells. Folacin is essential to your mental and emotional health.

Folacin deficiencies, particularly among women, are not uncommon. A U.S. Department of Agriculture survey revealed that many women get less than half the recommended level of folacin. If you're taking contraceptive pills, or if you've been taking aspirin because of its connection to mitigating the development of cardiovascular disease, you may need extra folacin in your diet. A number of health problems are related to folacin deficiencies, including depression, infections, cervical dysplasia in women on the pill, and cancer.

> Nutri-Tip: Folacin
> To retain the most folacin in your foods, cook vegetables in the least possible amount of water or oil. Stir-frying them in the smallest possible amount of oil is the best method. The best possible folacin boost is a spinach salad: a half cup of raw spinach gives you twice the RDA of folacin.

The emphasis on vegetables and legumes in the Nutripoint program will guarantee that you'll receive an adequate supply of folacin. Folacin is readily available in green, leafy vegetables. Those at the top of the Nutripoints list are rich in the vitamin. Even if you're among those who need extra folacin, you'll be more than adequately supplied by the Nutripoint program.

Calcium Calcium is one of the most abundant minerals in the body, and is essential to human life. Calcium sustains the maintenance and development of bones and teeth, and is critical to blood coagulation, muscle action, heartbeat, and nerve function.

Calcium has been a "hot" mineral for many years, and with good reason. A government survey revealed that 68 percent of Americans are deficient in calcium. Those especially vulnerable to calcium deficiency are women: adolescent girls and middle-aged women. The deficiency shows up in later years, when these women suffer from osteoporosis—a weak bone structure that can lead to dowager's hump and easily fractured bones.

One of the reasons people have become at risk for calcium deficiency is that many of the foods that have high levels of calcium also have high levels of fat. Milk and other dairy products, which are the most common sources of calcium, are often avoided by people on a low-fat diet.

> Nutri-Tip: Calcium
>
> A half cup of cooked broccoli or four ounces of nonfat yogurt will give you over a third of your daily requirement, while a half cup of cooked bok choy will give you well over a third. One-quarter cup of nonfat dry milk gives you over a third of your daily requirement, and it can be added to foods such as dressings, baked goods, and meat loafs to boost calcium supplies without adding many calories.

Unfortunately, many people have resorted to calcium supplements to try to increase their calcium intakes. Most are not absorbed nearly as well as calcium in foods, so I strongly recommend that you rely instead on the high-Nutripoint foods listed in the milk/dairy food group for the best low-fat sources of calcium. And keep in mind that weight-bearing exercise such as walking or jogging increases calcium absorption while caffeine, alcohol, and smoking decrease it.

Iron A trace mineral essential for life, iron is the "blood mineral." It's responsible for the transport of oxygen in the body by means of the hemoglobin in red blood cells. Iron deserves attention because it is so commonly deficient in the average diet. Nearly half of the population is deficient in iron. Women are often iron deficient, particularly because of their monthly blood loss during menstruation. But young children are also commonly iron deficient.

Of all the nutrient-deficiency diseases, anemia is the most common. And if you find it hard to translate a condition such as anemia into real-life problems, you'll be amazed to learn that one study of women found that their work performance quadrupled when they increased their iron intake.

> Nutri-Tip: Iron
>
> You can dramatically increase your iron intake by taking some vitamin C in the form of, say, orange juice with an iron-rich meal. Orange juice with breakfast, for example, can boost the absorbed iron by 200 percent. Avoid drinking coffee or tea with meals: they decrease iron absorption.

Magnesium Magnesium is essential for every biological process. It aids in the body's use of carbohydrates, fats, and proteins, and works in conjunction with other minerals, including calcium, phosphorus, and potassium. Many of us are deficient in magnesium because of our low-calorie diets of highly processed foods. A USDA food consumption survey revealed that only 25 percent of Americans get enough magnesium. Despite deficiencies, magnesium supplements are not the answer. Magnesium is a mineral that perfectly illustrates my contention that supplements are to be avoided because they're frequently unbalanced. Because magnesium works in conjunction with calcium, for example, if you increase your magnesium intake, you must increase your calcium intake at an even ratio, and vice versa if you take calcium supplements. Very few people are aware of this relationship between minerals. If you get your minerals from foods, however, Mother Nature takes care of the balance for you.

Nutri-Tip: Magnesium

A half cup of fresh, cooked spinach has about one-quarter of your daily magnesium requirement. Dried bran cereals such as All-Bran, Bran Buds, Bran Chex, and Bran Flakes are good sources of magnesium, with one ounce of many of them providing about one-quarter of your daily requirement.

Potassium Potassium is the third most abundant element in the body. It works with magnesium to help regulate the heart, and with sodium to help regulate blood pressure and send nerve impulses. Fortunately, potassium is abundant in the average diet and so rarely poses the problem of deficiency. People who might be in danger of potassium deficiency include those suffering from a digestive disease, those using diuretics, and those with uncontrolled diabetes. Athletes and others who sweat profusely may find that their potassium levels are low.

Nutri-Tip: Potassium

If you are an athlete, or if you exercise heavily in high temperatures, you should be wary of potassium depletion. Watch for weakness or fatigue over a longer than usual period. A quick recovery can be effected with a "natural potassium supplement": a glass of orange juice or a banana. Avoid potassium supplements, as overdoses pose serious risks.

Phosphorus You have a pound and a half of phosphorus in your body. Along with calcium, it's the most abundant mineral. Phosphorus, along with calcium, is responsible for the building of bones. It also plays a major role in other metabolic functions, including cell reproduction and conversion of foods to energy.

> Nutri-Tip: Phosphorus
> If you frequently take antacids that contain aluminum, they can block your absorption of phosphorus. Check with your druggist to find an antacid that doesn't contain aluminum, or try to boost your phosphorus intake.

Because phosphorus is so widely available in a variety of foods (dairy products, meats, fish, grains, nuts, and beans) you rarely have to worry about a phosphorus deficiency.

Zinc Zinc is a critical trace mineral that promotes growth and healing. It aids the immune system in its efforts to prevent disease, and is important in a wide range of metabolic activities.

Marginal zinc deficiencies seem to be a common price paid for today's style of eating. Low-calorie diets are the culprits. A USDA study revealed that only 8 percent of the surveyed groups achieved the recommended zinc levels. The typical woman eats only half the calories she would need to get sufficient zinc. Because of zinc's important role in boosting the immune system, this is a potentially dangerous nutritional situation. Zinc deficiencies also play a role in eating disorders such as anorexia nervosa and bulimia, osteoporosis, low sperm counts, gum disease, and fetal complications, including low birth weight and other disorders.

> Nutri-Tip: Zinc
> One ounce of the following cereals will provide you with nearly a third of your daily zinc requirement: All-Bran, Bran Buds, 40% Bran Flakes, Nutri-Grain, and Special K. Three ounces of lean pot roast will give you half your daily zinc requirement.

The Excessives

The excessives are the elements in our diet that there are just too much of. As I mentioned before, most of these items are not totally bad; indeed, all of them, with the exception of caffeine and alcohol, are essential to human life. It's just that our eating patterns have emphasized these elements to our detriment. We simply can't continue to eat diets high in fat, calories, cholesterol, sodium, and sugar without paying the price in both long- and short-term symptoms and diseases.

The following are the excessives that have been figured into the Nutripoint formula:

Total fat
Saturated fat Calories
Cholesterol Sodium
Sugar Caffeine
Alcohol

Fat Fat has become one of the biggest problems in our diet. While fat is essential for life (as a concentrated energy source, a carrier of fat-soluble vitamins, and a source of essential fatty acids), too much fat is ultimately life-threatening. Most of us are eating three to five times the amount of fat we need to keep our bodies functioning. We really only need the equivalent of one tablespoon of fat per day. All the excess fat we're eating is contributing to heart disease, colon and breast cancer, and obesity (which is linked to a number of other diseases).

Nutri-Tip: Fat

I think that one of the major "fat booby traps" is salad dressings. Salad dressings pose a problem because many people think they are eating better because they're eating more salads and vegetables on the Nutripoint program. But commercial salad dressings are loaded with fat, and most people don't realize that when you factor the fat and calories into the equation, it's negating much of the benefit of the vegetables. Even if you do virtually no cooking, you owe it to yourself to either find a good low-fat or non-fat commercial dressing, or to try one of our Nutripoint dressing recipes. You'll find such a dressing every bit as flavorful as those oily ones, and far more healthful. Make up a batch and keep it handy in your refrigerator. You can even bring a small amount with you to a restaurant and ask for a salad without dressing so that you can use your own.

Cutting down on fat is one of the most important things you can do to improve your diet and thereby extend your life. Nutripoints will make it easy for you, as fat is heavily weighted as a negative factor. By sticking to the foods that are at the high end of the Nutripoint food charts, and by being sure to limit your meat and dairy servings and portions to the Nutripoint recommendations, you'll be keeping your fat intake to 30 percent of your total calories, and your saturated fat to within 10 percent of your total calories that are well within the limit set by the American Heart Association. (We break out saturated fat from the total fat because while foods with saturated fat don't contain cholesterol, they cause the body to produce cholesterol and thereby raise serum cholesterol levels.)

Calories Hi-cal, low-cal, no-cal—calories have been the dominant issue in the way most of us have approached nutrition for the past thirty years. All we want to know about calories is how to avoid them, and this obsession has given us such a distorted picture of what nutrition is all about that far too many of us are actually malnourished. A recently published book, for example, is an endless listing of the calories in every imaginable food, the premise of the book being that you can lose weight by substituting low-calorie foods for high-calorie ones. But if you binge, as you no doubt will, you can catch up by eating next to nothing until you're back to your goal. This is all pretty basic, but the implication is that you can substitute, say, a candy bar for a tuna sandwich on whole wheat and get away with it if the calories in the two foods are the same. I'm surprised that this old-fashioned approach to nutrition is still given any credence at all. The fact is, calories are just one of many factors that need to be considered in the decision as to whether a food is good or bad, nutritious or not.

Strictly speaking, calories are units of heat measurement: a calorie is the amount of energy it takes to raise the temperature of 1 gram of water 1 degree centigrade. Calories are the fuel that enable our bodies to perform their endless metabolic tasks. The average adult man burns 1,500 to 2,000 calories per day, and the average woman, 1,200 to 1,800. You need to consume about that many calories for your body to function: less and you'll force your body to call on stored energy and thereby lose weight; more and you'll store the excess calories as fat and gain weight. It's that simple.

Many of us are overweight. Some of us are overweight to the extent that it seriously affects our health. Probably *most* of us believe we are overweight by at least five or ten pounds. Many of us think that if we could only restrict our caloric intake for a while we'd get back down to what we weighed in college, or high school, or eighth grade, or whatever our personal "golden age" was. But most of us hate diets because they're boring or hard to follow, or because they make us feel sick or dizzy. In fact, I can promise you that you don't have to restrict the amount of food you eat. With the Nutripoints program you'll find that you can eat far more than you might have thought, but lose or maintain your weight (depending on your goal) by eating foods that are more nutritious and lower in calories.

> Nutri-Tip: Calories
>
> I think the best thing you can do for yourself is to forget about calories. In the course of working with thousands of patients, I've found that the people who are the most knowledgeable about calories are also those with the most finely developed ability to "cheat" on a diet. If you can recite the number of calories in a Twinkie or chocolate cake, and think that if you skip a breakfast of equivalent calories you'll be back on track, you're only fooling yourself. *Don't worry about calories; focus instead on Nutripoints.*

Cholesterol There is a 50-percent chance that your blood cholesterol level is higher than desirable: half of all adult Americans have levels that are too high. There is a 25-percent chance that your blood cholesterol level is "high," meaning it's high enough to need intensive medical attention.

Although controversy continues on the precise meaning and implications of blood cholesterol levels, there is no doubt that a high level puts your life in danger. The tragedy of coronary heart disease—contributed to by high levels of blood cholesterol—certainly does that to 40 percent of its victims, the first warning sign being a fatal heart attack.

High levels of cholesterol have become the hidden time bombs in our postwar diet—a diet that's rich in fatty foods. We're now seeing the effects of a lifetime on such a diet: an increased risk of serious coronary heart disease, which is now the number one killer in this country. Indeed, among the people of the famous Framingham, Massachusetts, study, who have been tracked now for more than forty years, only those with a cholesterol level below 150 milligrams daily have been found to be free of risk from premature death due to clogged arteries.

Fortunately, the effects of a high-cholesterol diet can be mitigated and even reversed. When Nathan Pritikin completely changed his diet in middle age, as the result of serious heart disease, the results were dramatic. His autopsy revealed that his extremely low cholesterol diet had given him the unblocked, pliable arteries of a young child. More recently, Dr. Dean Ornish has shown that individuals on a near-vegetarian diet, using yoga-style relaxation techniques, and incorporating moderate exercise, can indeed slow or even reverse the process of atherosclerosis.

You've no doubt been reading a great deal about cholesterol for the past few years, but you may also be confused about how to translate research reports into your own "heart safe" diet. Nutripoints will eliminate this confusion because cholesterol is one of the major negative factors used in the Nutripoint analysis program. The higher the cholesterol level of a food, the lower in Nutripoints.

On the Nutripoint program, cholesterol intake is limited to 300 milligrams daily, which is in keeping with the recommendations of the American Heart Association. In addition to simply limiting cholesterol intake, Nutripoints lowers serum cholesterol levels by emphasizing fiber in the diet. This abundant fiber in the diet binds with bile acids that contain cholesterol, and thereby transports cholesterol out of the body.

The average person who follows the program will see a 14-percent reduction in two weeks, depending on how high his or her cholesterol was to begin with. (If it's very high, the reduction tends to be greater; in our live-in programs, I've seen drops of from 25 to 50 percent in people with high cholesterol. It wouldn't be unusual for someone to go from 250 to 180.)

If you are already suffering from coronary heart disease, the Nutripoints program is a safe and practical way to keep your cholesterol intake at the lowest possible level. Simply stick to the food items near the top of the list, and avoid those below the recommended level.

The following is a breakdown that you might find interesting. It identifies the worst offenders in terms of *both* cholesterol and calories. These foods show a high ratio of cholesterol to calories, and are thus double threats. Each entry has more than 1 milligram of cholesterol per calorie.

Cholesterol per Calorie

Food	***Cholesterol per Calorie***
Sweetbreads	10.2
Scrambled eggs	2.8
Fried eggs	2.7
Caviar	2.2
Wendy's green pepper, onion, mushroom omelet	2.2
Beef liver (fried)	2.1
Squid (boiled)	2.1
Carl's Jr. scrambled eggs	2.0
Pate (chicken liver, canned)	1.9
Wendy's ham, cheese, onion omelet	1.9
Omelet (ham and cheese)	1.8
Squid (raw)	1.8
Wendy's ham, cheese, mushroom omelet	1.8
Egg salad	1.7
Spinach salad (egg, bacon, ham)	1.5
Egg foo young	1.3
Wendy's Creamy Peppercorn dressing	1.3
Shrimp (steamed)	1.2

Wendy's ham and cheese omelet	1.2
Beef heart	1.1
Crabs (hard-shell, steamed)	1.0
Cheese sauce	1.0

Cholesterol is a waxy substance found only in animals. Cholesterol in food is referred to as *dietary* cholesterol, while cholesterol in our bodies is called *blood* or *serum* cholesterol. Although these substances are the same, they differ in origin: the body ingests cholesterol found in animal-based foods, and it manufactures its own cholesterol in response to consumed cholesterol. While the body needs cholesterol to function, it doesn't need to consume any. The body is capable of manufacturing enough cholesterol to fulfill all its needs. The trouble with consuming large amounts of cholesterol is that it reduces its ability to remove dietary cholesterol from the bloodstream.

The ultimate result of excess cholesterol, along with inflammation, is clogged arteries, as the cholesterol adheres to the walls of the arteries and impairs their ability to carry oxygen through the body. Among many things, blood carries a regular supply of oxygen to the heart. Without oxygen, the heart muscle weakens, causing chest pain, heart attacks, and eventually death.

The U.S. Department of Health and Human Services makes five recommendations to help reduce your blood cholesterol levels:

1. Eat less high-fat food, especially those foods high in saturated fat.
2. Replace part of the saturated fat in your diet with unsaturated fat.
3. Eat less high-cholesterol food.
4. Choose foods high in complex carbohydrates.
5. If you are overweight, reduce your weight.

Nutripoints is a simple way to help you achieve all five of these goals.

You'll notice as you look at the food rating charts that some foods have a notation regarding cholesterol. This is because some foods, such as organ meats, while very high in nutrients, are also very high in cholesterol. If you are on a diet that severely limits your cholesterol, you should avoid such foods, even though they may be high in Nutripoints. There is a further explanation of this on page 259 just before the charts.

The FDA has defined the terms used in cholesterol labeling on foods as follows:

Cholesterol free: less than 2 milligrams per serving.

Low cholesterol: less than 20 milligrams per serving.

Cholesterol reduced: products reformulated or processed to reduce cholesterol by 75 percent or more.

The list that follows is a complete breakdown of all the sources of cholesterol in your diet. When you see any of them listed on a food label, you know the food contains cholesterol, or is a vegetable product that doesn't contain cholesterol, but is high in saturated fat, which can raise your serum cholesterol levels. (Just one gram of saturated fat is equal to eating 20 milligrams of cholesterol in its effect on your serum cholesterol levels.)

Animal fat
Bacon fat
Beef fat
Butter
Chicken fat
Cocoa butter*
Coconut*
Coconut oil*
Cream
Egg and egg-yolk solids
Ham fat
Hardened fat or oil*
Hydrogenated vegetable oil*
Lamb fat
Lard
Meat fat
Palm kernel oil*
Palm oil*
Pork fat
Turkey fat
Vegetable oil*
Vegetable shortening*
Whole milk solids

Sodium Sodium is a mineral that helps regulate blood pressure, and is essential for the proper functioning of the nervous system. Sodium is essential to life and, indeed, there are traces of sodium in almost everything we eat. There is more than enough sodium occurring naturally in foods to fulfill our daily requirements. The problem is, many of us consume ten to twenty-five times the amount (about one-tenth of a teaspoonful) we need.

Excess sodium can cause serious health problems, including high blood pressure, which can lead to stroke, and heart and kidney disease. Almost 20 percent of us are genetically prone to developing high blood pressure if we eat a diet that is too high in salt.

***Contain no cholesterol, but are sources of saturated fat.**

How do we avoid excess salt? Well, of course, Nutripoints has made it easy for you. Just choose foods from the top of the list and you'll be eating a diet that is naturally low in sodium. In addition, I recommend that you avoid processed foods whenever possible. The simple fact is, salt is added to so many processed foods in such large amounts that if such foods are a mainstay of your diet it's very difficult to avoid sodium. For example, a recent article in *Consumer Reports* contained the following surprising facts:

- One ounce of Kellogg's Corn Flakes has almost double the amount of sodium of an ounce of Planters Cocktail Peanuts: 260 milligrams versus 132.
- Two slices of Pepperidge Farm white bread have more sodium than a one-ounce bag of Lay's potato chips: 234 milligrams versus 191.

These two examples demonstrate that if you need to restrict your sodium intake, you'll have to do more than simply shun table salt. For one thing, sodium by itself is tasteless; it's in the form of sodium chloride that it becomes the common table salt we think of. But sodium by itself is still added to foods. Fortunately, some manufacturers are now including labeling that will help you make low-sodium choices. The following are sodium-related labeling terms as defined by the Food and Drug Administration:

Sodium free: less than 5 milligrams per serving.

Very low sodium: less than 35 milligrams per serving.

Low sodium: 140 milligrams or less per serving.

Reduced sodium: 75-percent reduction in sodium from that usually found in a product.

Unsalted, no salt added, without added salt: foods processed without salt that would ordinarily have it; e.g., "no salt added" pretzels or potato chips.

You should also be aware of other sodium-containing ingredients that could be listed on a package, including monosodium glutamate, baking soda (also identified as sodium bicarbonate), garlic salt, brine, and sodium citrate.

What of the actual amounts of sodium in a product? The Center for Science in the Public Interest recommends that if a product contains less than 135 milligrams of sodium per serving, consider it safe. If it contains more than that amount, try to find a similar product with less salt, or look for a "without added salt" version.

Because so many of my patients and clients are concerned about sodium intake, I'm including a list of salt substitutes. I think you'll find these suggestions very useful.

Morton Lite Salt
Morton Salt Substitute
No-Salt
Nu-Salt
McCormick's salt substitutes:
  Salt-Free Parsley Patch
  All-Purpose
  Sesame All-Purpose
  Garlic Saltless
  It's a Dilly
  Lemon Pepper
  Popcorn Blend
Mrs. Dash
Spike
Sherry (avoid "cooking sherry," as it's high in sodium)
Lemon juice
Lime juice
Garlic powder
Onion powder
Vinegar (incl. balsamic, rice wine, apple, red wine, raspberry, blueberry vinegar)
Low-sodium soy sauce
Ginger
Cumin
Salsa
American Heart Association spices
Pepper
Green chili peppers
Gourmet Shop Saltless Seasonings
Low-sodium broths

Nutri-Tip: Sodium

There are a number of ways to reduce the sodium in your diet, such as simply cutting out table salt, which you may well be familiar with. But one that I always pass on to my patients is the following: if you rinse canned tuna with tap water for one minute you will remove 80 percent of the sodium. This is an especially useful tip because tuna packed in water is so high in Nutripoints. It's also wise to rinse canned vegetables before cooking.

Sugar Sugar, along with cellulose and starch, is a principal component of carbohydrates. The body does need glucose (one of the components of sugar) to function. But sugar, as opposed to starch or complex carbohydrates, is quickly digested (there's little or no fiber to slow its absorption), and gives you an immediate burst of energy. Complex carbohydrates, on the other hand, are usually rich in fiber. They burn more slowly and give the body a more stable energy supply, as well as providing nutrients.

The drawback of sugar as a source of energy is that it contributes far too many calories in return for a very small contribution in terms of nutrients. This drawback would make sugar enough of a nutritional waste, but it's also involved in other physical problems. There's no doubt, for example, that a high sugar consumption contributes to dental caries. There is also evidence linking excess sugar to diabetes and heart disease. Sugar is also a major culprit in causing obesity. It's so calorie-dense that it's very difficult for average people to burn off all the calories they're consuming in a day when sugar is a major component of their diet.

Despite sugar's poor nutritional value, most of us get an amazing 20 percent of our total daily calories from sugar. This means that we're eating twenty to thirty teaspoons of sugar *each day*. That's an incredible amount of sugar, and we just can't afford it in terms of weight control and in terms of the nutrients we need each day. Even if you never add sugar to any food you eat, you're still overdosing on it if you don't know how to read food labels. Did you know, for example, that some ketchups and salad dressings are about one-third sugar? Some of the mixes you use to coat meats before baking have the same percentage of sugar as a Hershey bar: 50 percent. Everything from bacon to soups, from gravy mixes to spaghetti sauces can have large amounts of hidden sugars. You probably know that some breakfast cereals have enormous amounts of sugar; indeed, a few cereals have so much sugar that it's actually the main ingredient. (And they'll still run ads claiming to be "part of a balanced breakfast"!)

Sugar is by far the most popular food additive. But if you learn its various disguises, you can avoid it. The following are the various forms of sugar you'll find listed on food labels:

Brown sugar	Turbinado sugar
Corn syrup	Caramel
Dextrose	Dextrin
Glucose	Fructose
Honey	Grape sugar
Lactose	Invert sugar
Maple sugar	Maltose
Sorghum syrup	Molasses

If you see any of these ingredients listed among the first few on a label, you know the product is high in sugar. Sometimes manufacturers will add sugar in a variety of forms. For example, you'll see corn syrup, dextrin, and molasses all listed in various places in the label. Even if they're not among the first ingredients, you can be sure that the product has plenty of sugar; if you added them all together, sugar might well be the first or second ingredient.

Of course, you don't really have to worry about reading labels because Nutripoints has done the work for you. The numbers have accounted for the amount of sugar in foods.

This seems like a good spot to talk about natural and artificial sweeteners. According to the Calorie Control Council in 2004, as many as 180 million Americans routinely eat and drink sugar-free food products. It is important for us to monitor the safety of these products long-term for health effects. Some choose to use these products sparingly in their diet since they are in many cases "man-made". Others choose to avoid them entirely as they feel they are guinea pigs whom the companies test them on, since initial studies to determine their safety cannot assess their effects over 10-20 years or a lifetime. Here is a summary of basic information on common natural and artificial sweeteners so you can get all the information to make your own decision on which ones are the best for you.

Blackstrap Molasses

- Contains many nutrients including iron, calcium, potassium, magnesium, niacin, pantothenic acid, B-6, and traces of other nutrients.
- It is the end product, or by-product of the production of refined sugar (and it's where all the nutrients are).
- Can be used in cookies, breads, other baked goods, sauces, and marinades. It can also be used as a general sweetener if you enjoy the flavor.

Sucanat® (sugar cane natural)

- Extracted from sugar cane and fresh juice is evaporated by a special Swiss process which only removes water and retains all of the molasses.
- Is organically grown with no added preservatives or additives.
- Has lower sucrose level than conventional sugar.
- Contains many of the same nutrients as blackstrap molasses to a lesser degree.
- Can be used just like white or brown sugar.

Brown Sugar

- Contains significantly more iron than white sugar, and most of the nutrients in Blackstrap molasses, but to a lesser degree.

Distilled fruit juice

- Fruit concentrates available in the frozen juice section of grocery.
- Pomegranates, peaches, grapes, apple are commonly used.
- Contain natural "fructose" along with some nutrients and antioxidants.
- Can make your own by cooking whole fruits at low temperature, creating a thick syrup.
- Work well in baked goods .

Honey

- Sweeter than sugar per volume, but more calorically dense.
- Contains fructose, not sucrose.
- Contains small traces of nutrients, is totally natural.
- Should be avoided by small infants due to possible minute amounts of contamination.

Fructose

- Does not require insulin to be used by the cells like sucrose does.
- Occurs naturally in fruits and vegetables, and in it's refined form retains some, but very little of the nutrients in the original food.
- Converted to glycerol by liver and can raise triglycerides.
- When in the form of corn syrup it is a highly refined sugar created in a lab which has no nutritional value other than pure carbohydrate.

White Sugar (sucrose)

- Refined sugar cane to the point there are virtually no nutrients left but sucrose.
- The most commonly used sweetener, used as a standard for sweetness.
- Increases glucose and insulin response.

- Recommendation: cut back on amount of sugar instead of using substitutes, use Sucanat® instead of sugar, or combine less sugar or Sucanat® with a substitute to compromise.

Xylitol (Xylosweet®)

- Discovered in 1891 and used as a sweetener in foods since 1960.
- FDA: safe
- Occurs naturally in fruits and vegetables, and in normal metabolism.
- Commercially derived from birch or other hardwood trees.
- Same sweetness and volume, but 40% less calories than sugar.
- May reduce the risk of cavities, ear infections.
- Heat stable
- Slightly "cool" flavor
- Expensive
- Too much may cause digestive distress, same for cousins—sorbitol, mannitol, maltitol, lactitol, isomalt, erythritol.
- Can't use it to make bread, yeast can't grow on it.

Sucralose (SPLENDA®)

- Discovered in 1976.
- Spun from regular sugar is a way the body doesn't recognize it, thus not absorbed.
- 600 times sweeter than sucrose.
- No calories, no effect on blood sugar, does not promote tooth decay.
- Blended with maltodextrins, so each packet has 0.5 grams of carbs.
- Heat-stable for cooking.
- Proponents claim over 100 studies over 20 years showing the safety of sucralose, however others cite research which showed shrunken thymus glands and enlarged liver and kidneys in animals.
- 50/50 split of Splenda®/sugar or Sucanat® recommended for baking.

Aspartame (NutraSweet®, Equal®)

- No calories, no carbs.
- Not heat stable, cannot be used in cooking.
- Contains natural proteins which are metabolized by the body, but they are in an unnatural form that is isolated from whole foods' amino acid complex.
- 200 times sweeter than table sugar, does not promote tooth decay, does not effect blood sugar.

- By far the most commonly used no-calorie sweetener it is found in more than 6000 products and consumed by over 200 million people around the world.
- Breaks down into phenylalanine and methyl alcohol (methanol). Methanol is toxic in large quantities, but our bodies can handle small amounts, fruits we eat produce more ethanol than aspartame in our bodies.
- Should not be used by people with phenylketonuria (PKU), who are unable to metabolize phenylalanine.
- FDA: approved in 1981 as safe after more than 100 scientific studies, when used in moderation. To surpass the FDA's Acceptable Daily Intake (ADI, set at 100 times less than that which could potentially cause harm in animals), a 150-pound adult would have to consume 20 12-ounce diet sodas or 97 packs of NutraSweet per day. Some conflicting evidence regarding whether it caused cancer in laboratory animals. There is no clear link to brain tumors in humans as yet according to the National Cancer Institute.
- Many reports have been made to the FDA regarding side effects in people using food products containing aspartame such as headaches, nervousness, dizziness, memory impairment, and depression. There is conflicting evidence thus far as to the cause and mechanism related to aspartame. Those who feel they are experiencing direct negative side effects of using aspartame should avoid its use.

Stevia (stevioside or steviol)

- Extract from a shrub native to South America.
- Virtually calorie-free.
- May help lower blood pressure.
- Not FDA approved, but sold as a dietary supplement.
- Used safely in other countries for years.
- Lab studies in rats showed lower sperm counts, fewer live babies, higher death rates and genetic changes. But doses were much higher than those humans consume.
- Bitter overtone
- 300 times as sweet as sugar (one teaspoon as sweet as a cup of sugar).

Saccharin (Sweet 'N Low®)

- FDA: safe
- Not metabolized in body—secreted
- Suspected link to bladder cancer, but just in rats at extremely high doses (750 cans/day human equivalent), now deemed safe.
- Used since around 1879.

- No calories.

Acesulfame-potassium or Ace-K (Sunette®, Sweet-One®)

- Discovered in 1967 and used in U.S. since 1988, Europe since 1983.
- Four calories per gram, 200 times sweeter than sugar.
- Not absorbed by body, excreted.
- Heat stable, does not promote tooth decay, no effect on glucose.
- Approved by FDA and many studies have shown it's safety. However some experts feel some of the studies were flawed and there may be a risk for cancer in animals which may carry over to humans.

Cyclamate (SugarTwin®, Sucaryl®)

- Discovered in 1937.
- Banned in U.S. since 1970, but available in Canada and 50 countries worldwide.
- 30 times sweeter than sucrose
- Some studies showed risk of bladder cancer in rats.
- Not used in commercial products, but available as a "table top" sweetener.
- Measured spoon for spoon like sugar.
- Heat stable, so OK for cooking.

Neotame

- New sweetener, approved by FDA in 2002.
- No calories, 7,000-13,000 times sweeter than sugar.
- Composed of the amino acids aspartic acid and phenylalanine, which are metabolized in the body.

> Nutri-Tip: Sugar
>
> Satisfy your sweet tooth nature's way, with fruits that are naturally sweet. Watermelon is a good choice, and frozen grapes, can make a great snack. Fresh strawberries are another an excellent choice, and high in Nutripoints.

Caffeine Caffeine is a stimulant that blocks the effects of our brain's natural tranquilizing agent, allowing the brain to temporarily move into a higher gear. It affects blood pressure and heart rate, and increases respiration. It's a diuretic as well as a vasoconstrictor and vasodilator: it allows the blood vessels of the brain to constrict, and those of the heart to dilate.

Caffeine is today's drug of choice among the vast majority of Americans. Its positive effects are undeniable: it gives a boost of energy and temporarily sharpens mental acuity; it allows you to concentrate on monotonous tasks; it's used in cold medications to counteract the sleep-inducing effects of antihistamines; and it can be useful in the treatment of certain types of headaches, as it constricts the blood vessels in the head.

But caffeine is a drug. The Department of Health, Education, and Welfare lists it, along with nicotine and heroin, as an addictive substance, and admits that if it were being introduced today, manufacturers would probably be unable to market it: caffeine would be available only by prescription.

The dangers of caffeine addiction are real. Although links between caffeine and heart disease and cancer have largely been disproven, there remains a real connection between caffeine consumption and birth defects, breast disease, digestive diseases, and anxiety. It's the more subtle effects of caffeine that are troublesome to most of us, often because we never make the link between caffeine consumption and our minor symptoms. If you suffer from insomnia, afternoon fatigue, tension headaches, and general anxiety, you might be suffering from the effects of caffeine addiction.

I suggest that you have no more than two caffeinated drinks per day, or a maximum of 200 milligrams of caffeine. I recommend you stick to decaffeinated soft drinks, coffee, and tea.

Nutri-Tip: Caffeine

I think water-processed decaffeinated coffee or Postum (either regular or coffee flavor) makes a good substitute for regular coffee. Just be careful not to lighten your coffee substitutes with cream. Go for skim milk, or try it black.

Alcohol Alcohol is both a toxin and a drug. It's a toxin because the liver must work to detoxify it. That's why you always hear of liver damage among alcoholics; the liver is simply exhausted from its labors to detoxify a constant intake of alcohol. Alcohol is also a carbohydrate, although it's almost an "antinutrient" because it increases your need for other nutrients while contributing almost nothing of any nutritional value of its own. Alcohol is also a drug that acts as a sedative. It anesthetizes the brain beginning with the frontal lobe (reasoning section) and moving on to the speech and vision centers.

Most of us have a schizophrenic view of alcohol: we accept, and perhaps enjoy, its regular use for ourselves and among friends, but we deplore the countless lives it's ruined when abused. The problem with alcohol, of course, is control, and there can be a fine line between "regular" and "addictive" consumption of alcohol.

In addition to the seriously dangerous properties of alcohol, many people don't realize that alcohol can be destructive of nutrients. It will deplete stores of or limit the body's absorption of nutrients, including calcium, riboflavin, folic acid, iron, zinc, thiamin, folacin, and vitamins B_{12}, C, D, and A. What this means to you is that if you regularly consume alcohol with meals, say, a glass of wine with lunch and dinner, you may be counteracting the benefits of many of the nutrients you're consuming with those meals.

As I mentioned earlier in the chapter, recent studies have shown that red wine contains phytochemicals which may help prevent heart disease, and even provide positive benefits from the alcohol itself. The other side of the story is that these same phytochemicals can be obtained by drinking red grape juice—without the negative effects or risks associated with alcohol consumption. As for the benefits of alcohol in general, every drug which has a positive effect—has a corresponding negative effect on the body. It's like trading off a benefit to one organ of the body to the detriment of another. Are the benefits worth the negatives? In my opinion—no.

I think the healthiest alternative is not to drink at all. But if you wish to drink, you should take the "damage control" approach: I suggest you limit yourself to one or two drinks daily. Avoid hard liquors that are at the bottom of the Nutripoints alcohol list, and stay with wines, wine coolers, beer, and near-beer.

Nutri-Tip: Alcohol

Why not try alcohol-free beer? Some brands have an excellent flavor and can help break a bad habit if you're accustomed to, say, having a beer when you get home from work. I also suggest that you try some of the mixed drinks without alcohol. A Virgin Mary is a good choice, it's spicy and has a lot of flavor.

PART IV

NUTRIPOINTS AT WORK

THIS SECTION OF THE BOOK IS DEVOTED TO EVERYTHING YOU NEED TO know to use the Nutripoints program in your daily life. It will answer all your questions, from "Can I get *too many* Nutripoints?" to "What foods on a Chinese restaurant menu are the best choices?"

First, let's examine a simple breakdown of how to make the most of Nutripoints.

If you only used Nutripoints to help you choose one food over another, for example, as a guide to selecting a vegetable with a higher score (spinach at 75 Nutripoints instead of a baked potato at 8.5 Nutripoints, or a chicken salad sandwich on whole wheat at 4 Nutripoints rather than a ham and cheese sandwich on whole wheat at 1 Nutripoint), you would improve your diet. But you would not ensure that you'd get all the RDAs of the essential vitamins and minerals, or that you'd get optimum amounts of protein, carbohydrates, and fiber. And it would not ensure that you'd avoid excess calories, cholesterol, total fat, saturated fat, sodium, sugar, alcohol, and caffeine.

If you only used Nutripoints to choose one food over another, and tried to get at least 100 Nutripoints per day from a variety of foods, you would upgrade your diet and you would get the RDA for every vitamin and mineral. But you would not get optimum amounts of protein, carbohydrates, and fiber. And you would not be avoiding excess calories, cholesterol, total fat, saturated fat, sodium, sugar, alcohol, and caffeine.

To get the full benefit of Nutripoints, you must select foods that will give you a daily score of at least 100 Nutripoints while staying within the serving limits for each group and meeting the minimum required servings for each Nutrigroup. This is the most complete and effective use of Nutripoints. This use of the system will ensure that you get 100 percent of the Recommended Dietary Allowances; that you get optimum amounts of protein, carbohydrates, and fiber; that you avoid excess calories, cholesterol, total fat, saturated fat, sodium, sugar, alcohol, and caffeine.

YOUR CURRENT NUTRIPOINT STATUS

Before you begin using the Nutripoints program, I recommend that you take stock of your current eating habits. The best way to do this is by keeping a food diary for three days. The most immediate benefit of making a three-day food diary is that it will allow you to analyze your current diet in terms of Nutripoints. It will instantly pinpoint the weaknesses in your diet, will give you a powerful incentive to get started on Nutripoints, and will serve as encouragement when you begin to see how quickly your diet improves, and your scores go up, with just a few basic changes in your diet.

Keeping a food diary is also a helpful way to get used to using Nutripoints in your daily life: you'll become familiar with the Nutrigroups and get a handle on the highly rated foods.

KEEPING A FOOD DIARY

When patients and clients first come to me for help, I always ask them to make a record of what they've been eating for three typical days. You have an advantage over these people: you can make more accurate records because you'll be doing it as it happens. (You'd be amazed at how much some of us can eat, almost unconsciously. If you tried to recall *everything you* ate two days ago, could you?)

Accuracy really counts, so please don't try to fool yourself. Remember that you don't have to show these lists to anyone if you don't want to. If you are tempted to skip this step of recording what you eat—remember this: research shows that the people who keep food diaries are the people who make the best progress. Take advantage of this valuable tool.

I suggest that you buy a new notebook just for your Nutripoint scores. You might abandon it after a while, but in the beginning, you'll find it very helpful. You need to jot down exactly *what* you ate and in *what amounts* for each meal. It's best to record *typical* days; they don't have to be consecutive. In other words, you can record a Wednesday (skip Thursday because you were on the road and not eating typically), a Friday, and a Saturday. It's a good idea to include one weekend day as well as two weekdays. Don't forget to record snacks, beverages, and condiments. Try to make your notes as soon as possible after a meal or snack so that you can remember whether it was really three or five crackers you had.

Try to get your portion sizes as accurate as possible. Typical portion sizes would be 1 cup, 1 teaspoon, 1 tablespoon, 4 ounces, 2 slices, and so on.

The following table will help you judge portion sizes:

Typical Portion Sizes

Meat, Poultry, Fish

3 oz. = size of palm of average woman's hand (exclude fingers)
= amount in a sandwich
= amount in a quarter-pound hamburger (cooked)
= chicken breast (3 inches across)
6 oz. = restaurant chicken breast (6 inches across)
= common luncheon or cafeteria portion
8 oz. = common evening restaurant portion

Cheese

1 oz. = 1 slice on sandwich or hamburger
= 1-inch cube or 1 wedge airplane serving
½ cup = 1 scoop cottage cheese

Salads

1 cup = dinner salad
2–4 cups = salad bar salad

Potato

1 small = 2 ½ inches long
1 medium = 4 inches long
1 large = 5 inches long (restaurant portion)
1 huge = 6 inches long (meal-in-one potato)

Vegetables

½ cup = cafeteria or restaurant portion
= coleslaw or beans at a BBQ restaurant

Fats

1 tsp. margarine/butter = 1 pat
3 tsp. = 1 Tbls.
1 Tbls. mayonnaise = typical amount in sandwich
2 Tbls. dressing = typical amount on a dinner salad
= 1 small ladle (restaurant)
= ½ large ladle (restaurant)

Beverages

1 ½ oz. = 1 jigger per alcoholic drink
6 oz. (¾ cup) = typical juice portion
= small glass of wine
8 oz. (1 cup) = common milk portion
12 oz. = 1 can of beer or soft drink

The following is a typical part of a daily record:

Meal	*Food*	*Serving Size*
Dinner	Chicken breast (baked, no sauce)	4 oz.
	Baked potato	1 medium
	w/margarine	2 pats
	w/cheese sauce	¼ cup
	Broccoli (steamed)	½ cup
	Apple (fresh)	1 large
	Dinner roll (no margarine)	1 small
	2-percent milk	8 oz.
Snack	Popcorn	3 cups
	Coke	12 oz.
	Chocolate candy bar w/nuts	2-oz. bar

After you have the three-day list, check each food portion with the Nutripoint values in this book. The easiest way to do this is to use the alphabetical listings in the back of the book.

You're going to want to know three things for each of your food diary entries:

1. Portion size
2. Nutripoints
3. Nutrigroup

The following is a sample Nutripoint Daily Record Sheet. You'll notice that this table includes an "Other" column. Use it to record points for foods in the Other Groups that you eat. These numbers are added or subtracted from your daily total along with the Nutrigroup totals. This record sheet will help you figure out how to list foods so that you can readily see how you're doing on points and portion sizes.

For a sample of how a record sheet is completed, see the Nutripoint menus on pp. 186-200.

You'll want to check each food you consumed to learn how many Nutripoints your serving had. The alphabetical listing of more than 3,600 foods will probably contain any food you might have eaten. Check it for each of the entries in your food diary. Be sure to check the portion size listed. If you ate a cup of something and the Nutripoints are calculated at a half cup, you must double your Nutripoints and count it for two servings. Conversely, if you ate a half cup of something and the Nutripoints are calculated at a cup, you would halve your Nutripoints for the particular food and count it for one-half serving. If you can't find a specific food listed, figure out the components of that food and make an estimate. For example, if you had a salad that was composed of rice, mayonnaise, and some cut-up vegetables, check the values of each of these ingredients and add them to arrive at a Nutripoint score for that food.

In addition to checking your daily Nutripoint scores, you want to determine the balance of your diet and whether you're getting the necessary variety. So, when you check the Nutripoint score for each food, also check each food's Nutrigroup, e.g., meat/fish, grain, vegetable, and so on.

Remember that the daily Nutripoint goal is at least 100 points divided among the six Nutrigroups as follows:

Daily Nutripoint Recommendations

Servings	*Nutrigroup*	*Nutripoints*
4	Vegetable	55
3	Fruit	15
2	Grain	10
1	Legume	5
2	Milk/dairy	10
1	Meat/fish	5
	Total:	**100**

Now it's time to analyze your scores. The following are the three factors you're looking at:

1. How many of the six Nutrigroups do you have points in? This will give you

an idea of how varied your diet is.

2. Did you achieve the recommended number of servings for each Nutrigroup? This will show you how well balanced your diet is.

3. Did you achieve your Nutripoint goal of at least 100 points for the day? This will show you how nutritionally sound your diet is.

The following is a chart that suggests a simplified way to analyze your daily score. You just fill in the Nutripoints for each of the required servings of each Nutrigroup. You can then readily see if you've reached your goal for that Nutrigroup and for the day. You may well find that when you make up your food diary your scores and/or servings are way off, but this chart will at least give you a very visual way of analyzing your numbers:

Nutrigroup	*Nutripoints/Servings*		*Group Totals*	*Goals*
Vegetable	☐☐☐☐	=	________	55
Fruit	☐☐☐	=	________	15
Grain	☐☐	=	________	10
Legume	☐	=	________	5
Milk/dairy	☐☐	=	________	10
Meat/poultry/fish	☐	=	________	5
			Total:	**100**

From the countless surveys I've done on the diet histories of patients, I've learned that there are certain patterns in the average diet. Most people find that their biggest weakness is that they don't get nearly enough variety and balance in their diet. Indeed, most people seem to choose nearly all their foods from only three out of the six Nutrigroups: meat/ poultry/fish, milk/dairy, and grains. Some people do even worse and omit grains as well. Most people get few, if any, legumes, and most people fall short on fruits and vegetables.

Many people have what I think of as "miscellaneous" diets: they eat a lot of meats and dairy foods, along with a lot of miscellaneous items that don't fall into any Nutrigroup, such as sugar, fat, and condiments.

NUTRIPOINT DAILY RECORD SHEET, DAY ____

Food Selection/Serving Size	Nutripoints							
	Veg.	Fruit	Grain	Leg.	Meat	Milk	Other	
Breakfast								
Lunch:								
Dinner:								
Totals:								
Goals:	55	15	10	5	5	10	0	100

The average person gets 50 to 100 Nutripoints daily, *even when eating considerably more than the allotted number of servings.* This means that the average person is getting a poor nutritional bargain in his or her daily diet: fewer vitamins and minerals—sometimes *far* less than the RDA—at a cost of more calories than they need.

By using the Nutripoints program, you can get 100 to 200 Nutripoints daily in *significantly* fewer calories, thus enjoying a more nutrient-dense diet. And you can achieve this usually without making noticeable cuts in the *amounts of* food you eat.

The following is a sample three-day record kept by one of my patients along with a detailed nutrient analysis:

Weekday 1*

		Nutripoints	Nutrigroup
Breakfast			
(7:30 a.m.)	1 cup Kellogg's Corn Flakes	18.0	Grain
	½ cup whole milk	2.5	Milk/dairy
	1 medium banana	7.5	Fruit
	1 cup coffee	−3.5	Misc.
	Subtotal:	**24.5**	
Lunch			
(12:00 p.m.)	Ham sandwich	1.0	Meat
	w/mayo	−1.0	Fat
	on rye	4.5	Grain
	½ cup coleslaw	3.0	Vegetable
	1 cup potato chips	0.0	Vegetable
	12 oz. iced tea	−4.0	Misc.
	Subtotal:	**3.0**	
Dinner			
(7:00 p.m.)	6 oz. breaded, fried flounder fillet w/lemon	−0.5	Meat
	1 cup broccoli w/butter sauce	26.0	Vegetable
	½ cup cooked carrots w/butter	10.0	Vegetable
	1 cup coffee	−3.5	Misc.
	Subtotal:	**32.0**	
Snack			
(10:00 p.m.)	2 chocolate chip cookies	−4.0	Grain
	Subtotal:	**−4.0**	
	Daily Total:	**55.5**	

Nutrigroup	*Points*	*Goal Met*
Vegetable	39.0	No
Fruit	7.5	No
Grain	18.0	Yes
Legume	0.0	No
Meat	0.5	No
Milk/dairy	2.5	No
Misc.	−11.0	–
Fat	−1.0	–

***Although on this day 56 percent of the 100-point daily total was met, the goal for only one Nutrigroup was met.**

WEEKDAY 1			
Male, age 40 Exercise Avg.: 0 calories/day	Present Wt. (lbs.): 185 Target Wt. (lbs.): 160		Body Fat (%): 20 Height (in.): 70
Nutrient Analysis **Nutrient**	**Present Daily Intake at 185 Lbs.**	**Assessment**	**Recommended Daily Intake at 160 Lbs.**
Calories	1,558 cal	OK	1,840 cal
Protein	71 gm	High	58 gm
Total fat	78 gm	High	41-61 gm (max.)
Polyunsat./sat. fat ratio	1.0	OK	1.0
Cholesterol (dietary)	234 mg	OK	100-300 mg
Complex carbohydrates	143 gm	Low	230-322 gm
Sugar	10 gm	OK	0 gm
Alcohol	0.0 gm	As per Dr.	As per Dr.
Fiber (dietary)	14 gm	Low	20-35 gm
Calcium	492 mg	Low	800 mg
Phosphorus	675 mg	OK	800 mg
Magnesium	256 mg	OK	350 mg
Sodium	2,785 mg	OK	2,000-4,000 mg
Potassium	3,045 mg	OK	3,750 mg
Zinc	6 mg	Very low	15 mg
Iron	11 mg	OK	10 mg
Vitamin A	12,354 IU	OK	5,000 IU
Thiamin (B_1)	2.3 mg	OK	1.4 mg
Riboflavin (B_2)	2.3 mg	OK	1.6 mg
Niacin (B_3)	26 mg	OK	18 mg
Pyridoxine (B_6)	2.7 mg	OK	2.2 mg
Pantothenic acid	2.8 mg	Low	5.5 mg
Folic acid	888 mcg	OK	400 mcg
Vitamin B_{12}	3.1 mcg	OK	3.0 mcg
Vitamin C	223 mg	OK	60 mg
Caffeine	473 mg	Very high	0-200 mg

Calorie Sources	**Present** (%)	**Goal** (%)
Protein	17	10-20
Fat	46	20-30
Complex carbohydrates (fruits, vegs., starches)	35	50-70
Simple carbohydrates	2	0-10
Alcohol	0	0

Weekday 2

		Nutripoints	Nutrigroup
Breakfast			
(7:30 a.m.)	1 boiled egg	−6.0	Milk/dairy
	1 blueberry muffin	0.0	Grain
	w/1 pat butter	−2.0	Fat
	1 cup coffee	−3.5	Misc.
	Subtotal:	**−11.5**	
Lunch			
(12:00 p.m.)	2 pc. pepperoni pizza	−8.0	Grain
	Tossed salad	33.0	Vegetable
	w/2 Tbls. Thousand Island dressing	−3.0	Fat
	Subtotal:	**22.0**	
Dinner			
(7:00 p.m.)	6-oz. pork chop	−2.0	Meat
	1 cup mashed potatoes	4.0	Vegetable
	w/gravy	−1.5	Fat
	½ cup green beans	12.0	Vegetable
	1 6-oz. glass of wine	−14.0	Alcohol
	1 pc. apple pie	−8.0	Fruit
	Subtotal:	**−9.5**	
	Daily Total:	**1.0**	

Group	*Points*	*Goal Met*
Vegetable	49.0	No
Fruit	−8.0	No
Grains	−8.0	No
Legumes	0.0	No
Meat	−2.0	No
Milk/dairy	−6.0	No
Misc.	−3.5	—
Fat	−6.5	—
Alcohol	−14.0	—

WEEKDAY 2			
Male, age 40	Present Wt. (lbs.): 185		Body Fat (%): 20
Exercise Avg.: 0 calories/day	Target Wt. (lbs.): 160		Height (in.): 70
Nutrient Analysis **Nutrient**	**Present Daily Intake at 185 Lbs.**	**Assessment**	**Recommended Daily Intake at 160 Lbs.**
Calories	2,437 cal	High	1,840 cal
Protein	88 gm	High	58 gm
Total fat	147 gm	Very high	41-61 gm (max.)
Polyunsat./sat. fat ratio	0.5	Low	1.0
Cholesterol (dietary)	723 mg	Very high	100-300 mg
Complex carbohydrates	147 gm	Low	230-322 gm
Sugar	28 gm	OK	0 gm
Alcohol	14.8 gm	As per Dr.	As per Dr.
Fiber (dietary)	9 gm	Very low	20-35 gm
Calcium	544 mg	OK	800 mg
Phosphorus	1,068 mg	OK	800 mg
Magnesium	196 mg	Low	350 mg
Sodium	4,403 mg	High	2,000-4,000 mg
Potassium	2,380 mg	Low	3,750 mg
Zinc	10 mg	OK	15 mg
Iron	10 mg	OK	10 mg
Vitamin A	3,072 IU	Low	5,000 IU
Thiamin (B_1)	2.2 mg	OK	1.4 mg
Riboflavin (B_2)	1.5 mg	OK	1.6 mg
Niacin (B_3)	18 mg	OK	18 mg
Pyridoxine (B_6)	1.3 mg	Low	2.2 mg
Pantothenic acid	4.3 mg	OK	5.5 mg
Folic acid	251 mcg	Low	400 mcg
Vitamin B_{12}	4.7 mcg	OK	3.0 mcg
Vitamin C	56 mg	OK	60 mg
Caffeine	175 mg	OK	0-200 mg

Calorie Sources	**Present** (%)	**Goal** (%)
Protein	14	10-20
Fat	55	20-30
Complex carbohydrates (fruits, vegs., starches)	23	50-70
Simple carbohydrates	4	0-10
Alcohol	4	0

Weekend Day

		Nutripoints	Nutrigroup
Breakfast			
(10:00 a.m.)	2 pancakes	1.0	Grain
	w/2 Tbls. maple syrup	−5.0	Sugar
	w/1 tsp. butter	−2.0	Fat
	2 sausages	−2.5	Meat
	8 oz. orange juice	15.0	Fruit
	1 cup coffee	−3.5	Misc.
	Subtotal:	**3.0**	
Lunch/Snack			
(3:00 p.m.)	Turkey sandwich	4.5	Meat
	on white bread	2.5	Grain
	w/mayo	−1.0	Fat
	w/lettuce and tomato	5.0	Vegetable
	Subtotal:	**11.0**	
Dinner		2.0	Meat
(7:30 p.m.)	1 6-oz. steak		
	½ cup scalloped potatoes	4.0	Vegetable
	Tossed salad	33.0	Vegetable
	w/2 Tbls. ranch dressing	−3.5	Fat
	Subtotal:	**35.5**	
Snack			
(9:00 p .m.)	½ cup Haagen-Dazs ice cream	−7.0	Milk/dairy
	Subtotal:	**−7.0**	
	Daily Total:	**42.5**	

Group	*Points*	*Goal Met*
Vegetable	42.0	No
Fruit	15.0	Yes
Grains	3.5	No
Legumes	0.0	No
Meat	4.0	No
Milk/dairy	7.0	No
Misc.	−3.5	—
Fat	−6.5	—
Sugar	−5.0	—

WEEKEND DAY			
Male, age 40	Present Wt. (lbs.): 185	Body Fat (%): 20	
Exercise Avg.: 0 calories/day	Target Wt. (lbs.): 160	Height (in.): 70	
Nutrient Analysis **Nutrient**	**Present Daily Intake at 185 Lbs.**	**Assessment**	**Recommended Daily Intake at 160 Lbs.**
Calories	2,430 cal	High	1,840 cal
Protein	108 gm	High	58 gm
Total fat	156 gm	Very high	41-61 gm (max.)
Polyunsat./sat. fat ratio	0.8	OK	1.0
Cholesterol (dietary)	409 mg	Very high	100-300 mg
Complex carbohydrates	103 gm	Very low	230-322 gm
Sugar	42 gm	OK	0 gm
Alcohol	0.0 gm	As per Dr.	As per Dr.
Fiber (dietary)	8 gm	Very low	20-35 gm
Calcium	621 mg	OK	800 mg
Phosphorus	1,169 mg	OK	800 mg
Magnesium	174 mg	Very low	350 mg
Sodium	3,034 mg	OK	2,000-4,000 mg
Potassium	2,346 mg	Low	3,750 mg
Zinc	12 mg	OK	15 mg
Iron	15 mg	OK	10 mg
Vitamin A	2,803 IU	*Low*	5,000 IU
Thiamin (B_1)	1.8 mg	OK	1.4 mg
Riboflavin (B_2)	1.8 mg	OK	1.6 mg
Niacin (B_3)	36 mg	OK	18 mg
Pyridoxine (B_6)	2.7 mg	OK	2.2 mg
Pantothenic acid	3.3 mg	Low	5.5 mg
Folic acid	254 mcg	Low	400 mcg
Vitamin B_{12}	6.4 mcg	OK	3.0 mcg
Vitamin C	47 mg	OK	60 mg
Caffeine	175 mg	OK	0-200 mg

Calorie Sources	**Present** (%)	**Goal** (%)
Protein	17	10-20
Fat	60	20-30
Complex carbohydrates (fruits, vegs., starches)	17	50-70
Simple carbohydrates	6	0-10
Alcohol	0	0

3-DAY AVERAGE

Male, age 40 | Present Wt. (lbs.): 185 | Body Fat (%): 20
Exercise Avg.: 0 calories/day | Target Wt. (lbs.): 160 | Height (in.): 70

Nutrient Analysis Nutrient	Present Daily Intake at 185 Lbs.	Assessment	Recommended Daily Intake at 160 Lbs.
Calories	2,142 cal	OK	1,840 cal
Protein	89 gm	High	58 gm
Total fat	127 gm	Very high	41-61 gm (max.)
Polyunsat./sat. fat ratio	0.7	Low	1.0
Cholesterol (dietary)	455 mg	Very high	100-300 mg
Complex carbohydrates	131 gm	Very low	230-322 gm
Sugar	27 gm	OK	0 gm
Alcohol	4.9 gm	As per Dr.	As per Dr.
Fiber (dietary)	11 gm	Very low	20-35 gm
Calcium	552 mg	OK	800 mg
Phosphorus	971 mg	OK	800 mg
Magnesium	209 mg	Low	350 mg
Sodium	3,407 mg	OK	2,000-4,000 mg
Potassium	2,590 mg	OK	3,750 mg
Zinc	9 mg	Low	15 mg
Iron	12 mg	OK	10 mg
Vitamin A	6,077 IU	OK	5,000 IU
Thiamin (B_1)	2.1 mg	OK	1.4 mg
Riboflavin (B_2)	1.8 mg	OK	1.6 mg
Niacin (B_3)	27 mg	OK	18 mg
Pyridoxine (B_6)	2.2 mg	OK	2.2 mg
Pantothenic acid	3.5 mg	Low	5.5 mg
Folic acid	464 mcg	OK	400 mcg
Vitamin B_{12}	4.7 mcg	OK	3.0 mcg
Vitamin C	109 mg	OK	60 mg
Caffeine	274 mg	High	0-200 mg

Calorie Sources	**Present** (%)	**Goal** (%)
Protein	16	10-20
Fat	55	20-30
Complex carbohydrates (fruits, vegs., starches)	24	50-70
Simple carbohydrates	4	0-10
Alcohol	1	0

In addition to the food records of this particular patient, I've included a breakdown of the nutrient content of his meals. You won't need such a breakdown because the Nutripoint numbers are really a simplified version of what those numbers tell you. But I think it's interesting to see just where the weaknesses were in this patient's diet. We can see from the nutrient analysis of the three-day food report that while the total calorie intake was fine, the protein was high, the fat total was very high, the cholesterol level was very high, and the complex carbohydrate and fiber levels were very low. A few of the vitamins and minerals were low as well.

I chose this particular patient's record because it is fairly typical. It's not a terrible diet (I have seen people who earn virtually *no* Nutripoints in a three-day food record), but it shows where typical weaknesses exist. It also very quickly, in a visual way, points out where improvement can be made. Instead of looking at just numbers of calories and not really learning very much from them, you can look at the low Nutripoint numbers and see where you need to boost your scores.

Well, how did you do?

Remember that 100 daily Nutripoints is the basic goal: you may fall far below it on some days and exceed it by a wide margin on others. The more Nutripoints you can get over the minimum 100 level, the better—within the allowed number of servings.

UPGRADING YOUR DIET

It's time to refocus your approach to food with the help of Nutripoints. Unless your diet is truly terrible, I think you'll find this an easy shift to make. Many people tell me that they're delighted to find that rather than being an "authoritative" diet plan that urges them to eat tons of lettuce or grapefruit, or some other food they might not like, Nutripoints leaves the choice *up to them.*

Your food diary has revealed where your diet is weak. You're probably not eating enough different kinds of foods. Most people find that just by paying attention to balancing their diet, they improve it enormously. So you'll probably need to work on getting sufficient servings from the various Nutrigroups. But how do you choose foods *within* each group? The following are the steps you need to take:

Step 1: First, I suggest you do your own personal food survey. Go through the lists by Nutrigroups and check the foods you eat regularly. Are they high in Nutripoints? If so, great. If not, it's time to think about eliminating the foods that are low in Nutripoints, or at least those that are below the recommended level for each Nutrigroup.

Step 2: Make a list of the foods you like and eat regularly that are high in Nutripoints. This will be the basis of your new, upgraded diet. These are the foods you can rely on because you already know that you like them and that they are high in Nutripoints.

Step 3: Now you need to focus on *variety. Go* through the lists by Nutrigroups again and look for foods you like or would probably like but rarely eat. Make sure you don't neglect the Nutrigroups you're weak on. (You'll know from your food diary if, for example, you rarely eat vegetables or fruits.) Perhaps you found that you *never* eat legumes. Well, now's the time to go through that Nutrigroup list and find some legumes you like. Figure out how you're going to work them into your diet. When you first begin with Nutripoints, you may find that it's difficult to work in a serving of legumes every day. This is perfectly OK. Many people make a transitional stage in which they substitute one meat serving for one of the legume servings. (You'll want to check the menus and recipes in Part VI for some good suggestions.)

Remember that *variety is* as important as a high Nutripoint score. This pertains to choosing foods *within* a Nutrigroup as well as to choosing foods *among* Nutrigroups. Remember that each food has a unique "fingerprint" of nutrients that identifies it: it will be strong in some, weak in others. If you consistently pick only the top four vegetables, for example, you'll be missing out on the nutrients available in other vegetables you need. Keep in mind that as long as you don't go below the recommended level of foods, it's better to have a variety within a list than an extremely high score.

Step 4: An excellent way to upgrade your diet is to use Nutripoints as the basis for making *substitutions in* your diet. You would do this between foods within a single Nutrigroup. For example, say you eat a lot of pork. You might want to scan the meat/poultry/fish Nutrigroup for a food with a higher Nutripoint level. Or perhaps you like spinach and romaine lettuce equally: the next time you make a salad, include a lot of spinach and you'll be boosting your score.

Substitutions can be particularly useful when cooking. The following table offers some effective alternatives.

Cooking Substitutions

To Replace	*Nutripoints*	*Replace With*	*Nutripoints*
Butter	−7.5 (per tbs.)	Safflower Oil	−2.5
		Low-cal. margarine	−2 to −1
Heavy cream	−56 (per cup)	Evaporated skim milk	19
Cream cheese	− 40 (per cup)	Yogurt cheese (see page 236)	12 to 18
Eggs	−11.5 (per egg)	Egg Beaters	9 (per ¼ cup)
		Egg whites	1 (per egg)
Whole milk yogurt	2.5 (per cup)	Nonfat yogurt	9 (per cup)
Sour cream	−14 (per cup)	New Way Sour Cream (see page 247)	26 (per cup)
Sugar	−1 (per teas.)	No-calorie sweeteners	0.0
Salt	0.0	Salt substitutes (see page 82)	0.0
Coffee/tea	− 3.0 to − -3.5	Decaf coffee/ tea, herb tea, or Postum	0.0 to 5.5

Step 5: Another way to upgrade your diet is to use Nutripoints to *alter your food choice.* For example, say you eat a lot of fried chicken. Why not stick with chicken if you like it, but instead of frying, try broiling? Or make your hamburgers with a leaner grade of beef. If you already eat broiled chicken, why not boost your score by taking the skin off before you broil it? If you love fruits, why not have some melon instead of your usual apple?

You can make these changes in each Nutrigroup. In the milk/dairy group you can change from regular mozzarella to low-fat mozzarella; and you can change from regular milk to 2-percent milk, from 2-percent to 1-percent milk, and then to skim milk. You can go from two eggs to one whole egg plus one egg white. Or you can switch to Egg Beaters.

Nutripoints makes it easy for you to upgrade your diet. Simply familiarize yourself with the lists. It's as easy as looking for a version of a food you like with a higher Nutripoint score.

How do you keep track of your Nutripoint scores through the day? You can continue with your food diary notebook, or you can use a sheet such as the one on page 112, which not only will help keep track of your scores but will make keeping track of your servings from the various Nutrigroups automatic. (This chart is for those who want to consume 1,000—1,200 calories per day; your chart can be personalized for your desired calorie intake, according to the guidelines on pages 118-123.)

Obviously, you might want to alter this pattern on some days. Perhaps you'll have a fruit snack instead of a fruit dessert, or perhaps you'll have a grain as a snack instead of with dinner.

A Note on Water...

There is one nutritional "essential" that I didn't include in the Nutripoint formula for obvious reasons: water. Your body is actually two-thirds water—40 to 50 quarts—and we can't forget that it's every bit as essential to life as food.

Most people don't give any thought to the amount of water they drink, but I think it's important to do so. You should be sure to drink six to eight 8-ounce glasses of water per day. Some people find it helpful to put six pennies in their right pocket in the morning and move one to their left pocket each time they drink a glass of water. It helps them keep track of what they're actually consuming. Following the Nutripoint guidelines for your servings of these liquids, you can substitute 100-percent juice for your water servings, but don't count caffeinated coffee or tea because they act as diuretics. If you exercise, of course, you should increase the amount of water.

NUTRIGROUP TRENDS

Many people have asked me what food types, in general, seem to be the best bets in terms of Nutripoints. It's interesting to point out that there are various trends in each Nutrigroup. If you're familiar with them, you'll be better able to choose high-Nutripoint foods, even if you don't have the charts at hand. I should mention again that you can only compare Nutripoint ratings *within* each Nutrigroup. While you *can* compare apples and oranges, you *can't* compare apples and spinach. The following are some of the major trends in the Nutrigroups.

NUTRIPOINT DAILY RECORD SHEET 1,000-1,200 CALORIES

	Nutripoints							
Food Selection/Serving Size	Veg.	Fruit	Grain	Leg.	Meat	Milk	Other	
Breakfast: 1 Grain 1 Milk/Dairy 1 Fruit								
Lunch: 1 Meat or Legume 2 Vegetables 1 Grain								
Dinner: 1 Meat or Legume 2 Vegetables 1 Milk/Dairy								
Totals:								
Goals:	55	15	10	5	5	10	0	100

Vegetables When you're looking for the top vegetables, think light and fluffy. Green, leafy vegetables such as turnip greens, spinach, watercress, and beet greens all have terrific scores. After the leafy vegetables, which you can readily see would be both low in calories and high in nutrients, we have asparagus as well as the chunkier cruciferous vegetables, such as broccoli, cauliflower, and Brussels sprouts, which are very high in vitamins A and C (the vitamins the American Cancer Society recommends you focus on as a step to reduce your risk of cancer), as well as fiber and calcium. Next, in terms of scores, we have carrots and the more watery vegetables, such as okra, tomatoes, and squash, which are also high in vitamins C and A, as well as fiber.

All the top vegetables have a tremendous ratio of nutrients per calorie, but as you continue down the list, you'll find that processing and the adding of salt and fat lower the scores of even a terrific vegetable. Keep in mind when choosing vegetables that *all* vegetables above the recommended line are really good foods and that there's no need to worry about sticking to the very top of the list for your four daily servings. As long as you are choosing from above the recommended line, you shouldn't have any trouble getting your 55 Nutripoints. You can easily surpass the 55 Nutripoints goal in this category in the required servings—and that's good! It's your chance to get more points toward your overall goal of at least 100, and give you chance to hit the Excellent level at 150, or Superior level of 200 or more points per day.

Fruit The first trend we notice in the fruits is that the tropical fruits top the charts. Cantaloupe is right at the top, along with papaya, guava, mango, and kiwi. These fruits are packed with nutrients, including vitamin C, and fiber, and are extremely low in calories for their volume. After the tropical fruits we find the citrus fruits, including the orange, mandarin orange, tangerine, and grapefruit. Then come the berries, including raspberries, blackberries, and cranberries. Most of the fruits are high in vitamins A and C and fiber, with moderately high levels of other nutrients. Again, once we get below the recommended line, the addition of sugar, salt, or fat lowers the scores. Foods such as banana cream pie (−1 Nutripoint) get about as far as you can from the basic nutritional appeal of the banana. All-American apple pie does even worse (−2 Nutripoints). Jams, jellies, and preserves hit rock bottom because virtually all nutrition, including fiber, has been processed out of them, and tons of sugar has been added. Smucker's Concord Grape Jelly (−6 Nutripoints) represents the decline of the grape to the absolute bottom of the fruit chart.

Before we move on to the Grain section, I want to mention something about "juicing". Juicing fruits and vegetables is a great way to get your Nutripoints for the following reasons:

- Makes it convenient to get the recommended 5-9 servings of fruits and vegetables per day in a beverage when you would not be likely to eat them in their raw form.
- Retains all of the vitamins, minerals, enzymes, and phytonutrients in the food—especially if you use a high-powered blender (such as the Vita-Mix® which I personally own and highly recommend) which blends the whole food including the pulp.
- Breaks down the cell walls of the foods so all of the nutrients are more easily available and absorbed—so well that they are absorbed much better than when eating the food through chewing.
- Helps cleanse and detoxify the body, especially when used in conjunction with fasting. A great book on this subject is Dr. Don Colbert's "Toxic Relief" which I recommend for those wanting specifics on doing this safely and effectively.

There are many different types of juicers and prices can range up into the hundreds of dollars. A less expensive juicer such as the Juice Man is available for under $100. The Champion juicer is more expensive and will last for many years. The Vita-Mix is a different type of juicer that is really a powerful blender. It can completely juice and liquefy the entire fruit or vegetable. So you get the added benefit of the fiber in addition to the vitamins, minerals, antioxidants, enzymes and phytonutrients. The price is over $400, but I believe it is the best one to use since it keeps all parts of the whole food so you get all of the benefits possible. For information on the Vita-Mix® go to **www.VitaMix.com** or call 1-800-848-2649. I have made arrangements with Vita-Mix to offer you Free Ground Shipping in the U.S. or Canada ($25 US or $35 CN value) by using this code: **06-001375** when placing your order via the web or by phone.

Grains At the top of the grains list you find the highly fortified cereals. There's some controversy about fortification but, in order to keep the system honest, I had to put the cereals where they fell. (Please note the caveat about fortification on page 152.) The very best cereals are those with the most balance in their fortification, as well as those that began with a quality natural food with plenty of fiber and complex carbohydrates. Whole Wheat Total is at the top of the list at 64.5 Nutripoints. As we go down the line, we'll find cereals that are less balanced in terms of fortification, or cereals with less fiber or more sugar. The top-rated natural (unfortified) cereal is wheat bran (26.5 Nutripoints), followed by wheat germ (10.5 Nutripoints) and oatmeal (4.5 Nutripoints).

A breakdown of the cereals shows that fortified whole grains top the list, followed by bran, germ, and other whole grains, and then, as you begin processing and reducing the amount of whole grain and adding sugar, salt, and fat, the scores decline. You'll find that a terrible choice for breakfast is that "health" food of the sixties and seventies—granola the form of Nature Valley Oats 'n Honey Granola Bar, at −2 Nutripoints.

As you move down the grain list, you find the various breads (topped by Wonder Hi-Fiber bread at 6.5 Nutripoints), rices, and pastas. Pizza makes a respectable showing and allows those who must eat at fast-food restaurants to make a choice that will give them a grain serving as a positive contribution to their daily Nutripoint score, especially if they choose the lower fat versions. One slice of Pizza Hut's Chicken Supreme Thin 'N Crispy Pizza, for example, weighs in at 5 Nutripoints a slice. They also have a Fit 'N Delicious Pizza and Veggie Lover's Thin 'N Crispy Pizza, both at 3.5 Nutripoints per slice. Any good cereal for breakfast that scores above 6.5 Nutripoints (and most do), followed by a Pizza Hut lunch, would give you more than your two grain servings and above your 10 required Nutripoints for that Nutrigroup for the day.

Legumes Legumes are strangers to many people, though it's time you became familiar with them. They're a good protein alternative to meat and they're high in fiber, high in complex carbohydrates, low in fat and cholesterol, and high in nutrients. In our legume Nutrigroup, we include not only peas and beans but nuts and seeds. Bean sprouts top the list at 18 Nutripoints. It's easy to keep them on hand to put on sandwiches in place of lettuce, and to add to salads. Sprouting increases the nutritional value in the bean. Peas follow sprouted beans on the list. They're high in fiber, protein, and complex carbohydrates, as are the next items on the list, navy beans.

Down a bit from the beans is an excellent meat substitute: the vegeburger, which is usually made from soy, other legumes or grains. Sometimes they also contain vegetables. Since the first publication of this book, there have been so many new varieties that have popped up, you now have a great deal of flavors and brands to choose from. Also available now are many vegetarian meatless breakfast foods which are much lower in fat and calories than their meat counterparts, and contain fiber as an additional bonus.

After beans, peas, and tofu come nuts. They provide protein, but they're rated lower because they're high in fat (although it's not as saturated as the fat in meat). Remember, by the way, that there's no cholesterol in any vegetable product. As you descend the list, you find the adulterated foods, which have been processed and have suffered the addition of salt and sugar. Even some of the major brands of peanut butter make a dismal showing because of the addition of salt and sugar (Skippy at 0 Nutripoints, followed by Jif and Peter Pan at the same score), while a healthier choice for peanut butter shows up as Health Valley No Salt Chunky peanut butter (1.5 Nutripoints).

Milk/Dairy Because milk is an animal product, it's a good source of complete protein. It contains all the essential amino acids the body can't produce. And, of course, it's high in calcium and complex carbohydrates, as well as some of the B vitamins normally associated with beef or meat products. At the top of the milk Nutrigroup we find some interesting man-made creations, such as Egg Beaters, a fortified egg substitute that has no fat because all of the yolk has been removed. It's an especially good choice for cooking. The best natural food on the list is nonfat dry milk (12.5 Nutripoints). All of the fat and cholesterol has been removed, and what's left is protein, complex carbohydrates, and calcium. You can use nonfat dry milk in cooking: add some to meat loaf, casseroles, and other such dishes. You can, of course, also mix it with water to use in place of whole milk in baking, on cereals, and so on.

The major trend in milk foods, aside from the man-made foods, is that as the fat and cholesterol are eliminated, the Nutripoints go up. Dannon has an excellent product in nonfat yogurt, which is just as flavorful as regular yogurt, but a much better nutritional choice because of its reduced fat. (You can always add a dash of vanilla to nonfat yogurt to give it more flavor.) With fresh fruit, yogurt makes a terrific breakfast dish, and it's great for cooking.

You can readily see how the addition of fat changes a Nutripoint score: Fleischmann's Egg Beaters are rated at 21 Nutripoints, but when they become Fleischmann's Egg Beaters with Cheez, the score plunges to 8 Nutripoints. Cheese is a problem food because of its high fat content. Formagg Cheese Substitute gets around the fat problem and weighs in at 10.5 Nutripoints. Cottage cheese is the best natural cheese choice at 5.5 Nutripoints, followed by Laughing Cow Reduced Calorie Cheese at 2.5 Nutripoints.

Near the bottom of the list you find the foods that are egg, or primarily egg, with McDonald's scrambled eggs trailing the list at −19.5 Nutripoints, the second-lowest all-time low Nutripoint score (only sweetbreads, from the meat Nutrigroup, score lower, at −52).

Meat/Fish/Poultry At the top of the meat Nutrigroup we find raw clams (13.5 Nutripoints) and raw oysters (13 Nutripoints), but the problems with contamination of shellfish make these poor choices (thus the comment on the charts, and the warning on page 259). The very lean, red meats, with their high protein and nutrient content, follow the shellfish, followed by baked and grilled fish. We're happy to see tuna in water (8 Nutripoints) rating so high, as it's such an inexpensive and readily prepared food. You'll notice that the lean beefs are right up there with the lean chicken. You don't have to eliminate red meat if you stick with the very leanest cuts. The nutrients per calorie in beef can make it a good nutritional choice. After the lean beefs we find the lean chicken and turkey choices. As with the other Nutrigroups, as you process, and add salt and fat, the Nutripoints go down. The very worst choices are fatty meats, such as bacon and the lunch meats. The organ meats above the recommended line all have a comment on them concerning cholesterol because while they're high in nutrients, and thus have relatively high Nutripoint scores, they're also very high in cholesterol, and therefore are not really good nutritional choices, especially if you're concerned about cholesterol.

Fast Foods In general, the best choice at a fast-food restaurant is the salad bar—but that's providing you go easy on the salad dressing. For example, the new salads available at Wendy's range from 1 to −1.5 Nutripoints due to the high fat dressings included on them. Following that, a stuffed potato, if not too much fat in the form of cheese or butter has been added, is a good choice.

Taco Bell offers some good choices in terms of Nutripoints. Their bean burrito with green sauce weighs in at 4 Nutripoints, which is below your daily goal of 5 Nutripoints from the legume Nutrigroup, but is still better than a Taco Bell Light Taco (−1.5 Nutripoints). The best Taco Bell has to offer is in their new Fresco Style offerings of burritos, tacos, and tostadas. They range from 1.5 to 4 Nutripoints, which are good scores for fast foods. Del Taco also has some good scores for their entire lineup of food offerings, ranging from .5 to 3.5 Nutripoints. The reason these Mexican-style chains do better than the hamburger ones is due to use of beans and vegetables, vs. meat, cheese and bacon in the hamburgers.

As mentioned in the Grain section, pizza can also be a good nutritional choice, if you go with the thin crusts, lower fat versions, and use more vegetable toppings. Scores of these range from 1.5 to 5 Nutripoints.

It's nearly impossible to get a good breakfast at a fast-food restaurant, as the choices are usually loaded with fat: butter, cheese, eggs, and sausage. Wendy's various omelets, scoring around −10 Nutripoints, are among the worst of all possible fast-food choices.

PERSONALIZING THE NUTRIPOINT PROGRAM

Thus far we've been talking about the basic Nutripoints program, which requires a minimum of 100 Nutripoints per day. This level of Nutripoints is geared to someone who requires 1,000−1,200 calories per day. This is the level of Nutripoints we use in the Cooper Wellness Programs at the Aerobics Center. We do so because many of our participants are trying to lose some weight. After they've finished two weeks at the center on this level, we recommend that when they go home they move up to Level 2 of the program, at 1,500 calories and, in some cases, 1,800 calories. In *no* case do we recommend that anyone go below 100 Nutripoints daily because you really cannot expect to get adequate nutrients at this level. Moreover, such a low level of calories would have a negative effect on your metabolism. (We don't pinpoint the calories precisely for two reasons: first, we want to de-emphasize the importance of calories as a measure of foods, and second, we can't specify any more precisely without losing the element of choice that you enjoy with Nutripoints.)

This basic level of Nutripoints we use at the Center isn't right for everyone. Daily nutritional needs depend on age, sex, frame size, weight, and activity level. Obviously, a small woman who weighs 103 pounds, and who is totally sedentary, is going to need fewer calories than a 200-pound football player in training.

In general, you may well find that you need fewer calories on Nutripoints than you might think. We've had many individuals on the 1,000−1,200 regime who begin, thinking that they wont be satisfied with this number of calories. But because so much fat is eliminated from their diets, 1,000 calories turns out to be far more food than they imagined. My suggestion is to begin at a level of the system a bit lower than what you think your daily caloric needs are. If you find you're not getting enough food, move up to the next level of Nutripoints. There is an element of trial and error in choosing the right level for you. If, after being on one level for a couple of weeks, you find it's too much or too little food, adjust to the next level accordingly.

The following is a breakdown of the three levels of Nutripoints to help you figure out where you might need to personalize the system and adjust your daily total goals:

Level 1: 100 Nutripoints daily/1,000—1,200 calories

This basic level of 1,000—1,200 calories per day is adequate for those on a weight-loss program, or for a basically sedentary woman of 125 pounds or less on a weight maintenance program.

The serving recommendations are those we've already looked at:

Nutrigroup	*Servings*	*Goal*
Vegetable	4	55
Fruit	3	15
Grain	2	10
Legume/nut/seed	1	5
Milk/dairy	2	10
Meat/fish/poultry	1	5
Total		**100**

See page 112 for the chart to use for this level.

Level 2: 150 Nutripoints Daily/1,500—1,800 calories

This level is appropriate for the following individuals: active women; inactive, heavier women; inactive to moderately active men; and men over 200 pounds who are trying to lose weight.

Nutrigroup	*Servings*	*Goal*
Vegetable	6	85
Fruit	4	20
Grain	3	15
Legume/nut/seed	2	10
Milk/dairy	2	10
Meat/fish/poultry	2	10
Total:		**150**

Level 3: 200 Nutripoints Daily/2,000+ calories

In this level we've increased the vegetable, fruit, and grain servings in order to increase complex carbohydrates. On Level 3, you don't have to be so particular about shooting for the top of the lists to keep calories under control; there's more margin for error when you need more calories per day. But you should still avoid any foods below the recommended level.

Nutrigroup	*Servings*	*Goal*
Vegetable	8	120
Fruit	6	30
Grain	4	20
Legume/nut/seed	2	10
Milk/dairy	2	10
Meat/fish/poultry	2	10
Total:		**200**

NUTRIPOINT DAILY RECORD SHEET 1,500-1,800 CALORIES								
	Nutripoints							
Food Selection/Serving Size	Veg.	Fruit	Grain	Leg.	Meat	Milk	Other	
Breakfast:								
1 Grain								
1 Milk/Dairy								
2 Fruit								
Lunch:								
2 Meat or Legume								
3 Vegetables								
1 Grain								
1 Milk/Dairy								
Dinner:								
2 Meat or Legume								
3 Vegetables								
1 Grain								
Totals:								
Goals:	85	20	15	10	10	10	0	150

NUTRIPOINT DAILY RECORD SHEET 2,000+ CALORIES

	Nutripoints							
Food Selection/Serving Size	Veg.	Fruit	Grain	Leg.	Meat	Milk	Other	
Breakfast:								
2 Grain								
1 Milk/Dairy								
2 Fruit								
Lunch:								
2 Meat or Legume								
4 Vegetables								
1 Grain								
1 Milk/Dairy								
2 Fruit								
Dinner:								
2 Meat or Legume								
4 Vegetables								
1 Grain								
2 Fruit								
Totals:								
Goals:	120	30	20	10	10	10	0	200

Don't be overwhelmed by the number of servings for, say, vegetables in this level of Nutripoints: you can simply increase the amounts of a serving of a single food instead of having so many different foods. For example, instead of a half cup of sliced carrots for one serving (30 Nutripoints), have a full cup for two servings (60 Nutripoints). Remember that with the fruit Nutrigroup, you can make fruit juice a serving. Many people who are on this level of Nutripoints are very active and require a fair amount of liquids throughout the day. If you are careful to have a no-sugar-added 100-percent fruit juice instead of a soft drink, it will fulfill some of your fruit servings. Instead of a Coke (−6 Nutripoints), have some orange juice (11 Nutripoints), or some orange-pineapple juice (9.5 Nutripoints).

THE VEGETARIAN OPTION

It wasn't so long ago that vegetarians were considered at best off-beat, at worst nuts. But just as people are now willing to face the fact that smoking can cause lung cancer, and that high-fat and -cholesterol diets can cause heart disease, they are also willing to entertain the notion that meat may not always be the best and only source of protein in our diets. Even groups such as the American Dietetic Association and other health organizations are saying that not only is a vegetarian diet safe (people used to worry that you couldn't get sufficient protein from it), it can also be a healthier option than a diet that includes meat.

Solely on the basis of nutritional factors, including avoidance of excessives such as cholesterol and fat, and in an effort to increase fiber, Nutripoints has already incorporated some vegetarian principles. We've decreased the number of recommended meat servings to one a day, which is fewer than most people currently eat, and we've switched the main source of protein from meat/fish/poultry to a combination of meat/ fish/poultry and legumes.

The advantage of getting some of your protein from plant sources rather than solely from meat/poultry/fish is that along with protein you're getting more complex carbohydrates, more fiber, less saturated fat, and less cholesterol. As you already know, the reduction of these elements in your diet will make you less susceptible to cancer and heart disease.

In addition to avoiding the lifestyle diseases, there's another factor that argues in favor of shifting the emphasis from meat as the primary source of protein in your diet: by "eating low on the food chain," as vegetarians refer to this option, you lessen your chances of accumulating toxic substances. Any drug that livestock are treated with eventually winds up in their meat. A diet very high in meat is eventually introducing these toxins into your body, and no one knows what the ultimate effect of these toxins will be. In addition to toxins introduced by man in the form of drugs, animals are also more likely to harbor organisms or pathogens that can be passed to man. In general, animal diseases can be passed to us, while plant diseases cannot. When you weigh all the factors, from drug contamination to contaminants that regularly affect animal foods such as oysters and clams, it seems clear that you're going from increased potential for harm to decreased potential for harm when you shift your emphasis from meat to other sources of protein.

I've been a vegetarian for over thirty years now, and I guess I'm living proof of what a vegetarian diet can mean in terms of health: my cholesterol runs around 180, and my recent best time on the treadmill was rated "superior." I also feel that my energy level is terrific and that my general state of health is excellent.

If you're interested in vegetarianism, you might want to consult some of the excellent books that have been published on the subject, including *The Vegetarian Alternative* by Vic Sussman and *The Gradual Vegetarian* by Lisa Tracy.

There are various types of vegetarians, identified as follows:

Strict vegetarian (vegan): This is the most restricted level of vegetarianism. Vegans eat no animal products, including dairy.

Lactovegetarians: These vegetarians eat milk, cheese, and other dairy products, with the exception of eggs. They also refrain from eating meat, fish, and poultry.

Ovolactovegetarians: These vegetarians eat animal protein in eggs and dairy products, but no meat, fish, or poultry. This is the type of vegetarian that I am. Remember, the *white portion* of eggs provide high quality protein and have a positive Nutripoint score, as well as *low-fat* dairy products.

There is a new type of vegetarian these days who doesn't eat any red meat. This isn't an official category of vegetarianism, but it's quite popular. While such people are not really vegetarians, they still represent a trend I think is good because they're avoiding a major source of fat and cholesterol, as well as any potential toxins.

The Nutripoint Vegetarian option is geared to the ovolactovegetarian option because I believe it's the safest type of diet: you're totally eliminating all flesh food (meat), but you're still getting complete protein in the form of whole dairy products and low-fat cheeses and yogurts. The protein level (which many people worry about) is completely adequate at 75 grams a day—clearly more than the 56 grams recommended for men and the 46 recommended for women per day.

Adequate protein has always been the controversial point of vegetarian diets, and many people have been turned off to vegetarianism by "food combining." There's something about having to worry about eating rice with beans to get certain nutrients, for example, that discourages people. They think that if they don't eat the right foods together in the precisely correct combinations, they'll wither and die. The fact is, you *do* need to pay attention to getting adequate amounts of certain foods, but this is very easy to do, and it soon becomes second nature. Most important, you don't have to combine all of these foods *in the same meal.*

The reason that animal protein is an excellent source of protein for the human body is that it contains high concentrations of essential amino acids your body needs but cannot produce on its own. Foods that are high in these essential amino acids are called "complete," or high quality. Meats are high in these amino acids because the animal has put them together from the plants it's eaten: the balance is already achieved. Meats are therefore a "complete," or high-quality, protein. To get a balance of high-quality protein without meat, you have to do the combining yourself. Some plant foods are high in one amino acid, and some are high in others: by combining them you achieve a complete protein. And, as I mentioned, you don't have to make the perfect combination at each meal; the body is far more adaptable than that. Your body has an amino acid pool that stores amino acids for future use. As long as you eat, within a period of a few days, a variety of foods that complement one another, you'll achieve the effect of high-quality protein.

Some examples of foods that in combination provide complete protein are:

Cereal w/milk
Rice w/sesame seeds
Rice/cheese casserole
Legume soup w/bread
Macaroni and cheese
Corn tortillas and beans
Cheese sandwich
Pea soup and bread
Rice/bean casserole
Lentil curry w/rice

On page 126 you'll find a graphic summary of how to achieve complete protein with combinations of foods. You should know that a vegetarian diet is high in fiber, and you might have an adjustment period during which you'll experience

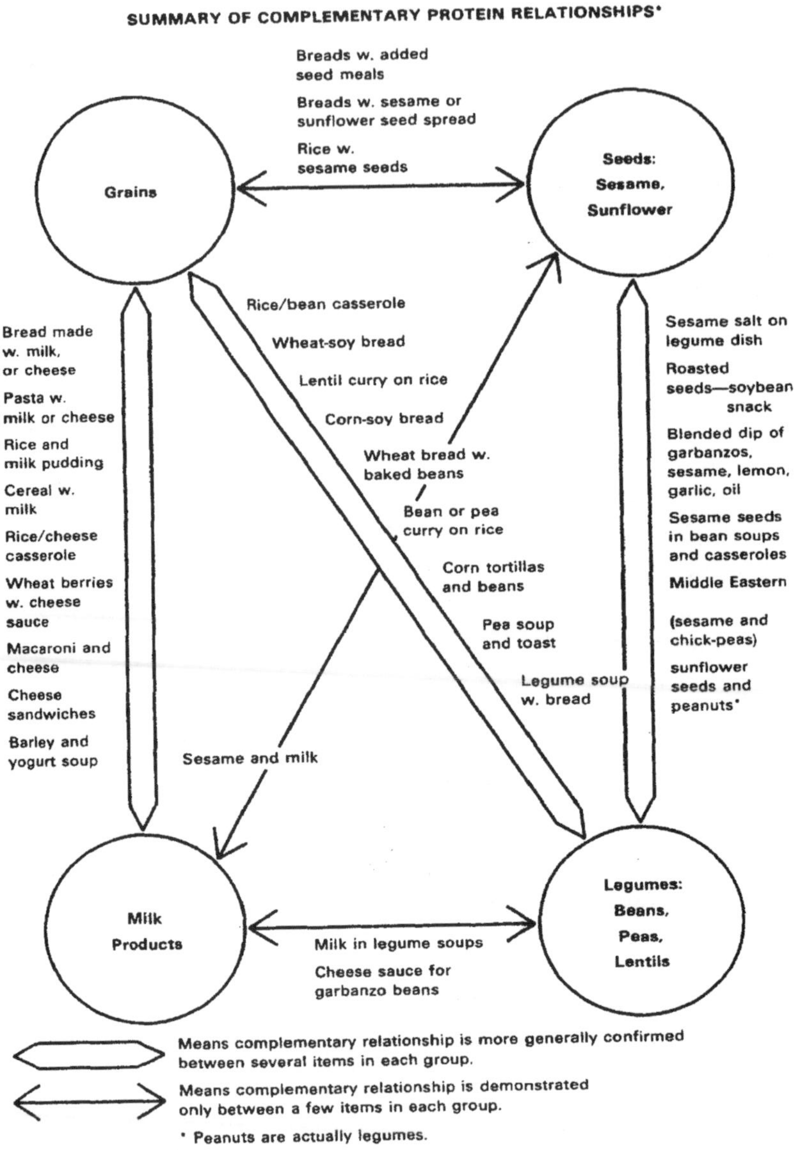

*Adapted from Frances M. Lappé, *Diet for a Small Planet.*

excess gas and bloating. This is due to the fact that certain bacteria work to break down fiber and, in the process, give off gas. The body eventually adjusts and produces less gas, although it will still produce a bit more than when on a low-fiber diet. There are various methods to cut down on this gas.

First, be sure to cook all beans thoroughly; they're supposed to be soft, and if they're too chewy, they probably haven't been well cooked and are therefore likely to cause more gas. It often helps to soak beans in plenty of water overnight, and then discard the water and add fresh for cooking. Don't eat beans with other gaseous vegetables, such as cabbage. If you have a serious problem with gas and bloating from beans, you might want to stick to the beans that are least likely to cause gas, including lentils, black-eyed peas, lima beans, chick-peas, and white beans. There is also a good product called "Beano", which are tablets that eliminate the after-effects of eating beans and other gas-producing foods. You should be able to find them at your local grocer's or health food store.

You might also notice that your body produces more frequent, and looser, bowel movements while on a high-fiber diet. This is actually good: your digestive system is getting waste out of your body as quickly as possible, and the fiber is absorbing water, which helps dilute carcinogens and excrete them. More frequent bowel movements also keep fat from sitting in the colon and causing a risk for cancer. In addition, frequent bowel movements help to flush cholesterol out of the system.

The Vegetarian option for the 1,000—1,200 calorie version of Nutripoints breaks down as follows:

Nutrigroup	*Servings*	*Goal*
Vegetable	4	55
Fruit	3	15
Grain	2	10
Legume/nut/seed	2	10
Milk/dairy	2	10
Total:		**100**

You'll notice that this version of the vegetarian option simply substitutes one additional legume serving for the meat/poultry/fish option. If you prefer, instead of the two legume servings, you can have one legume serving and one additional milk/dairy serving.

The 1,500—1,800 calorie version is:

Nutrigroup	*Servings*	*Goal*
Vegetable	6	85
Fruit	4	20
Grain	4	20
Legume/nut/seed	3	15
Milk/dairy	2	10
Total:		**150**

The 2,000+ calorie vegetarian option is:

Nutrigroup	*Servings*	*Goal*
Vegetable	8	120
Fruit	6	30
Grain	4	20
Legume/nut/seed	3	15
Milk/dairy	3	15
	Total:	**200**

As with the other higher-calorie versions of Nutripoints, you don't have to always depend on a huge number of servings from one Nutrigroup: you can sometimes simply increase the serving sizes to double the Nutripoints in a single serving. And you can get some of your vegetables, as well as fruits, in juices.

NUTRIPOINT RECOVERY

I have always found that a great limitation of a traditional "diet," which was most commonly a weight-reduction diet, was that you had to stick pretty strictly to the prescribed food choices and menus. This is not a whim of the diet-creators; in the best diets, it's done to ensure that you get an adequate balance of proteins-carbohydrates-fats, and that you get sufficient nutrients. In order for these diets to fulfill their promise of weight loss *and* adequate nutrition, they had to insist on strict compliance with the recommended menus.

What this meant in practical terms was that once you "cheated" and put butter on your toast, or ate a cookie, you were lost. You'd failed. Most people felt that following such a diet was walking a tightrope: one slip and they might as well throw in the towel. Patients had often presented their "diet histories" as a series of failed diets. Or they would lose some weight on a particular diet and then gain it all back, or gain it back with interest.

Nutripoints is different. *It puts the control back in your hands because it puts the information in your hands. You* don't have to rely on a menu plan or a list of food choices devised by someone else; you make the foods choices you like. And if you follow the system, you'll achieve your goal.

And what about those "failures"? They don't exist on Nutripoints. That's because you have the means, to *quantify* your food choices yourself. This doesn't mean that you won't sometimes get fewer Nutripoints than you should, or perhaps too few or too many servings in one or more of the Nutrigroups, but when you *do* stray from the system, you can recover. This is because Nutripoints is a system of numbers. If you get fewer points on one day, you can redouble your efforts on the next day and get a higher score.

I tread lightly here because some people look upon the recovery feature of Nutripoints as a license to binge. In other words, they think that if they get 200 Nutripoints on Tuesday, they can go wild on Wednesday and get only 10 Nutripoints and still be on top of things: the extra 100 Nutripoints on one day will help make up for the missing 90 the next. It doesn't work this way.

The basic premise of Nutripoints is that you want to improve your nutrition and your health. You know that it's not good to eat three slices of bacon and two fried eggs. Even if you eat the best diet in the world the following day, that overload of fat, cholesterol, and sodium is going to take its toll. No system can tell you that it won't. The difference with Nutripoints is that if you don't reach your goal one day, you can still recover the next by trying harder.

The way I explain this to my patients is that they don't have a license to eat a bowl of ice cream. But if they find themselves at a dinner party and the main course is cooked crab in a mayonnaise-based sauce, with broccoli in cheese sauce, and with chocolate pie for dessert, they don't have to refuse to eat. They can eat some of their meal, figure on getting a low Nutripoint score for that day, and move on the next day to choose from the tops of the Nutrigroups so that their daily "atonement" score will be particularly high. They'll be helping their bodies by making an extra effort to reduce the fat, cholesterol, and calorie intakes that were exceeded the previous day.

Because Nutripoints is a numbers system, it gives you the power to improve your overall nutritional status when circumstances have forced you into a situation that will produce a low score.

SHOPPING FOR NUTRIPOINTS

Now that you know where you stand before you embark on the Nutripoint program, I hope you're inspired to jump right in. You can start immediately, with your next meal, if you wish. Or you can take a day or two to familiarize yourself with the charts and stock your kitchen with foods that are high in Nutripoints, while you discard those that could sabotage your score.

One patient told me after he had been on Nutripoints for a month that the biggest change in his life was the volume of food in his refrigerator—and it wasn't what you might think. Before Nutripoints, he said, his refrigerator frequently looked half empty. That's because it was filled with processed and frozen prepared foods. After all, a box of frozen carrots in butter sauce doesn't take up as much room as a bunch of fresh carrots, and a frozen pot pie doesn't take up as much room as some fresh chicken and fresh vegetables. He now says, after Nutripoints, when he opens his refrigerator he sees the colors of real foods instead of a lot of packages, and his refrigerator always looks jammed.

The following are some tips on shopping that will help you through the supermarket maze:

Prepare to Shop

1. Amazingly enough, *47 percent of all food purchases are impulse buying.* This means that nearly half of what we buy is just something that looks good at the moment. It may not be a good nutritional value, or it might not even fit our personal "food-style." Many of us go into a "supermarket trance" the minute we hit the aisles, and begin buying for a fantasy family. When we unload the grocery bags at home, we too often realize that we didn't get half of what we needed, and what we did get we don't have much use for. The cure for this is a shopping list. Yes, it's basic, but it works. Buy only what's on your list, and perhaps other items that you regularly use, or that are on sale. Use the Nutripoint "shopping lists" (see page 161) to help you find the best nutritional bargains. If you take the time to check these lists, you may well find that you can improve your nutritional status just by making a few wise choices among brands.

2. Keep a list hanging in your kitchen, perhaps attached with a magnet to your refrigerator door, so that every time you notice you need something you can jot it down. Take the time to check Nutripoints for foods that could be substituted for foods that are lower in Nutripoints.

3. If you have some recipes you're going to try, be sure to check them over and add all necessary ingredients to your shopping list. It's amazing how often we never get around to preparing a certain recipe because we keep forgetting to buy that one critical ingredient.

Time Your Shopping Trips

1. Shop when your energy level is high and your temptation level low. You probably already know that you shouldn't shop when you're hungry. Don't shop when you're tired, either. One patient told me that her husband could always tell when she was exhausted: she came home from her usual after-work shopping trip with nothing but frozen entrees. If you *are* going to buy nothing but frozen entrees, at least make sure in advance that they're entrees that are high in Nutripoints.

2. If at all possible, avoid taking small children to the supermarket with you. It's terribly distracting to have to argue with a three-year-old who wants candy and sugared cereals and keep your mind on your list at the same time. If you must bring children with you, plan ahead and bring something—a small toy or healthful snack packed in a margarine tub—that will keep them occupied. One patient told me that she had her two kids help out at the market: she would instruct them to find certain items they were familiar with and praise them lavishly when they did. They enjoyed helping and were distracted from the usual supermarket temptations.

3. Frequent the biggest and best-stocked supermarket in your area. I recommend that you look for a supermarket with the best and most extensive produce section and adopt it as your regular shopping place. The advantage of frequenting the same supermarket is that you can develop a relationship with the manager and request that they carry certain items. Some high-Nutripoint frozen dinners, for example, might not be available in your local markets, but if you request them, many managers will be happy to stock them.

Shop Wisely

1. Buy fresh fruits and vegetables in season. They're almost invariably tastier and more nutritious.

2. Never buy junk foods! If you have them in the house you'll probably eat them. Many people use guests as an excuse to buy things they ordinarily never have around. If you're having guests, prepare snacks and meals that are high in Nutripoints. They'll enjoy them as much as you, and you'll be doing them a favor by sparing them the chip and dip routine. If you must have some kind of snack food around, buy it in the smallest possible size and, if possible, in individual packages.

3. If you're buying convenience foods, make sure they're high in Nutripoints.

EATING OUT

Many of my patients ask me for tips on dining out. I wish I could evaluate all of the various restaurant preparations so that I could give you Nutripoints for each menu entry, but because of the endless variations in restaurant recipes, even for identical items, that's impossible. What this means is that a familiarity with the Nutripoint charts will help guide your food choices so that you can maintain your optimum diet. But, to some degree, without Nutripoints to guide you, you're back into the old days of watching fats and other negatives in order to eat well. The following are general tips that should help you eat well in restaurants:

• If possible, choose a restaurant in advance—a place that you know has some good Nutripoint choices on the menu. If you become a regular, many restaurants will be happy to fulfill certain requests, such as a vegetable combination dish that's not on the menu; plain, grilled fish; or meat cooked without butter. We're lucky today in that many restaurants have responded to consumer demand and become health conscious: they routinely offer grilled or baked foods, salads without dressing, vegetarian dishes, and low-fat entrees.

• Chinese, Japanese, and Indian restaurants are good choices for restaurants that tend to serve healthful foods. They use plenty of grains and vegetables, and the meat or fish portions of meals tend to be relatively small.

• If you're with a group that's ordering cocktails, stick with a carbonated soda water with a twist of lemon or lime, or perhaps a Virgin Mary or another mixed drink without alcohol. An orange juice spritzer of carbonated water and orange juice is refreshing, and is a good nutritional choice. Cranberry juice is always a good choice to fall back on, which I personally use often.

• If the restaurant puts bread and rolls on the table, unless others at your table object, ask them to remove the butter. It's too easy to find yourself slathering a piece of roll with butter or dabbing it on your potatoes or vegetables. You'll find that good, crusty rolls and bread really don't need butter, and the savings in terms of calories and cholesterol will be well worth it. If the restaurant doesn't serve the bread warm, you can always ask them to heat it. This brings out the natural flavors and makes it more satisfying.

• Always be sure to order salad without dressing or with dressing on the side. As we've seen, salad dressings can be a major source of fat and cholesterol if they're made with cheese or cream. Have your salad with just a bit of olive oil and vinegar, or ask if the restaurant has a low-fat or low-calorie dressing option.

• Be sure to order special dishes in advance when traveling by air. The fruit plates, vegetarian plates, and diabetic plates that most airlines serve are excellent choices, offering a delicious, fresh meal that's largely free of excess fat and sodium.

The following are tips for specific types of restaurants:

Chinese Chinese food can be an excellent choice, as it relies on a lot of vegetables cooked quickly to retain nutrients. Stir-frying is a terrific method of cooking, and is a fixture in most Chinese restaurants. It uses very little oil, and therefore adds little fat to foods. Most Chinese vegetable and fish dishes are good choices. The only drawback to Chinese restaurants is their liberal use of MSG (which some people are allergic to), and their use of salty and/or sugary sauces. Fortunately, most Chinese restaurants are responsive to requests and quite willing to eliminate MSG, sugar, and salt from their cooking. Whole, steamed fish with sauce on the side is an excellent choice, and simple, stir-fried chicken and vegetable dishes are also good. The white or brown rice that help to round out the meal are good choices, as are the following selections: moo goo gai pan, mixed vegetables, won ton soup, and steamed dumplings. Avoid foods such as crispy fried beef, fried won tons, and any sweet and sour dishes. Yes, you can splurge on a fortune cookie. At 19 calories and very little fat, one or two won't do you too much harm.

French French food can be difficult because of the use of sauces. If you stick with plain grilled meat or fish and simple salads, you'll be fine. Avoid anything prepared *remoulade,* because that refers to a mayonnaise sauce. Be sure to steer clear of vichysoisse and other cream-based soups, and onion soup with cheese on top. (You can ask for the onion soup without the cheese as an alternative.) Clear soups are the best choices. Stick with green salads, avoid anything that might be prepared with mayonnaise, and ask that dressing or sauce be served on the side. Bread is fine, but avoid butter, and stay away from croissants, which are loaded with butter. The best dessert bets include fresh berries, but pass up the cream.

Indian Indian restaurants provide some excellent choices because of their traditional reliance on legumes, vegetables, and yogurt-based sauces and dips. Some of the foods that are particularly good choices on an Indian menu include dal, vegetarian curries, raita, pulka (unleavened bread), basmati rice with vegetables, lentil soups, and tandoori baked chicken (which has been marinated in yogurt and roasted). Avoid puri (fried bread), samosa (fried appetizers), and any foods served with muglai (creamy curry sauce) or coconut-milk curry sauce. Be sure to avoid egg-based dishes. The biggest problem with Indian food is that many restaurants use ghee (which is clarified butter) or coconut oil (one of the few vegetable products that is a saturated fat) for cooking. Be sure to ask about this. Many restaurants will now use other oils for cooking if you so request.

Japanese Japanese restaurants can offer a good array of choices high in Nutripoints. The cuisine of Japan is low in fat, and makes good use of a variety of vegetables. Miso soup is a good choice, as it's based on soy with vegetables. Udon (noodles) served with broth and various meats and vegetables is a good main course, as are the yakitori (chicken or beef) preparations, which are meats broiled on a skewer. Be sure to avoid any fried dumplings, and any smoked or pickled foods. Tempura, which is fried, is not a good choice, and tonkatsu (fried pork) and torikatsu (fried chicken) are also to be avoided. Because of problems with seafood contamination, be very careful that the sushi you eat is from a highly reputable restaurant that serves only the freshest fish from the best sources.

Italian We traditionally think of Italian food as being heavy, and it can be. But the fact is, southern Italian cuisine is now recognized as among the healthiest in the world. You just have to be careful to avoid northern Italian cuisine, which is rich in fat. Cioppino (seafood soup) is a good appetizer, as is minestrone soup. Steamed mussels in a red sauce can make an appetizer or a meal. Pasta with vegetable and/or tomato sauces is a good choice. Just be careful to avoid pasta selections that have cream-based sauces, or ones that are loaded with cheese. Avoid fettucini Alfredo, lasagna (except vegetable lasagna), cannelloni, and garlic bread. Plain, grilled fish or meats can be good choices.

Mexican You have to pick and choose your way through a Mexican menu to get good nutritional value. While a dish such as chicken tostada would be a good choice, something such as a beef burrito with cheese and sour cream (heavily laden with fat and cholesterol) wouldn't. Rice, corn, and bean-based dishes can be good choices, but you must steer clear of cheese. Make sure refried beans aren't cooked in lard (which is high in saturated fat and cholesterol). Steamed corn tortillas, soft chicken tacos, black bean soup, gazpacho, and beans in a soft tortilla are all good choices. Choose the soft tacos over the crisp, as the crisp ones are fried. You can dip a plain corn tortilla in salsa, but avoid overly salted chips that are routinely served with salsa. If you can afford a dish high in fat (but low in cholesterol), you can try guacamole.

THE PERFECT MATCH: BOOSTING YOUR NUTRITION

Good nutrition depends on careful shopping, careful food storage, the best cooking techniques, and on the chemistry of the foods themselves as they work in your body. The absorption of certain nutrients can be improved when certain foods are eaten in combination; conversely, some foods inhibit the availability of nutrients when eaten with certain other foods. Alcohol, for example, impedes the body's absorption of various vitamins and minerals, including thiamin, calcium, vita-min D, folacin, and vitamin B_{12}. The following are some examples, adapted from the very informative *Jean Carper's Total Nutrition Guide,* of how you can get the best nutritional value from your foods by mixing and matching:

- Boost your iron absorption (this is particularly important for women) by adding vitamin C to any meal or food that's rich in iron. Just one glass of orange juice can boost the absorption of non-heme (nonmeat) iron by 200 to 500 percent.

- Avoid drinking tea with meals. Excess tea can help induce iron-deficiency anemia. It takes only two mugs of strong tea to reduce the amount of non-heme (nonmeat) iron you can absorb from a meal.

- Megadose supplements of vitamin C (one gram per meal) can impair vitamin B_{12} absorption to the point at which a deficiency can develop.

- Fruits and vegetables that are high in potassium (including spinach, beet greens, bok choy, tomatoes, beets, and cantaloupe) can help counter the effect of excess sodium in the diet. This is helpful to people who have a genetic disposition for hypertension.

- Many medications block or inhibit the absorption of various nutrients. Antibiotics, for example, can have an effect on your absorption of vitamins K and B_{12}. If you take a medication regularly, including birth control pills, check with your doctor to see if that medication has any effect on your nutritional status.

- Never add baking soda when cooking vegetables, as the alkaline solution thus created can destroy riboflavin (vitamin B_2).

ANSWERS TO COMMON QUESTIONS ABOUT NUTRIPOINTS

I've tried to cover every aspect of Nutripoints you need to know. But sometimes information is more accessible in a question-and-answer format. Also, there are certain common questions my patients ask that don't fit into neat categories. The following are the most common questions people ask about Nutripoints:

How does Nutripoints™ differ from the Weight Watchers® Points® system?

Nutripoints has been used in the U.S. since 1988 and in 10 countries worldwide since 1990. It is a *positive* approach to better nutrition—you try to get *more* points, not less. So it's not about depravation and limiting—it's about getting more good foods. It is based on analysis of *26 factors* in foods, so it is very *comprehensive.* Over 3600 foods are analyzed, so you can find nearly any food you are interested in. Nutripoints is *not* a weight-loss program—it's a healthy eating plan for everyone, although most people lose weight and fat on it, simply by making better food choices and eating less calories naturally.

Why do I want to get more, rather than fewer, Nutripoints? Isn't this different from traditional programs that recommend you eat the least amount of calories?

For some people, adjusting to a positive goal (Nutripoints), rather than a negative one (calories), takes a bit of a psychological shift. But in the long run, as my patients tell me, it's far more appealing, and far easier to live with.

Yes, Nutripoints is different. A Nutripoint number assigned to a food is not, like a calorie, a one-dimensional number. Rather, it's an *overall quality rating* of the food that considers a number of factors—both positive and negative. You want to get more Nutripoints because the better a Nutripoint score, the higher the quality of a given food. The numbers are based on nutrients per calorie and the least excessives (bad elements) per calorie. The more Nutripoints you get, the more nutrition you get with the least excessives.

You might think of a Nutripoint as one point toward your vitamin quota for the day, 100 of which will give you 100 percent of the RDA, provided the points are distributed over the six Nutrigroups.

What happens if you eat too many points for the day, or for one Nutrigroup?

If you stick with the recommended number of servings for each Nutrigroup, you can't get too many Nutripoints. Anything over 100 Nutripoints for a day, or for the goal for a given Nutrigroup, is that much more nutrition you are concentrating into the food you eat. Remember that this "excess" good nutrition is fine because you are getting it in a natural form; it's nothing like taking megadoses of vitamins.

There is one problem with getting too many Nutripoints within one group. In some Nutrigroups, the only way to get super-high levels of Nutripoints, while staying within the recommended number of servings, is to pick most of your servings from the very top of the list. If you do this, it's at the expense of variety, and variety, I must stress, is very important.

Remember that each food has a "fingerprint" of nutrients that distinguishes it from other foods. If you choose all of your servings in vegetables from, say, turnip greens, you won't be diversifying your portfolio of vitamins and minerals. It would be much better to get one serving of turnip greens, and the other servings from vegetables below turnip greens that are still within the recommended area of the list.

If I eat more than 100 Nutripoints for the day, doesn't that mean that I've eaten too many calories?

Remember, the higher the Nutripoint score, the higher the nutrient density. This means the more nutrition per calorie. A high Nutripoint score means that you are getting a higher quality of food, while the number of servings you have determines the number of calories. If you get 300 Nutripoints within the recommended number of servings, you'll be within calorie limitations, and the quality of your food will be excellent.

How do you figure your score for a food item listed in the charts when you eat more or less than the serving-based points for that item? For example, if you eat an entire Arby's roast beef sandwich, but the points are only given for half a sandwich, what do you do?

Whether the points are negative or positive points, you double them if you eat double the portion listed. But don't forget that you must count that food item as *two* servings from that Nutrigroup. If you eat half the portion listed, you get half the Nutripoints, and you count that food as half a serving.

You'll notice that some foods list portion sizes that may be half of what you'd expect. For example, some of the slices of pizza are rated for half a slice. This is a tip-off that the food is calorie-dense. A large portion size is a sign that the food is a low-calorie, high-quality food, as it takes so much volume to fulfill the calorie requirement for a serving.

What happens if I eat more than the recommended number of servings per day?

There are two purposes in having a recommended number of servings per day. First, they provide the formulation within the Nutrigroups for balance between the various vitamins and minerals. Second, they provide the proper mix of carbohydrates, protein, and fats for overall daily totals. After you pick the Nutripoint level that suits you (see page 118), if you eat any more than the recommended number of servings, you will not be guaranteed your level's caloric limit.

The point I make over and over to my patients is this: when you stay within the recommended boundaries of Nutripoints, everything works. When you abandon those boundaries, you have to begin worrying about all of the old problematic factors: calories, cholesterol, sugar, fat, sodium, and so on.

If I can get my 100 Nutripoints in one serving before I fulfill the serving requirements, either for a Nutrigroup or for the day, why should I eat more food and more calories?

There are two components to an optimum diet: one is total calories, and the other is the right mix of carbohydrates, fat, and protein. Even though you get off to a good start by eating a food high in Nutripoints, you won't achieve all the requirements of your body unless you eat at least the specified number of servings per day. The goal of Nutripoints is to pick the highest-quality foods you like within each group, thus getting all of your calories, or thus limiting your calories to the right number—at *the same time* getting the proper mix of carbohydrates, protein, and fat, as well as the highest level of other nutrients, including vitamins and minerals.

What if I try to eat just foods that are high in Nutripoints, and don't bother with the serving requirements?

To get the full benefit of Nutripoints, you must consider the serving requirements along with the food scores. Think of it this way: the food scores take care of getting the best; the serving requirements take care of limiting the worst. If you pay attention just to getting foods with high scores, your nutritional status will no doubt be improved, but that's only half the picture.

You still need to limit the excessives, including fat, saturated fat, cholesterol, sugar, sodium, alcohol, and caffeine. Nutripoints can assure you of achieving all these goals only if you follow the system as it was designed: high food scores in conjunction with the correct serving requirements.

I'm forced, because of business, to eat out a lot. What if I can't get in my legume serving for a day because I can't find anything appropriate on a restaurant menu?

This is a common problem, even if you don't eat out at restaurants. Many people are simply not used to buying and cooking legumes. Indeed, in the menus and recipes provided, I've assumed that you won't be able to get in the legume serving every day, and I've allowed for it by occasionally substituting a meat/poultry/fish serving.

If you miss a serving from the legume Nutrigroup, the best alternative is to substitute a serving from the meat/poultry/fish Nutrigroup. Naturally, you should try to make your substitution from the top of that Nutrigroup. You'll want to get at least a 5-Nutripoint meat/poultry/fish serving so that your total in the meat Nutrigroup for that day would be 10 rather than 5. This substitution will ensure that you're getting adequate protein for the day without too many extra calories.

What would happen if I occasionally ate a few foods from below the recommended line? What, really, is the reason for a cutoff point?

If you dip below the recommended levels on the charts, it will be more difficult to achieve the goals of the system, and it will be impossible to guarantee the results promised by Nutripoints. If you try to balance a poor choice with foods that are very high in Nutripoints, it will help you regain your balance. It's possible that the poor food choice is so high in one of the excessives that it causes you to exceed the limit for that excessive. Your other good choices are therefore limited in how much they can redeem you: they can give you optimum nutrients for that day, but they can't take away the excessive amounts of whatever excessive you've eaten.

What if I'm short in Nutripoints for one Nutrigroup, but over the goal in another: is that OK?

There's a simple answer to many questions about Nutripoints: once you abandon the program, you forfeit what it promises. I don't mean to make this sound bleak. It's just that the system has been designed to work as it's laid out. Once you begin to modify it, results can't be guaranteed. This doesn't mean that you need to abandon hope if you are short a few Nutripoints. The fact is, most people find that they're eating better on Nutripoints than they ever have in their lives, even if they don't follow the system religiously. It's impossible to say what your status would be if you were off in one Nutrigroup. If you're short by just a few points, you're probably OK. If you're short in one or two Nutrigroups every few days, you're less likely to be OK.

If you go over your Nutripoint goal for the day—say, 200 Nutripoints—how bad could it be to eat a food with a −3, which only pulls your score down a little bit?

It's difficult to appreciate at first why it's such a big deal to cut a few points off your daily score unless you understand how the numbers and servings function as *limits* as well as guidelines. If you eat a negative food when you've achieved a high Nutripoint score for the day, it means that while you've achieved all your *essential* goals, you haven't stayed within your *excessive* limits. In other words, you've probably eaten too much fat and/or cholesterol, sugar, sodium, calories. So, while you've gotten all of your vitamins and minerals, you could be harming yourself by consuming, say, too much cholesterol. You can more easily understand why this would be so just from a logical standpoint: would it make sense for someone to get a high Nutripoint score—say, 350 Nutripoints—and then eat 150 points worth of negative foods to get their final score down to 200? Of course not!

Why is there so much difference between the ratings for one Nutrigroup and another? In other words, why is the highest-rated vegetable 79 Nutripoints, while the highest dairy product gets only 23.5 Nutripoints? Does this mean we'd be better off eating just vegetables, or does it mean that a different standard was used for different Nutrigroups?

The same standard—the Nutripoint formula—was used to rate *all* foods. We can see from the ratings that, in general, vegetables offer more nutrition per calorie than milk and dairy products. So you can compare foods from Nutrigroup to Nutrigroup *in general,* but you can't finally say that because vegetables are better foods, that's all you should eat. Balance is a critical part of an optimum diet, and the only way to achieve balance is to choose foods from various Nutrigroups. The reason for this is that each Nutrigroup has its own nutrient profile, which distinguishes it from every other Nutrigroup. Although we know a great deal about the nutrients in foods, there are probably things yet to be discovered concerning micronutrients. Given this, there may be micronutrients in, say, grains, that your body requires to function. Therefore, even though a grain food has a lower score than a vegetable food, you'll be avoiding grains to your peril. The only situation in which foods from different Nutrigroups can be interchangeable is between the legume/nut/seed and meat/poultry/fish groups. This is because the basic nutrient profile critical to the human body in these groups seems to concern protein. As it's possible to get sufficient protein from plant sources, it's possible to make exchanges between these two Nutrigroups.

How can all the complex information we have about vitamins and minerals, in particular, be reduced to one number? How can you compare apples and oranges? Aren't oranges high in vitamin C while bananas are high in potassium? Can't you eat carrots because they're high in vitamin A?

While it is true that certain foods are high in specific nutrients, many of our beliefs about eating a certain food for the sake of a certain nutrient reveal more about our past inability to accurately compare foods than about the food's usefulness.

In fact, while there are about fifty nutrients, including water, that are needed daily for optimum good health, the list can be narrowed down, for practical purposes, to the ten most important, or "leader," nutrients. If you are careful to consume these leader nutrients, the other forty or so will be present in sufficient amounts to meet your nutritional needs. A study was done that demonstrated this. The study tried to discover if foods rated solely on eight vitamins and minerals (protein, vitamin A, vitamin C, niacin, riboflavin, thiamin, iron, and calcium) were valid guides to improved food choices. The foods were analyzed in various ways, and finally demonstrated that nutrient-density scores, even when based on only eight nutrients, do in fact serve as valid indicators of the overall nutritional worth of a food. They also found that high nutrient-density scores are a good measure of the nutritional complexity of a food. *Foods with the highest scores are high not just for one or two nutrients but for most nutrients.* Of the fifty foods in this study, for example, forty-three had high scores for six or more of the eight nutrients measured. Foods in the middle of the ratings had good scores for only two to five of the eight nutrients measured, and most of the bottom fifty foods failed to have a decent score for even a single nutrient.

In fact, nature, with the help of Nutripoints, has made it easy for us: you don't have to eat two dozen foods to cover all of the major and minor nutrients, you just have to eat foods that are high in Nutripoints.

How did you arrive at the line that defines the recommended level in the lists? Why isn't it just the point at which the numbers become negative, which seems more logical?

The Nutripoint scores for foods had to take into account not only the absolute value of each individual food but how that food would fit into the pattern of balance in a daily diet. The numbers are not intended to reflect a perfect gradient; there's no point at which a food becomes taboo. My effort was, as much as possible, to eliminate the excessives and promote the essentials. It's all a question of relative values. So, as you reach the bottom of the lists, the food choices simply become comparatively poorer. If you choose too many of those poor foods, you won't meet the goals of Nutripoints. The recommended line reflects an effort to guide your choices to a point at which you can choose near the bottom of the list, *but above the recommended level,* and still achieve your Nutripoint goals.

As to why the cutoff point is not simply all negative numbers: there are some foods that are negative but that are OK to eat sometimes. Fat, for example, can be a part of your diet, but all the fats have negative numbers.

Why is it that sometimes there may be five or ten foods with the same rating? Are they all exactly the same?

When we figured out the Nutripoint scores, we carried out the numbers to the nearest one-hundredth. This means that a food might have, for example, wound up with a rating of 4.26. To avoid confusion with too many numbers (and, from a practical standpoint, because these differences are really quite minor) we rounded off these numbers. The food rated at 4.26 would have become 4.5.

If there are a number of foods listed at the same number, the order of listing reflects the small fractional differences in their ratings. They are listed in descending order. A food that appears, for example, at 4 is better than any food at 4 beneath it. Remember that these differences are so minor that, for practical purposes, foods at 4 can be considered equal.

Is a food with a score of 20 twice as good as a food with a score of 10?

Yes and no. Yes, it is twice as nutritious per calorie when adjusting for negative factors (excessives) that help determine the ratings. But no, it may not have double the nutrition. A food with a score of 10 may have nearly as much nutrition as a food with a score of 20, but the lower score may reflect the presence of negative factors that drop the rating. Hence a food with a rating of 20 is twice as good as a food with a rating of 10, *based on the criteria we have set in the Nutripoint formula.*

If a food has negative Nutripoints, does that mean it contains no nutrition?

Not necessarily. A food with negative Nutripoints may contain no nutrition plus some excessives that pull it down, or it may be extremely nutritious but be pulled down by a lot of excessives. You can't tell just by looking at the Nutripoint number. In these cases, its negative score is used to tell where it stands in comparison to other foods.

If something has 100 Nutripoints, does that mean it's a perfect food?

Not necessarily. It's possible that a food with an extremely high Nutripoint rating is high in nutrition per calorie, but it doesn't mean that it's perfectly balanced over the eighteen essentials. There really is no perfect food. Good nutrition comes from a balance that you achieve by choosing from the six Nutrigroups.

Are you absolutely positive that I'll get 100 percent of the RDA for all vitamins and minerals if I get 100 Nutripoints per day?

If you get 100 Nutripoints per day following all the guidelines of the Nutripoints program, you can be reasonably assured that you're getting 100 percent of the RDA for all of the essential vitamins and minerals. If, however, you make many of your food choices from near the bottom of the lists, it is possible that you will occasionally be slightly below 100 percent on some of the nutrients. The system has to take this very small risk if it's to allow you to make the food choices yourself. If you try to choose many of your foods from the higher portion of the list, you'll have no trouble getting 100 percent of RDAs. If you get over 100 Nutripoints, there's no doubt that you'll be reaching, and probably surpassing, the RDAs for all the essential vitamins and minerals.

Also, since your body can store nutrients for some time and can vary its ability to absorb them, it is not necessary to meet precisely all the RDAs every single day. The National Research Council that set up RDAs says, "RDA(s) are presented as *daily* allowances in order to simplify dietary calculations.

Nevertheless, the various protective mechanisms of the body are such that if the recommended dietary allowance for a nutrient is not met on a particular day, a surplus consumed shortly thereafter will compensate for the inadequacy for normal individuals. In estimating dietary adequacy it would seem entirely acceptable to average intakes of nutrients over a 5–8 day period." Thus over a five- to eight-day period, a Nutripoint score of 100 each day achieved by using a variety of foods would meet the RDA standards.

Why are some foods that are high in cholesterol at the top of the list? I thought cholesterol was a negative factor and would therefore pull that food's score down.

You'll notice that there are some foods near the top of the list, particularly in the meat/poultry/fish Nutrigroup, that have a symbol identifying them as a high cholesterol food. What this means is that these foods, although high in Nutripoints, are also high in cholesterol. This occurs because these foods are extremely high in vitamins and minerals. They earned their scores honestly according to the Nutripoint formula, but their cholesterol level is nonetheless extremely high.

Most of the foods that fall into this category are organ meats, such as liver. The liver acts as a storage system in the body to store vitamins and minerals, and that's why it's so rich in nutrients. But it also produces cholesterol. About 70 to 80 percent of cholesterol is produced by the liver; the rest is gained from dietary sources. About 1,000 milligrams of cholesterol is produced by the human body each day. As animal livers also produce cholesterol, if you eat liver, you're eating a concentrated source of cholesterol. By the way, not all organ meats are rich in nutrients, and the Nutripoint charts reflect this. Sweetbreads, for example, are an organ meat, but they're not high in nutrients, and you'll find them at the very bottom of the meat/poultry/fish list.

Another reason that liver, despite its high nutritional content, may not be a good food choice is that one of the functions of the liver is to detoxify the blood. Any contaminants in the body are processed by the liver, which becomes a concentrated storage house of such toxins, which, obviously, are not a positive element in any diet.

All foods on the Nutripoints list above the recommended line that are high in cholesterol have daggers (†) next to them. By "high in cholesterol" I mean foods that have a cholesterol per calorie ratio of 1 or above; in other words, for every calorie there is one or more milligrams of cholesterol. From a practical standpoint, this means that while these foods are high in nutrients they should be avoided, despite their high Nutripoint scores. Just one three-ounce serving of liver, for example, would have approximately 400 milligrams of cholesterol, which would put you well above the American Heart Association guidelines of 300 milligrams of cholesterol per day.

What about the fact that oxalic acid, which is a component of green, leafy vegetables, binds the calcium in greens so that it is not available and not readily absorbed by the body? Do you take this sort of thing into account in the formula?

While it's true that oxalic acid does interfere to some degree with the absorption of calcium by the body, it doesn't have as negative an effect as some people believe. Certain foods contain oxalic acid, which combines with calcium and magnesium to form insoluble compounds that are thus unavailable to the body. But most foods simply don't contain *enough* oxalic acid to bind with any significant amount of calcium or magnesium in the food. Thus, green, leafy vegetables can still be considered a good source of calcium in the diet when supplemented with a variety of low-fat dairy products.

Absorption levels could not be taken into account in the Nutripoints formula because there are simply too many variables connected with absorption that can't be quantified. In the section on food combinations (page 158), however, you'll find some helpful information on how you can boost absorption of nutrients. The section on essentials (page 64) will give you tips if you're concerned about a particular nutrient.

How does the Nutripoint program assure me that I get my citrus fruit and my green, leafy and yellow/orange vegetables every day?

The beauty of Nutripoints is that it automatically fulfills the requirements suggested by nutritionists over the years. The reason we've heard citrus fruit so highly recommended is that it's very high in vitamin C. But Nutripoints also identifies other foods that are high in C. If you choose foods from the top of the list, you'll be getting foods, citrus or not, that are most likely very high in vitamin C.

As for the green, leafy and yellow/orange vegetables, Nutripoints rates these vegetables very highly in the first place. These foods are high in vitamin A.

(Green, leafy vegetables are also high in vitamin C and calcium.) The vitamin A you get from yellow/orange vegetables is in the form of beta carotene, which we've all heard about is so important in preventing disease and maintaining health. The body does not care whether it gets its beta carotene from green, leafy vegetables or from yellow/orange vegetables. Either one will fill the bill. Picking foods high on the Nutripoint lists will assure you that you're getting foods high in all your vitamin/mineral requirements.

Remember that it's an old-fashioned concept to assign one vitamin or one mineral to a single food. Nature has made it easy for us, as Nutripoints reveals: most foods that are generally high in one vitamin or mineral are also high in others. In other words, the good foods are usually very good, and the bad (or unnatural) ones are awful!

How does getting 100 Nutripoints assure me that I'm getting 100 percent of RDAs and limiting calories, cholesterol, sodium, sugar, caffeine, and alcohol?

The formula for Nutripoints does this by identifying foods that are simultaneously highly nutritious and low in excessives. Foods that appear below the recommended level are really the other half of the equation. If you avoid them, you'll be steering clear of foods that would put you over the limit on any one of the excessive factors. By avoiding the negative and getting the positive, you achieve your goal.

How can you say that following the program will meet, or exceed, recommendations of the American Dietetic Association, the American Heart Association, the American Cancer Society, and the National Cancer Institute?

The American Dietetic Association officially recommends the use of USRDAs for every adult. Nutripoints is designed to fulfill this requirement. The American Dietetic Association also makes the following recommendations, which are virtually identical to the USDA dietary recommendations. You'll readily see that each of these recommendations is reflected in the Nutripoint formula:

1. Eat a variety of foods.
2. Maintain a desirable weight.
3. Avoid fat, saturated fat, and cholesterol.
4. Eat foods with adequate starch and fiber.
5. Avoid too much sugar.
6. Avoid too much sodium.
7. If you drink alcohol, do so in moderation.

The American Heart Association recommends a limit of 300 milligrams of cholesterol per day and a limit of 3,000 milligrams of sodium per day. The recommended limits are part of the formulation of Nutripoints, and are the limits set in the formula.

The American Heart Association and the American Cancer Society also recommend 30 percent or less fat consumed as calories in the diet as a preventive measure against coronary heart disease and many types of cancer, particularly colon and breast cancer. Nutripoints sets 30 percent of fat as calories as the upper limit in its formulation.

The American Cancer Society recommends getting a high amount of vitamins A and C in foods, as these vitamins have been correlated with lower rates of cancer. This is one of the strengths of Nutripoints: it identifies foods highly concentrated with vitamins A and C, and thus is a cancer-prevention diet.

The National Cancer Institute recommends 25 to 35 grams of dietary fiber per day. Nutripoints sets 35 grams as the recommended amount per day in its formulation.

Picking foods from the top of the Nutripoint lists could result in a diet that *betters* these various guidelines.

Will the Nutripoint program help prevent cancer?

There are still many questions about the causes of cancer, but there's no doubt that there are steps you can take, in terms of nutrition, that will decrease your risks for certain types of cancer. Nutripoints will certainly lower your risk for various types of cancers, as it incorporates the basic recommendations of the American Cancer Society into the tenets of the system. These seven recommendations include:

1. Avoid obesity.
2. Cut down on total fat intake.
3. Eat more high-fiber foods.
4. Include foods rich in vitamins A and C in your daily diet.
5. Include cruciferous vegetables in your diet.
6. Eat smoked, salt-cured, and nitrite-cured foods in moderation.
7. Keep alcohol consumption moderate, if you do drink.

You'll recognize that each of these recommendations is reflected in the basic Nutripoint formula.

Does your system take into account the nutrient losses from transportation, storage, and cooking?

In general, no. It's simply impossible to account for all these factors, with the exception of cooking. You'll notice that many of the fresh foods are listed raw and cooked. This will give you an idea of how the nutrition might vary from one state to another, although sometimes the variation is simply a reflection of amounts. Raw cabbage, for example, has greater volume than cooked cabbage.

The effects of transportation and storage are too variable and can't be measured. Some of these issues are discussed on page 50.

Why did you put certain foods, such as lemons, in the condiments section when they would seem more logically placed in the fruit section?

Most of the items in the condiments group are the foods you'd expect to find there, including spices and seasonings. Other foods are listed there because they're normally eaten in such small quantities that the calorie level for a given portion would be less than 20. They couldn't logically fit into the regular fruit Nutrigroup because the serving size would have to be so large that it simply wouldn't make sense. The average number of calories for the portions in the fruit Nutrigroup are 50 to 100. For lemons to fit there, I'd have to suggest that you eat two whole lemons to count as a serving. So, one-quarter lemon at 5 or 6 calories fits logically in the condiment section. In the condiment section I've adjusted the calorie portion of the formula so that the portion sizes fit normal eating patterns.

Why do you include foods such as legumes in your system? Many people never eat them. And why is Nutripoints geared toward massive amounts of fruits and vegetables?

As Willie Sutton replied when asked why he robbed banks, "Because that's where the money is." Legumes, fruits, and vegetables are highly nutritious foods, and they should play a large role in our daily diet. It's unfortunate that legumes are unfamiliar to so many people (though I think that's changing). Legumes are an excellent source of protein with no cholesterol, a lot of fiber, and complex carbohydrates. If we replaced one-quarter to one-half of our meat consumption with legumes (the Nutripoint program is designed to do this), we would be avoiding the major causes of the most prevalent lifestyle diseases, including cancer and heart disease.

As to massive amounts of fruits and vegetables, again, that's where the nutrients are! One of the major revelations of Nutripoints is that the best value in nutrition lies in *fruits and vegetables*. That's where we get the most nutrition for the fewest calories. The bonus of fruits and vegetables in terms of nutrition is that these foods are also high in complex carbohydrates and simple *bulk:* if you're dieting, they fill you up while giving you good nutrition. This is the exact opposite effect of junk foods, which *don't* fill you up and give you *nothing* in terms of good nutrition.

Why are some brand-name foods rated higher, and some lower, than their corresponding basic foods? For example, why are basic beans with pork rated 3 Nutripoints while Campbell's beans with pork is rated 2 Nutripoints?

The ratings of basic, generic foods came from USDA data. USDA data analyzes virtually every nutrient in a food. Manufacturers, however, analyze for basic nutrients, and their analyses can be variable and spotty. Therefore, when I plugged information from manufacturers into the system, I had to put a 0 for nutrients they don't provide (except cholesterol, fiber, fat, saturated fat, and sugar—all of which, when not available, I estimated using the best available parameters). It would be conjecture on my part to make estimates of other nutrients because they're highly variable from food to food and depend on food processing methods.

You, the reader, need to compare the numbers of brand-name foods separately from basic foods. In other words, you can't compare basic beans with pork to Campbell's beans with pork, although you can compare Campbell's beans with pork (2 Nutripoints) with Bush's beans with pork (1.5 Nutripoints) or Van Camp's vegetarian beans (3 Nutripoints).

In some cases, brand-name foods could exceed basic foods in Nutripoints because they're fortified. In most of those cases, you will see an asterisk next to the food in the chart that indicates fortification.

What about combination foods, such as lasagna, that have meat, a grain, and a vegetable in them—how did you determine which Nutrigroup to put them in?

You'll notice that I've categorized combination foods according to their major component, either by volume or calories, whichever made more sense. In the case of lasagna, it's in the grain Nutrigroup because the largest ingredient is pasta. I couldn't break down these combination foods because manufacturers provide data only for the entire dish, not the parts of the dish.

Does the Nutripoint formula take into account food additives and contaminants?

No, it doesn't. I would love to be able to do so, but there simply is no reliable, standardized way of measuring these elements in various foods. (For a fuller discussion of this subject, see pages 45-46).

How did you gather your data?

About half my information was from the Cooper Clinic Data Base, which is based on USDA information, for which millions of dollars went into research. I feel it's the most reliable data available. In their analyses they go as far as to indicate the number of samples they tested, and the range is usually from 10 to 200. That means for some bits of information—say, the amount of vitamin A in a carrot—they might have tested 200 carrots. In most cases, they've done enough to assure accuracy, but in an occasional case I found some margin for error. For example, in a few instances I found data that was based on only one sample. This single sample disagreed with data from either a manufacturer or from another source. In those cases, I went with common sense and used my own judgment to ascertain which data made the most sense. For each food, I've looked at from one to four sources to corroborate evidence.

With brand-name foods and fast foods I've had to rely on manufacturers. In most instances, manufacturers send out samples to reliable laboratories to get their nutritional data. In most cases, these manufacturers sent me copies of the reports as they came from the labs, or they gave the name of the lab or the research company. Some manufacturers don't have their foods analyzed and have no nutritional data whatsoever. Some manufacturers based nutritional information for their products on the USDA data for basic foods and extrapolated to arrive at their own "analyses." Whenever there was doubt, inaccuracy, or contradiction, I sifted through the available evidence to come up with what I believe is the most fair and accurate interpretation of the data.

Foods are constantly changing. How can you keep up with brand names and fast foods that come out after your list was compiled?

It's true that food formulations change constantly, but I am constantly adding to the 3,600+ foods, and I'd like to solicit manufacturers to send me information on their new foods, especially if they're formulating "light" or more healthful foods. We'd love to include such foods in new editions of *Nutripoints*. This is our

5th Edition of Nutripoints—we are constantly adding and deleting foods as the times change. I'd also like to think that with the advent of Nutripoints, manufacturers will have all the more reason to create more healthful foods. If consumers know which foods are better for them, surely it's an incentive to buy, and there's nothing like consumer pressure, or the pressure of the marketplace, to convince manufacturers to create more healthful formulations of foods.

Why are supplemental foods rated higher than natural foods? For example, I noticed that most of the cereals that are fortified have much higher scores than the natural, unfortified cereals. I thought you believed in getting vitamins naturally.

Yes, I do believe in getting vitamins naturally. That's why we have an asterisk next to a food that is significantly fortified. *Significantly fortified* means that 50 percent or more of the nutrition comes from fortification. In these cases, when foods are highly fortified, we have to take a look at the basic food that existed before the fortification. For example, Whole Wheat Total is basically a good food. Everything from the whole wheat is there, including the fiber and other basic nutrients. The fortification is added to something real. But if you look at Cap'n Crunchberries, you'll see a different story. In that case, there's no real basic food at all. You simply have to use common sense. If Cap'n Crunchberries is the only thing the kids will eat, you could do worse (although I do believe it's best to avoid such foods from the beginning so that kids don't get used to having them). A helpful way to judge a cereal that's highly fortified, and therefore high in Nutripoints, is to check the ingredients list on the box: if sugar is listed near the beginning of the ingredients, you'll know that the cereal is highly sweetened and, despite the fortification, not a good nutritional bet.

Is Whole Wheat Total at 64.5 Nutripoints better than Shredded Wheat at 5 Nutripoints? That's a toss-up. I think that Total might be considered marginally better because it does start with something good and adds vitamins to that basic food, but it's certainly not ten times better than Shredded Wheat, as the Nutripoint numbers might suggest. If you're looking at cost, it could well be that if you're following Nutripoints and thereby getting at least 100 percent of your RDA for all the vitamins and minerals, you're paying too much for Whole Wheat Total, which is charging you for vitamins you're already getting.

What about oysters and clams? I notice they're high on the list, but are they good food choices?

While it's true that oysters and clams are high on the list, you'll notice that they're marked with a double dagger (††) indicating caution. I had to grant them their high number of Nutripoints because that's how the system worked out. They're very high in certain minerals, including calcium, iron, zinc, phosphorus, and potassium, but I don't believe they're particularly good food choices because of the problems with shellfish contamination. Pollution of our coastal waters seems to be a sad fact of contemporary life, and shellfish, as bottom feeders, are more likely than other fish to become heavily contaminated. Moreover, when we eat shellfish, we eat the entire animal, not just a gutted fillet (which has had the liver and other repositories of many harmful pollutants removed). A recent publication from the National Centers for Disease Control pointed out that while certain diseases, including typhoid fever, hepatitis A, and cholera, have long been associated with shellfish ingestion, today we're finding that certain viruses are being transmitted by consuming them. As it's simply too difficult to monitor the harvesting and distribution of shellfish, I think that your best bet is to avoid eating shellfish, particularly raw shellfish.

What if someone doesn't have problems with cholesterol, high blood pressure, or weight control, but wants to get good nutrition? Your system has a built-in bias against cholesterol, sodium, sugar, and fat—but foods that are high in these elements can also be very nutritious, right?

Nutripoints rates the food, not the eater. Foods that are highly rated are the best available for the body, based on today's scientific research. We know that excess cholesterol, sodium, sugar, and fat are not good for the body. If you're lucky enough not to have a problem with any lifestyle diseases today, that, unfortunately, doesn't mean you won't be facing them tomorrow. A prudent diet is also *a preventive* diet. All people have an "excessive threshold" that seems to allow them to consume a certain amount of food that isn't good for them, but they then reach a point at which they're trying to *reverse* a problem such as high blood pressure, overweight, or diabetes. A prudent diet, one that follows Nutripoints, is going to protect you in the future, as well as make you feel good today.

Is Nutripoints for everyone?

Nutripoints is primarily for healthy adults. It's not designed for anyone under age eighteen who might need additional calcium and protein in his or her diet. Nutripoints is designed for people who are sedentary to moderately active, with no special medical problems that might involve diet. It's wise to check with your physician if you have any medical condition that might require special attention before you embark on the

Nutripoints program.

Can I follow Nutripoints if I have food allergies?

If you have any particular medical condition, you should consult with your doctor before beginning Nutripoints. A doctor or nutritionist could help you adapt Nutripoints to suit your particular condition.

Is there a Nutripoint program for kids or for people with special needs, such as pregnant women and athletes?

Not right now, although we're working on such a program and hope in the future to come up with various versions of Nutripoints that will accommodate people with special needs.

Can Nutripoints be used as a weight–loss program?

Nutripoints is designed as an optimal nutrition program for healthy adults. It can easily be adapted to be weight and fat-loss program by simply using the lower-calorie versions of the program (Levels I and II). Most people lose weight naturally using the system even when they are not trying to limit calories simply due to the healthier food choices it allows them to make—particularly if their diet was poor. It can also benefit those with diabetes, and people with hypertension or hyperlipidemia (high blood fats). It's best to work with a physician or dietitian in these cases to monitor your overall program, especially medications—which may need to be decreased or otherwise modified.

Why didn't someone think of Nutripoints before?

It took the happy marriage of computer technology and the latest nutritional data to produce Nutripoints. I have to assume that it wasn't done before because it never occurred to anyone that it *could* be done. Point systems that rate foods had been designed, but no one had developed a system that so exhaustively quantifies every element of a food, as well as putting that food into a total system that assures optimum nutrition. Certainly no nutrition plan has ever been offered that allows you complete freedom to choose, given only the limitations of the foods' Nutripoint scores.

Do you use the Nutripoint program yourself?

Of course! One of the reasons I developed the program is to help me reach my goal of living to be over 100. Because I am a nutritionist and a vegetarian, my diet was already pretty good to start: low in fat and high in fiber, vitamins and minerals. As I have done my research over the years and gotten more information on different foods, I've gradually been incorporating more and more high-Nutripoint foods into my diet. My personal diet survey revealed that I was getting between 150 and 200 Nutripoints daily and about 1,500 to 2,000 calories. Now, over time with Nutripoints, I'm getting between 200 and 300 Nutripoints daily, and I'm eating roughly the same number of calories.

Do you plan on creating a computer program to make it easier to compute daily running tallies of Nutripoints in each Nutrigroup?

Yes. We have already developed the *Planning and Tracking Software for Nutripoints* that you can use in your personal computer. If you're interested in this program, see the handy order form at the back of this book, or check our website at *www.Nutripoints.com*. The program has the following features:

- *Quick Lookup* feature for all 3600+ foods listed in Nutripoints. You can change the serving sizes and the right Nutripoint score is calculated for you.
- *Daily Diary, Charts and Graphs* display total scores, serving sizes and averages to track your Nutripoint progress.
- *Shopping List* feature helps you quickly incorporate your favorite high-Nutripoint foods into a convenient report.
- *Standard Meal* feature allows you to save time by entering your favorite groups of foods.
- *Meal Planner* helps you plan for the future and see how close you are to reaching your goals.

PART V

SPECIAL LISTS

TO MAKE NUTRIPOINTS EVEN MORE USEFUL, WE'VE CREATED SOME SPECIAL lists that highlight certain features of the system. They include:

- Top-Ten Nutripoint Foods
- Shopping Lists
- Bang-for-the-Buck Lists

TOP-TEN NUTRIPOINT FOODS

The following lists are a handy breakdown of the top ten foods in each of the Nutrigroups:

Vegetables
Turnip greens
Spinach
Bok choy
Mustard greens
Beet greens
Parsley
Broccoli
Watercress
Romaine lettuce
Dandelion greens

Fruits
Cantaloupe
Guava
Papaya
Strawberries
Black currants
Mango
Kiwi
Litchi
Mandarin oranges
Honeydew melon

***Grains* ***

Wheat bran
Wheat germ
Whole wheat crackers
Oat Bran/oat bran cereal
Rice Bran
Whole wheat pancakes
Quinoa
Oatmeal
Wild rice
Amaranth

*This list excludes fortified cereals.

Legumes

Bean sprouts
Green peas
Minestrone Soup
Navy beans
Green pigeon peas
Split Pea Soup
Lima beans
Black-eyed peas
Kidney beans
Vegetarian burger
Lentils

Milk/Dairy

Nonfat dry milk, prepared
Skim milk
Evaporated skim milk
Skim buttermilk
Nonfat plain yogurt
Lowfat 1-percent milk
Lowfat plain yogurt
Egg whites
Nonfat cottage cheese

Meat/Fish/Poultry
Tuna, baked or canned in water
Baked pike
Baked salmon
Baked halibut
Baked red snapper
Baked freshwater bass
Baked abalone
Baked swordfish
Quail without skin
Baked sole

NUTRIPOINT SHOPPING LISTS

Using Nutripoints well means shopping wisely. The food rating lists, both the Nutrigroup lists and the alphabetical lists, will be enormously helpful to you when you compare foods by type or by brand. But there are certain items we buy frequently, so I have provided lists comparing these by Nutripoints. This will save you searching through the lists to look for, say, the highest-rated spaghetti sauce. I think you'll find these lists enormously helpful, and I suggest that you draw up the same lists for food items you frequently buy, which I might not have included.

I have omitted from these lists items that have a dagger indicating cholesterol in the Nutrigroup and alphabetical lists, as I don't recommend you choose them. I have also omitted, for the same reason, items that fall below the recommended level for each Nutrigroup. I have also left out some generic foods because the point of these lists is to help people shop and compare, and in some cases the generic food ratings are meant more as a general reference. I've included some Nutripoint recipe foods where appropriate as a basis for comparison.

You'll also notice that I've only rated foods in the six major Nutrigroups and in the fat/oil group.

Vegetables

Frozen Vegetables	*Nutripoints*
Birds Eye spinach (whole leaf)	**57.0**
Birds Eye broccoli spears	**46.0**
Birds Eye cauliflower and red peppers	**41.5**
Whole Foods 365 Organic Chopped Spinach	**41.5**
Cascadian Farm Organic Broccoli	**39.0**
Pictsweet broccoli, carrots, and cauliflower	**36.0**
Green Giant broccoli, cauliflower, and carrots	**33.0**
Birds Eye baby carrots w/water chestnuts	**31.0**

Canned Vegetables	*Nutripoints*
Del Monte Early Garden spinach	**35.5**
Libby's mixed vegetables (natural pack)	**18.5**
Green Giant 50-percent Less Salt asparagus	**14.5**
Green Giant asparagus cuts	**14.0**
Green Giant mushrooms	**13.0**
Del Monte whole green beans	**13.0**
Green Giant 50-percent Less Salt green beans	**8.0**
Del Monte Golden Family-Style corn (no salt)	**6.0**
Green Giant Kitchen-Cut green beans	**4.5**
Green Giant whole kernel corn	**2.0**

Soups	*Nutripoints*
Nutripoint clear spinach	**23.5**
Health Valley no-salt vegetable	**13.0**
Health Valley vegetable	**12.5**
Health Valley no-salt tomato	**12.0**
Health Valley tomato	**11.5**
Health Valley chunky 5-bean vegetable	**11.0**
Progresso tomato w/vegetables	**6.5**
Pritikin vegetable	**6.5**
Campbell's chunky vegetable	**5.0**

Campbell's vegetarian vegetable	**4.5**
Campbell's minestrone	**3.5**

Spaghetti Sauce	*Nutripoints*
Pritikin	**9.5**
Aunt Millie's meatless	**4.0**
Prego no-salt	**4.0**
Aunt Millie's w/peppers and sausage	**3.5**
Ragu home-style w/ mushrooms	**3.0**

Fruits

Juices/Fruit Drinks	*Nutripoints*
Fuze White Tea fruit drink	**26.5**
V8 Diet Splash juice (all flavors)	**24.5**
Naked Juice Blue Machine juice	**22.5**
Kombucha Organic juice	**22.0**
SoBe Synergy Organic Elixir	**22.0**
ViaViente Nutritional drink	**22.0**
Fuze Green Tea fruit drink	**22.0**
Tropicana Light 'n Healthy orange juice	**22.0**
Fuze Replenish fruit drink	**18.0**
Minute Maid Light orange juice	**17.5**
Nutripoint Sunrise Cooler	**15.5**
Minute Maid Orange Juice w/C, E, Zinc	**15.0**
Fuze Refresh fruit drink	**15.0**
Slim-Fast Optima Smoothie	**15.0**
Nutripoint Strawberry Smoothie	**13.0**
Tropicana Healthy Heart orange juice	**13.0**
Naked Juice Just Apple juice	**13.0**
Naked Juice Red Machine	**13.0**
Tropicana Immunity Defense orange juice	**13.0**
Glaceau Stress-B Lemon-Lime vitamin water	**12.5**
Ocean Spray low-cal. Cranapple	**12.5**
Minute Maid Kids+ orange juice	**12.0**

Naked Juice Just Grapefruit juice	**12.0**
Tropicana Healthy Kids orange juice	**12.0**
V8 Splash Mango Peach juice	**11.5**
Fresh squeezed orange juice	**11.5**
Vruit Tropical Blend juice	**11.5**
Minute Maid Home Squeezed orange juice w/C, D	**11.5**
Naked Juice Just Fresh O-J juice	**11.5**
Minute Maid Heartwise orange juice	**11.5**
Minute Maid orange juice w/calcium)	**11.0**
Tropicana orange juice	**11.0**
Naked Juice Just O-J juice	**11.0**
Fuze Vitaboost fruit drink	**11.0**
Tropicana Low Acid orange juice	**11.0**
Naked Juice Green Machine juice	**11.0**
Minute Maid Tangerine juice	**11.0**
Unsweetened grapefruit juice	**11.0**
V8 Splash Tropical Blend juice	**11.0**
Snapple-A-Day Meal Replacement fruit drink	**11.0**
Citrus Hill orange juice (w/calcium)	**10.5**
Ocean Spray low-cal. cranberry	**10.5**
Minute Maid orange juice (frozen)	**10.0**
Fuze Focus fruit drink	**9.5**
V8 Splash Smoothies (all flavors)	**9.5**
Ocean Spray grapefruit juice	**8.0**
Ocean Spray cranberry juice cocktail	**7.0**
Fuze Lemon AID fruit drink	**6.5**
SoBe Elixir 3C fruit drink	**6.5**
Ocean Spray pink grapefruit juice	**6.0**
Welch's unsweetened grape juice (frozen)	**5.5**
SoBe Lean fruit drink	**5.5**
Dole pineapple juice	**5.0**
Fuze Energize fruit drink	**5.0**
Seneca apple juice (frozen)	**4.5**

Frozen Fruit	***Nutripoints***
Budget Gourmet apples glazed w/raspberry sauce	**10.5**
Birds Eye frozen strawberries (light syrup)	**8.5**
Birds Eye frozen strawberries (heavy syrup)	**5.0**

Dried Fruits	***Nutripoints***
Sun Maid dried apricots	**8.0**
Del Monte dried apricots	**7.5**
Sunsweet whole prunes	**6.0**
Sunsweet pitted bite-size prunes	**5.0**
Sun Maid dried peaches	**5.0**
Sun Maid mission figs	**4.5**
Sun Maid calimyrna figs	**4.0**
Sun Maid dried mixed fruits	**3.5**
Sun Maid dried fruit bits	**3.5**
Sun Maid zante currants	**3.5**
Sun Maid golden raisins	**3.0**

Grains

Breads	***Nutripoints***
Natural Ovens Bakery Hunger Filler bread	**10.5**
Natural Ovens Bakery Health Max bread	**6.5**
Wonder Hi-Fiber	**6.5**
The Sourdough whole wheat stone-ground	**6.0**
Roman Oat Bran and Honey Light	**5.5**
Fresh Horizons wheat	**5.0**
Pepperidge Farm whole wheat thin	**4.5**
Earth Grains wheat Lite 35	**4.5**
Roman Meal	**4.5**
Country Hearth stone-ground whole wheat	**4.5**
Wonder 100% whole wheat	**4.0**
Earth Grain honey wheatberry	**4.0**
Oroweat Bran'nola	**3.5**
Thomas' Protogen Protein	**3.5**

Earth Grain stone-ground wheat	**3.5**
Home Pride 100% whole wheat	**3.5**
Earth Grain salt-free sandwich	**3.5**
Arnold original Bran'nola	**3.5**
Arnold honey wheatberry	**3.5**
Earth Grains honey wheatberry	**3.5**
Roman Meal honey nut and oat bran	**3.5**
Oatmeal Goodness oatmeal and bran	**3.5**
Oatmeal Goodness oatmeal and sunflower seeds	**3.5**

Crackers	***Nutripoints***
High Fiber Ryvita	**9.0**
Wasa Crispbread (fiber plus)	**7.5**
Ralston Rykrisp	**5.0**
Wasa Golden Rye crispbread	**4.0**
Wasa Hearty Rye crispbread	**3.5**
Ryvita Dark Rye crispbread	**3.0**
Ralston Rykrisp seasoned	**3.0**

Prepared Pasta	***Nutripoints***
Nutripoint Angel Hair w/Sunshine Sauce	**10.0**
Nutripoint Fresh Pasta Salad	**4.5**
Green Giant Pasta Accents w/Cheddar	**4.0**
Green Giant Garden Gourmet Cheddar Rotini	**4.0**
Green Giant Pasta Accents w/Garlic	**3.5**
Morton spaghetti and meatballs frozen dinner	**3.5**

Unprepared Pasta	***Nutripoints***
Prince enriched macaroni and spaghetti	**4.0**
Buitoni Hi-Protein spinach linguine	**3.5**
Muellers macaroni (all types)	**3.5**
Prince Superoni	**3.0**
Buitoni linguine	**3.0**
Creamette Rainbow rotini	**3.0**

San Giorgio spaghetti	**3.0**
Celentano frozen cavatelli	**3.0**
Ronzoni spaghetti	**3.0**
No Yolks cholesterol-free egg noodles	**3.0**
Borden's Creamette spinach macaroni ribbons	**3.0**
San Giorgio linguine	**2.5**
Borden's Creamette elbow macaroni	**2.5**
Borden's Creamette spaghetti	**2.5**

Muffins	***Nutripoints***
Nutripoint Muffin	**10.5**
Whole wheat English muffin	**6.0**
Health Valley raisin oat bran muffin	**5.0**
English muffin w/raisins	**4.5**
Roman Meal English muffin	**4.5**
Pepperidge Farm English muffin	**4.0**
Nutripoint oat bran muffin	**3.5**
Arnold Extra Crisp muffin	**3.5**
Oroweat Health Nut English muffin	**3.0**
Thomas' regular English muffin	**2.5**
Arrowhead Mills oat bran wheat-free muffin	**2.5**
Thomas' honey wheat English muffin	**2.0**

Pancakes/Waffles	***Nutripoints***
Kashi Heart to Heart Honey Oat waffles	**15.5**
Aunt Jemima Whole Wheat pancakes	**8.5**
Aunt Jemima Lite Buttermilk pancakes	**8.0**
Aunt Jemima Buckwheat pancakes	**6.0**
Nutripoint Whole Wheat Orange pancake	**5.5**
Eggo Common Sense oat bran waffle (frozen)	**3.5**
Aunt Jemima Complete Buttermilk pancake mix	**3.5**
Aunt Jemima Original Complete pancake mix	**2.5**
Aunt Jemima blueberry waffles	**2.0**

Rice	*Nutripoints*
Wild rice (no salt)	**5.5**
Green Giant frozen wild rice w/sherry	**4.5**
Brown rice (no salt)	**4.0**
Spanish rice	**4.0**
Mahatma brown rice	**3.5**
Pritikin brown rice pilaf w/vegetables	**3.0**
Quaker Rice Cakes	**3.0**
White rice (no salt)	**3.0**
Minute Rice	**2.5**
Arrowhead Mills Quick brown rice	**2.5**
Uncle Ben's converted white rice	**2.5**
Mahatma long grain enriched rice	**2.0**
Carolina long grain enriched rice	**2.0**

Legumes/Nuts/Seeds

Soups	*Nutripoints*
Nutripoint French Market	**17.0**
Health Valley minestrone	**14.0**
Nutripoint lentil	**13.5**
Health Valley split pea	**10.0**
Health Valley lentil	**8.0**
Health Valley black bean	**7.5**
Nile Spice Foods lentil curry couscous	**6.5**
Wolfgang Puck's hearty lentil and vegetable	**6.0**
Imagine Foods creamy organic broccoli	**5.0**
Hain Natural split pea	**4.0**
Nutripoint Hot and Sour	**4.0**
Progresso minestrone	**4.0**
Alessi Lenticchie lentil (dry mix)	**3.0**
ZonePerfect beef lentil	**3.0**
Campbell's green pea	**2.5**
Progresso split green pea	**2.5**
Campbell's Chunky Old-Fashioned Beans 'n Ham	**2.0**

Milk/Dairy

Yogurt	*Nutripoints*
Yoplait Yogurt Drink, Nouriche Light (all flavors)	**10.5**
Dannon plain nonfat	**9.0**
Yoplait Yogurt Drink, Nouriche (all flavors)	**6.0**
Dannon plain low-fat	**5.5**
Yoplait Light yogurt (all flavors)	**5.5**
Dannon Light 'N Fit Smoothie yogurt	**5.5**
Dannon Light 'N Fit Creamy yogurt	**5.0**
Dannon Light 'N Fit yogurt	**4.5**
Weight Watchers nonfat peach	**4.5**
Columbo Fat-Free Light yogurt	**4.0**
Yoplait Ultra Low-Carb yogurt (all flavors)	**3.5**
Dannon Light 'N Fit Smoothie Carb Control	**3.0**
Dannon Light 'N Fit Carb Control yogurt	**3.0**
Dannon Natural Flavors yogurt	**2.5**
Dannon low-fat Fresh Flavors (all flavors)	**2.0**
Blue Bell frozen low-fat peaches and cream	**2.0**
Blue Bell frozen low-fat fruit (all flavors)	**2.0**
Borden low-fat Swiss Style Lite-Line plain	**1.5**
Dannon low-fat Fruit on Bottom (all flavors)	**1.0**
Dannon Dan'Up low-fat yogurt drink	**0.5**
Dannon low-fat with nuts, raisins, and fruit	**0.5**

Milk Drinks	*Nutripoints*
Spiru-Tein (w/skim milk)	**34.0**
Juice Plus+ Complete® (w/water)	**31.0**
MET-Rx White Box Protein Powder (w/water)	**23.0**
MET-Rx Total Nutrition Drink Powder (w/water)	**22.5**
Shake Mix, ZonePerfect	**22.5**
MET-Rx RTD-51	**18.5**
Smart Fuel Protein Anytime Mix	**17.5**
Slim-Fast Optima	**16.0**

Ready to Drink, ZonePerfect	**15.0**
Atkins Ready to Drink Shakes	**13.5**
Diet, Lite, Sego	**13.5**
Slim-Fast	**13.0**
Nestle Sweet Success	**13.0**
Soy Protein, Health Source	**12.5**
Glucerna	**12.5**
MET-Rx RTD-40	**12.0**
Ultra Slim-Fast	**11.5**
Balance 40-30-30 (mixed w/water)	**11.0**
Boost High Protein	**10.0**
Ensure Light	**9.5**
Ensure High Protein	**8.5**
MET-Rx Carb Count RTD	**8.0**
Ensure w/Fiber	**8.0**
Ensure	**8.0**
Carnation Instant Breakfast	**8.0**
Boost Breeze	**7.5**
Diet, Sego	**7.5**
Resource	**7.0**
Resource Plus	**6.5**
MET-Rx RTD Lite	**6.5**
MET-Rx Protein Plus Powder (w/water)	**6.0**
Muscle Milk, Cytomax	**6.0**
NutraStart	**5.5**
Sustical High Protein	**5.5**
Ensure Plus	**5.0**
Nutrament	**4.5**
Sustical Plus	**4.5**
Alba	**4.0**
Gatorade Nutrition Shake	**4.0**

Cheeses	*Nutripoints*
Formagg cheese substitute	**10.5**
Precious Ricotta Fat Free cheese	**5.5**
Dry cottage cheese	**5.5**
Nutripoint Honey Cream Cheese	**5.5**
Low-fat cottage cheese (1-percent)	**4.5**
Wendy's imitation Parmesan	**4.5**
Non-fat process American or Swiss cheese	**4.0**
Low-fat cottage cheese (2-percent)	**3.0**
Laughing Cow reduced-calorie	**2.5**
Cottage cheese	**1.5**
Wendy's imitation cheese	**1.5**
Weight Watchers low-fat cottage cheese	**1.5**
Borden sharp cheddar flavor	**1.0**
Low-fat ricotta	**0.5**
Low-fat mozzarella	**0.5**
Grated Parmesan	**0.5**
Kraft reduced-fat Swiss	**0.5**
Land O' Lakes skim mozzarella	**0.5**

Eggs	*Nutripoints*
Nutripoint Garden Scrambled Egg Beaters	**23.5**
Better 'n Eggs egg substitute	**23.5**
Fleischmann's Egg Beaters	**17.5**
Fleischmann's Egg Beaters Vegetable Omelette Mix	**13.5**
Weight Watchers Tofutti egg substitute	**10.0**
Scramblers egg substitute	**10.0**
Fleischmann's Egg Beaters w/Cheez	**6.0**
Egg white	**6.0**
Nutripoint Garden Scrambled Eggs	**5.5**
Second Nature egg substitute	**4.5**

Dinner Entrees	*Nutripoints*
Celentano cannelloni Florentine	5.5
Nutripoint Five-Cheese Casserole	5.5
Celentano manicotti (frozen)	2.0
Celentano stuffed shells (frozen)	2.0
Celentano broccoli-stuffed shells (frozen)	1.5
Le Menu stuffed three-cheese shells (frozen)	1.0
Weight Watchers baked cheese ravioli (frozen)	1.0
Patio cheese enchilada dinner (frozen)	1.0
Budget Gourmet cheese manicotti w/meat sauce	0.5
Le Menu three-cheese manicotti in tomato sauce	0.5
Budget Gourmet Slim cheese ravioli	0.5
Stouffer's Lean Cuisine cheese cannelloni	0.5
Weight Watchers frozen cheese manicotti	0.0

Seafood	*Nutripoints*
Nutripoint Scallop Kabob	16.5
Nutripoint Red Snapper Veracruz	13.5
Nutripoint Lettuce-Wrapped Salmon	10.5
Chicken of the Sea chunk-light low-sodium tuna in water	8.0
Pike (baked)	7.5
Salmon (steamed)	7.5
Halibut (baked)	7.5
Red snapper (baked)	7.0
Bumble Bee tuna, chunk-light, in water	7.0
Freshwater bass (baked)	7.0

Poultry preparations	*Nutripoints*
Nutripoint Chicken Stir-Fry	8.5
Nutripoint Chicken Salad	6.5
Quail (no skin)	6.0
Nutripoint Cajun Chicken Breast Sandwich	5.5
McDonald's chicken salad oriental	5.0
Nutripoint Chicken Enchiladas	5.0

Nutripoint Grilled Chicken w/Mango Sauce	4.5
Light meat turkey (baked, no skin)	4.5
Chicken breast (baked, no skin)	4.0
Chicken salad sandwich on whole wheat	4.0
Nutripoint Turkey Sandwich	4.0

Beef	*Nutripoints*
Nutripoint Beef Asada	7.0
Nutripoint Aerobics Hamburger	5.0
Chung King frozen beef teriyaki	5.0
Lean beef round steak (broiled)	4.0
Lean beef flank steak (broiled)	4.0
Lean beef top loin (broiled)	4.0
Lean beef tenderloin fillet (broiled)	3.5
Lean beef chuck roast (braised)	3.5
Lean hamburger (broiled)	3.0
Beef, macaroni, and tomato sauce	3.0
Beef jerky	2.5
Lean beef rib-eye steak (broiled)	2.5
Lean porterhouse steak (broiled)	2.5
Lean T-bone steak (broiled)	2.5

Tuna *	*Nutripoints*
Chick/Sea chunk-light, low-sodium, in water	8.0
Bumble Bee chunk-light, in water	7.0
Bumble Bee solid white, in water	6.5
Fresh broiled tuna	6.5
Chick/Sea chunk-light, in water	6.5
Chick/Sea chunk-light, in water and oil	6.0
Star Kist solid white, in water	6.0
Chick/Sea solid white, in water	5.5
Chick/Sea chunk-white diet albacore, low-sodium, water	5.0

***You can improve the points on almost any tuna by rinsing it in water to remove salt.**

Chick/Sea tonno solid light, in oil	4.0
Chick/Sea albacore solid white, in oil	4.0
Chick/Sea chunk-light, in oil	3.5

Soups	*Nutripoints*
Progresso Home Style chicken	5.5
Pritikin chicken w. ribbon pasta	4.5
Campbell's chunky beef	4.0
Campbell's turkey vegetable	2.5
Nile Spice Foods chicken vegetable couscous	2.0

Frozen Dinners	*Nutripoints*
Celentano frozen chicken primavera	6.0
Chung King beef teriyaki	5.0
Morton sliced beef	4.0
Morton frozen turkey dinner	4.0
Healthy Choice chicken oriental	3.5
Healthy Choice chicken Parmigiana	3.5
Healthy Choice sweet and sour chicken	3.0
Healthy Choice beef sirloin tips	3.0
Dining Lite chicken a la king	3.0
Chung King beef pepper oriental	3.0
Chung King frozen imperial chicken	3.0
Gorton's frozen ocean perch fillet	2.5

Fats/Oils

Spreads	*Nutripoints*
Smart Beat Squeeze margarine-like spread	1.0
Take Control Light margarine	0.0
Benecol Light margarine	0.0
Take Control margarine	-1.0
Weight Watchers reduced-calorie no-salt margarine	-2.0
Promise margarine	-2.0
Mrs. Filbert's family spread margarine	-2.0

Smart Balance Omega Plus w/Flax margarine	-2.5
Brummel & Brown margarine spread	-2.5
Hain safflower margarine	-2.5
Blue Bonnet reduced-calorie spread	-2.5
Mazola unsalted margarine	-2.5
Mazola Lite corn oil margarine	-2.5
Parkay soft diet margarine	-2.5
Kraft diet Touch of Butter spread	-2.5
Weight Watchers reduced-calorie margarine	-2.5
Fleischmann's diet margarine	-2.5

Dressings	*Nutripoints*
Nutripoint Lite Blue Cheese	8.0
Nutripoint Slim Guacamole Dip	7.5
Nutripoint Lite Ranch	3.5
Nutripoint Lite Orange Vinaigrette	2.5
Nutripoint Lite Caper Dressing	2.0
Nutripoint Lite Mayo Mix	1.5
Healthy Sensation non-fat dressing (all flavors)	0.0
Wish-Bone Lite Red French dressing	0.0
Kraft Free non-fat dressing (all flavors)	-0.5
Hidden Valley Take Heart non-fat dressing (all flavors)	-0.5
Wish-Bone Lite Italian dressing	-0.5
Nutripoint Lite Vinaigrette	-1.5
Kraft Catalina French	-2.0
Kraft French	-2.5

Sports Drinks/Snack Bars

Sports Drinks	*Nutripoints*
Motion Potion	24.5
Zing	13.5
AminoVital Fast Charge Sports Powder	8.5
GU Energy Gel	5.5
AminoVital Shake Mix	5.0

Accelerade Accel Sports Gel	**4.5**
Bodyfuel	**4.0**
Cytomax Energy and Recovery Drink	**3.5**
LowOz	**3.0**
Gatorade Energy Drink	**2.5**
Accelerade Powder Mix	**2.0**
AminoVital Ready to Drink	**1.5**
Exceed	**1.5**
Recharge	**1.0**
Endurox R4	**0.5**
Power Bar Sports Power Gel	**-1.5**
All Sport	**-2.0**
Lucozade	**-2.0**
Power Bar Recovery Drink	**-2.0**
Powerade	**-3.0**
Accelerade Ready to Drink	**-4.0**
Gatorade Endurance Hydration Formula	**-5.5**
Gatorade	**-6.5**

Snack Bars	***Nutripoints***
DrSoy Protein Bar	**34.5**
Pounds Off Bar	**29.5**
Clif Luna Bar	**28.5**
Pure Protein	**25.5**
Tiger's Sports Bar	**25.0**
Snickers Marathon	**23.5**
Energia	**23.0**
Power Bar, all flavors	**22.5**
Power Bar Pria	**21.0**
Power Bar Protein Plus, all flavors	**19.5**
Barbell Energy Bar	**18.5**
Power Bar Pria Carb Select	**16.5**
Bio-X Bar	**15.0**
ZonePerfect	**14.5**

PR Nutrition Bar	**14.0**
Breakthrough Honey Graham	**13.0**
Glucerna Meal Bar	**12.5**
MetaForm	**10.0**
Atkins Advantage Bar	**9.5**
Tiger's Milk	**9.0**
VO2 MAX	**9.0**
Balance Bar 40-30-30	**8.5**
Clif ZBar	**8.5**
Slim-Fast Optima Meal Bar	**8.5**
MET-Rx Big-100 Meal Replacement	**7.5**
Genisoy Xtreme	**7.0**
DrSoy Healthy Snacker Bar	**6.5**
Genisoy	**6.5**
Hershey's SmartZone	**6.5**
Think! Bar	**6.5**
FIBAR (all flavors)	**6.0**
MET-Rx Protein Plus	**6.0**
Nutra Blast	**6.0**
Promax Carb Conscious	**6.0**
Clif Bar	**5.5**
Clif Builder's Bar	**5.5**
Promax	**5.5**
South Beach Diet Meal Bar	**5.5**
Slim-Fast Optima snack bar	**5.0**
Ensure	**4.5**
SnackWells	**4.5**
Nutri-Grain, Kellogg's (all flavors)	**3.5**
GOLEAN Crunchy, Kashi	**3.0**
Melaleuca Fruit & Fiber Bar	**2.5**
Melaleuca Access Activity bar	**-1.0**
GOLEAN, Kashi	**-2.0**

A NUTRIENT BANG FOR THE BUCK

The lists that follow give you a way of stretching your food dollars by listing foods that are extremely high in nutrients while low in cost. We figured out the "Nutripoints per dollar" for each food and list the highest foods in each Nutrigroup here. The cost was based on the average price in local markets: some foods, particularly fruits and vegetables, may differ in cost in your area. They will, of course, be cheaper when in season.

Vegetables
Bok choy
Turnip greens
Cabbage
Parsley
Broccoli
Birds Eye whole leaf spinach
Mustard greens
Brussels sprouts
Cauliflower
Romaine lettuce
Raw spinach
Asparagus
Birds Eye broccoli, carrots, and red peppers (frozen)
Watercress
Red peppers

Fruits
Cantaloupe
Watermelon
Mandarin oranges (canned)
Orange juice
Orange
Kiwi fruit
Plums (canned, unsweetened)
Peach (fresh)
Honeydew melon
Papaya
Nectarine (fresh)
Grapefruit

Strawberries (fresh)
Casaba melon
Apricots (dry)
Apricot (fresh)
Mango
Guava

Grains

All Bran, Extra Fiber
Whole Wheat Total
Total Corn Flakes
Total Oatmeal
Product 19
Just Right
Just Right w/Fruit and Nuts
Fiber One
100% Bran
Bran Buds
Total Raisin Bran
All Bran
Kretschmer Toasted Wheat Bran
40+ Bran Flakes Fruitful Bran
Kellogg's Corn Flakes
Post Natural Bran
Grape-Nuts
Honey Buc Wheat Crisp

Legumes/Nuts/Seeds

Split peas
Mung bean sprouts
Arrowhead Mills dry soybeans
Navy beans
Pinto beans
Garbanzo beans
Baked beans w/tomato sauce
Kidney beans
Lentils
Peas (frozen)
Black-eyed peas (canned)

Birds Eye frozen peas
Health Valley split pea soup
Tofu
Health Valley minestrone soup
Health Valley black bean soup

Milk/Dairy

Carnation instant nonfat dry milk
Evaporated skim milk
Fleischmann's Egg Beaters
Carnation Instant Breakfast (no sugar)
Nonfat yogurt
Diet Sego
Egg white
Fleischmann's Egg Beaters w/Cheez

Meat/Fish/Poultry

Chick/Sea chunk-light tuna, in spring water
Salmon
Halibut
Raw oysters
Raw clams
Red snapper
Swordfish
Flank steak
Fresh tuna

PART VI

NUTRIPOINT MENUS AND RECIPES

THIS IS THE PART OF NUTRIPOINTS THAT'S DESIGNED TO GET YOU INTO THE kitchen. You'll find sample menus that cover fourteen days. For all the menu items that are identified by "Nutripoint"—for example, Nutripoint Grilled Cajun Chicken Breast or Nutripoint Caper Dressing—you'll find recipes in the recipe section. The page number following each dish on the menu refers to the page where the recipe appears.

The menus really serve two purposes. They're meant to be *used.* If you're the type of person who likes to have things spelled out, who likes to shop in advance and plan ahead, you'll love the menus because they'll answer all your questions about what you should be eating on Nutripoints.

The menus are also meant to serve as inspiration. You might want to mix and match various foods on different days. As long as you stick with the correct number of servings for each Nutrigroup, this is fine.

Kathleen S. Duran, R.D., the Director of Nutrition for the Aerobics Center Cooper Wellness Programs, developed our recipes. In developing the menus and recipes, we focused on taste, variety, and practicality. These menus and recipes are ones that we've used with great success with participants of the Residential Wellness Programs. As you'll see, the recipes taste great! We've received countless compliments on them from people who asked for recipe printouts to bring home. While aiming for high Nutripoint scores, we also kept in mind that a food not widely available or terribly expensive is not a good choice. We tried to use foods that are readily available in your supermarket, and we tried to make the recipes simple and easy to follow. Our goal was an eating program that would be high in Nutripoints, satisfying, tasty, and easy to live with.

As for Nutripoint scores, you can think of the two-week sample menus as a standard, optimum diet. The Nutripoint totals for each day range from 200 to 300 points for a 1,000 to 1,200 calorie diet. It's possible to get even higher scores than this, but, as I've said, we were concerned with practicality, and we wanted a meal plan that was easy and fun as well as nutritious. We analyzed the nutrients in Day 1 of the menus just to give you an idea of how the numbers might work out on a typical Nutripoint menu. You can see that they're well within the guidelines for an optimum diet.

If you need to increase your calorie level from the basic level of the menus and recipes, please refer to page 118 of Part IV for information on how to do this. The simplest way is to increase the serving sizes or to have additional portions of the suggested foods.

You may notice that we strayed from the serving recommendations in some cases, and you'll find it instructive to learn why because it may affect the way you use Nutripoints in your daily life.

We used a legume serving about half the time in place of a meat serving. We found that most people find it much easier to adapt to Nutripoints when they begin with roughly half the legumes in their diet that we ultimately recommend.

In some cases we used a grain entree with some low-fat cheese for protein instead of a meat or legume serving. On Day 6, for example, we have a grain serving (Nutripoint Spinach Lasagna) at lunch and omit a legume serving. Because the high-quality protein in the Nutripoint Red Snapper Veracruz more than satisfies our protein requirements, we went for additional complex carbohydrates in place of the legume serving. You might want to do this once or twice in the course of a two-week program. On Day 7 we skipped a grain serving because of the rice in the Nutripoint Herbed Lentils and Wild Rice casserole.

On some days we might skip a serving of vegetables if there is a good quantity of vegetables in another dish. On Day 4, for example, we skipped the vegetable at lunch because of the vegetables in the Nutripoint Chicken Stir-Fry. By making such substitutions, you'll find Nutripoints very easy to live with.

You'll notice that we used skim milk every day. You can use 1-percent or 2-percent milk if you prefer, but you should avoid whole milk entirely: it simply has too much fat.

You can mix and match recipes. For example, the Nutripoint Blackberry Freeze can be used along with the Nutripoint Banana Gladje. Some people find the Blackberry Freeze too strong on its own, but just delightful with the Banana Gladje.

I hope you'll be creative with your own combinations of Nutripoint foods. I'd welcome any recipes that you might care to share with me. I'd like to use any especially good ones, with proper credit of course, in future editions of this and other Nutripoint books.

NUTRIPOINT MENUS

NUTRIPOINT 1,000-1,200 CALORIE MENU								
Day: 1	Nutripoints							
Food Selection/Serving Size	Veg.	Fruit	Grain	Leg.	Meat	Milk	Other	
Breakfast:								
Whole Wheat Total cereal, 1 cup			64.5					
Skim milk, 1 cup						9.5		
Cantaloupe melon, ¼ melon		29						
Lunch:								
Nutripoint Cajun Chicken Breast Sandwich, 3 oz.					5.5			
Tomato, ¼ tomato	7.5							
Loose-leaf lettuce, 1 leaf	3							
Whole wheat bun, 1 bun			6					
Nutripoint Spinach Salad, 2 cups	65							
Nutripoint Lite Zero Dressing, 2 Tbls							1	
V-8 Spicy Vegetable Juice, 6 oz.	26							
Fresh orange, 1 whole		13.5						
No-calorie beverage							0	
Dinner:								
Nutripoint French Market Soup, 1 cup				17				
Nutripoint Tossed Salad, 2 cups	51.5							
Nutripoint Lite Caper Dressing, 2 Tbls.							2	
Lowfat (2%) cottage cheese, ½ cup						3		
Nutripoint Fresh Fruit Platter, ½ cup		17						
No-calorie beverage							0	
Totals:	153	59.5	70.5	17	5.5	12.5	3	321
Goals:	55	15	10	5	5	10	0	100

Nutrient Analysis: Nutripoint 1,000-1,200 Calorie Menu, Day 1

Nutrient	
Calories	1,214.0 cal
Protein	89.0 gm
Total fat	17.0 gm
Saturated fat	2.5 gm
Cholesterol (dietary)	99.0 mg
Complex carbohydrates	176.0 gm
Sugar	3.0 gm
Alcohol	0.10 gm
Fiber (dietary)	33.0 gm
Calcium	1,090.0 mg
Phosphorus	1,292.0 mg
Magnesium	452.0 mg
Sodium	1,988.0 mg
Potassium	4,508.0 mg
Zinc	25.0 mg
Iron	36.0 mg
Vitamin A	27,284.0 IU
Thiamin (B_1)	7.3 mg
Riboflavin (B_2)	3.7 mg
Niacin (B_3)	43.0 mg
Pyridoxine (B_6)	3.9 mg
Pantothenic acid	16.3 mg
Folic acid	1,676.0 mcg
Vitamin B_{12}	8.2 mcg
Vitamin C	429.0 mg
Caffeine	0.0 mg

Calorie Sources

Sources	*Percentage*
Protein	29
Fat	12
Complex carbohydrates (fruits, vegs., starches)	59
Simple carbohydrates (sugar)	0
Alcohol	0

NUTRIPOINT 1,000–1,200 CALORIE MENU								
Day: 2	Nutripoints							
Food Selection/Serving Size	Veg.	Fruit	Grain	Leg.	Meat	Milk	Other	
Breakfast:								
Nutripoint Fruited Cinnamon Cereal, 1 cup			5					
Skim milk, 1 cup						9.5		
Fresh blueberries, ½ cup		7						
Lunch:								
Nutripoint Beef Asada, 1 serving					7			
Nutripoint Tossed Salad, 2 cups	51.5							
Nutripoint Lite Ranch Dressing, 2 Tbls.							2	
Nutripoint Fresh Fruit Slices, 1 cup		23.5						
No-calorie beverage							0	
Dinner:								
Nutripoint Crunchy Fish, 3 oz.					6.5			
Nutripoint Vegetable Medley, 1 cup	48.5							
Nutripoint Spinach Salad, 2 cups	65							
Nutripoint Lite 16-Island Dressing, 2 Tbls.								
Nutripoint Wild Rice Soup, 1 cup			10.5					
Skim milk, 1 cup						9.5		
Nutripoint Blackberry Freeze, ¾ cup		8.5						
Totals:	165	39	15.5	0	13.5	19	3	255
Goals:	55	15	10	5	5	10	0	100

NUTRIPOINT L000-1,200 CALORIE MENU								
Day: 3	Nutripoints							
Food Selection/Serving Size	Veg.	Fruit	Grain	Leg.	Meat	Milk	Other	
Breakfast:								
Eggo Common Sense Oat Bran Waffles, 1½ waffles			3.5					
Dannon Lowfat Yogurt, 1 cup						5.5		
Nutripoint Hot Peach Topping, ½ cup		7						
Lunch:								
Nutripoint Lettuce-Wrapped Salmon w/Herb Sauce, 4 oz.					10.5			
Nutripoint Salad Greens with Balsamic Vinegar, 2 cups	42							
w/mushrooms (⅓ cup)								
w/tomato (⅓ pc.)								
w/carrots (⅓ pc.)	33							
Nutripoint Fresh Pasta Salad, ½ cup			4.5					
Nutripoint Banana Gladje, ⅓ cup		6						
No-calorie beverage							0	
Dinner:								
Nutripoint South-of-the-Border Vegetarian Chili, ¾ cup				13				
Nutripoint Tossed Salad, 2 cups	51.5							
w/broccoli (½ cup) and cauliflower (½ cup)	41							
Nutripoint Lite Ranch Dressing, 2 Tbls.							2	
Skim milk, 1 cup						9.5		
Nutripoint Rainbow Compote, ½ cup		18						
Totals:	167.5	31	8	13	10.5	15	2	247
Goals:	55	15	10	5	5	10	0	100

NUTRIPOINT 1,000-1,200 CALORIE MENU								
Day: 4	Nutripoints							
Food Selection/Serving Size	Veg.	Fruit	Grain	Leg.	Meat	Milk	Other	
Breakfast:								
Nutripoint Bran Muffin, 1 muffin			10.5					
Nutripoint Garden Scrambled Egg or with Egg Beaters egg, ¾ cup						5.5/ 23.5		
Fresh grapefruit, ½ fruit		13						
Lunch:								
Nutripoint Chicken Stir-Fry, 1 cup					8.5			
Nutripoint Tossed Salad, 2 cups	51.5							
Nutripoint Hot and Sour Soup, ½ cup				2				
Fresh sliced pineapple, ½ cup		8						
No-calorie beverage							0	
Dinner:								
Nutripoint Venison w/Juniper Berry Sauce, 6 oz.					6.5			
Nutripoint Spinach Salad, 2 cups	65							
Nutripoint Lite Orange Vinaigrette Dressing, 2 tbs.							2.5	
Cooked broccoli flowerettes w/Butter Buds	38.5							
Orzo pasta, 1 cup			5					
Skim milk, 1 cup						9.5		
Nutripoint Poached Pears, ½ pear		4						
Totals:	155	25	15.5	2	15	15/ 33	2.5	230/ 248
Goals:	55	15	10	5	5	10	0	100

NUTRIPOINT 1,000-1,200 CALORIE MENU								
Day: 5	**Nutripoints**							
Food Selection/Serving Size	**Veg.**	**Fruit**	**Grain**	**Leg.**	**Meat**	**Milk**	**Other**	
Breakfast:								
Product 19 cereal, 1 cup			56					
Skim milk, 1 cup						9.5		
Banana, ½		7.5						
Lunch:								
Health Valley 5-Bean Minestrone Soup, 1½ cups				14				
Ryvita High Fiber Crackers, 2 pcs.			2					
Wasa Fiber Plus Crackers, 2 pcs.			5					
Nutripoint Tossed Salad, 2 cups	51.5							
w/green peppers, alfalfa sprouts, red cabbage	28							
Nutripoint Lite Ranch Dressing, 2 tbs.							2	
Nutripoint Sunrise Cooler, ½ cup		15.5						
Dinner:								
Nutripoint Chicken Salad, ¾ cup (on a bed of lettuce)					6.5			
Nutripoint Tossed Salad, 2 cups	51.5							
Nutripoint Lite Orange Vinaigrette Dressing, 2 tbs.							2.5	
Carrot sticks, 1 med. Carrot	35.5							
Plain, lowfat yogurt, ½ cup						3.5		
Nutripoint Fresh Fruit Platter, 1 cup		34						
Totals:	166.5	57	63	14	6.5	13	4.5	322.5
Goals:	55	15	10	5	5	10	0	100

NUTRIPOINT 1,000-1,200 CALORIE MENU								
Day: 6	Nutripoints							
Food Selection/Serving Size	Veg.	Fruit	Grain	Leg.	Meat	Milk	Other	
Breakfast:								
Nutripoint Whole Grain Pancakes, 4 pcs.			5.5					
Skim milk, 1 cup						9.5		
Nutripoint Hot Blueberry Topping, ½ cup		2.5						
or Nutripoint Hot Red Raspberry Topping, ½ cup		9						
Lunch:								
Nutripoint Spinach Lasagna, 1 cup			10					
Nutripoint Vegetable Medley w/Butter Buds, 1 cup	48.5 51.5						-1.5	
Nutripoint Tossed Salad, 2 cups								
Nutripoint Lite Vinaigrette Dressing, 2 tbs.								
Nutripoint Strawberry Smoothie, 1 cup		13						
Dinner:								
Nutripoint Red Snapper Veracruz, 3 oz.					13.5			
Nutripoint Spinach Salad, 2 cups	65							
Nutripoint Lite Caper Dressing, 2 Tbls.							2	
Cooked peas and carrots, ½ cup	28							
Skim milk, 1 cup						9.5		
Peach Vitari Soft Serve, ½ cup		6.5						
Totals:	193	22/ 28.5	15.5	0	13.5	19	.5	263.5 /270
Goals:	55	15	10	5	5	10	0	100

NUTRIPOINT 1,000-1,200 CALORIE MENU								
Day: 7	Nutripoints							
Food Selection/Serving Size	Veg.	Fruit	Grain	Leg.	Meat	Milk	Other	
Breakfast:								
Whole Wheat Bagel			4					
Nutripoint Honey Cream Cheese, ¼ cup						5.5		
Skewer of fresh fruit, 1 cup (pineapple, cantaloupe, strawberries)		52						
Lunch:								
Nutripoint Herbed Lentils and Wild Rice, 1 cup				6.5				
Baked potato with Nutripoint New Way Sour Cream, ¼ cup	17					6.5		
Nutripoint Tossed Salad, 1 cup	26							
Nutripoint Lite Ranch Dressing, 2 Tbls.							2	
Natural Fruit-flav. no-cal Soda, 12 oz.							0	
Dinner:								
Nutripoint Grilled Chicken w/Mango Sauce, 4 oz.					4.5			
Nutripoint Vegetable Medley, 1 cup	48.5							
Nutripoint Tossed Salad, 1 cup w/Balsamic vinegar, 1 Tbls.	26						0	
Fresh strawberries, 1 cup		19						
No-calorie beverage							0	
Totals:	117.5	71	4	6.5	4.5	12	2	217.5
Goals:	55	15	10	5	5	10	0	100

NUTRIPOINT 1,000–1,200 CALORIE MENU								
Day: 8	Nutripoints							
Food Selection/Serving Size	Veg.	Fruit	Grain	Leg.	Meat	Milk	Other	
Breakfast:								
40+ Bran Flakes, ¾ cup			21					
Skim milk, 1 cup						9.5		
Fresh-squeezed orange juice, 6 oz.		11.5						
Lunch:								
Nutripoint Aerobics Burger					5			
Whole wheat bun			6					
Nutripoint Tossed Salad, 2 cups	51.5							
Nutripoint Lite Blue Cheese Dressing, 2 Tbls.							4	
V-8 juice, no salt, 6 oz. (w/lemon)	28.5							
Nutripoint Fruit Salad Plate, 1 cup		28.5						
Dinner:								
Nutripoint Grilled Salmon w/Yellow Bell Pepper Sauce, 4 oz.					7			
Nutripoint Marinated Asparagus, 8 pcs.	38.5							
Nutripoint Spinach Salad, 2 cups	65							
Nutripoint Lite Orange Vinaigrette Dressing, 2 tbs.							2.5	
Nutripoint Key Lime Mousse, ½ cup						5.5		
Totals:	183.5	40	27	0	12	15	6.5	284
Goals:	55	15	10	5	5	10	0	100

NUTRIPOINT 1,000—1,200 CALORIE MENU								
Day: 9	Nutripoints							
Food Selection/Serving Size	**Veg.**	**Fruit**	**Grain**	**Leg.**	**Meat**	**Milk**	**Other**	
Breakfast:								
Instant Total Oatmeal w/skim milk, ½ cup			51					
Hot Kashi cereal (pilaf), ¼ cup			3					
Skim milk, 1 cup						9.5		
Raisins, ¼ cup		4						
Lunch:								
Nutripoint Chicken Enchiladas, 2 pcs.					5			
Cooked frozen corn, ½ cup	8							
Nutripoint Tossed Salad, 2 cups	51.5							
w/fresh red peppers (½ pc.) and fresh green peppers (½ pc.)	20							
Nutripoint Lite Ranch Dressing, 2 Tbls.							2	
Fresh fruit salad, ½ cup		13						
Dinner:								
Nutripoint French Bread Pizza, 1 pc.			6					
Nutripoint Coleslaw, ¾ cup	15							
Skim milk, 1 cup						9.5		
Mandarin orange in juice, ½ cup		15.5						
Totals:	94.5	32.5	60	0	5	19	2	213
Goals:	55	15	10	5	5	10	0	100

NUTRIPOINT 1,000–1,200 CALORIE MENU								
Day: 10	Nutripoints							
Food Selection/Serving Size	Veg.	Fruit	Grain	Leg.	Meat	Milk	Other	
Breakfast:								
Just Right cereal w/fruit/nuts, ¾ cup			36.5					
Skim milk, 1 cup						9.5		
Fresh raspberries, ½ cup		12.5						
Lunch:								
Nutripoint Tuna Salad, ½ cup					5			
Raw vegetables: Carrots (1 pc.)	35.5							
Celery (2 pcs.)	7							
Radishes (1/3 cup)	10							
Whole wheat bread, 2 pcs.			6					
Fresh apple (½ pc.)		2						
Orange slices (½ pc.)		7						
Dinner:								
Nutripoint Lentil Soup, 1 cup				13.5				
RyKrisp crackers, 2 pcs.			2					
Nutripoint Spinach Salad, 2 cups	65							
Nutripoint Lite Ranch Dressing, 2 tbs.							2	
Raw cauliflower, 1 cup	40.5							
Low-fat (2%) cottage cheese, ½ cup						3		
Fresh papaya, ½ pc.		20.5						
Totals:	158	29.5	44.5	13.5	5	12.5	2	265
Goals:	55	15	10	5	5	10	0	100

NUTRIPOINT 1,000-1,200 CALORIE MENU								
Day: 11	Nutripoints							
Food Selection/Serving Size	Veg.	Fruit	Grain	Leg.	Meat	Milk	Other	
Breakfast:								
Quaker Puffed Wheat, ½ cup			3					
Kretschmer Honey Wheat Germ, ¼ cup			8					
Skim milk. 1 cup						9.5		
Nutripoint Fresh Fruit Slices, 1 cup		23.5						
Lunch:								
Nutripoint Jambalaya, 1 cup			7.5					
Cooked kidney beans, ½ cup (mix with Jambalaya)				8.5				
Nutripoint Tossed Salad, 2 cups	51.5							
Nutripoint Lite Vinaigrette Dressing, 2 tbs.							-1.5	
Cooked okra. ½ cup	31							
Sliced tomatoes, ¼ pc.	7.5							
Orange Passion Juice, 6 oz.		9.0						
Dinner:								
Pan-fried bass (Pam w/olive oil) w/lemon					7			
Nutripoint Home-Style Potatoes, ½ cup	5.5							
Nutripoint Tossed Salad, 1½ cups w/cooked green beans, ½ cup	45							
Nutripoint Lite Orange Vinaigrette Dressing, 2 tbs.							2.5	
Dannon low-fat yogurt w/vanilla and sweetener to taste, 1 cup						5.5		
Fresh apricot pieces (added to yogurt), 3 pcs.		13.5						
Totals:	140.5	42	18.5	8.5	7	15	1	232.5
Goals:	55	15	10	5	5	10	0	100

NUTRIPOINT 1,000-1,200 CALORIE MENU								
Day: 12	Nutripoints							
Food Selection/Serving Size	Veg.	Fruit	Grain	Leg.	Meat	Milk	Other	
Breakfast:								
Whole wheat English muffin, 1 pc.			5.5					
Laughing Cow Reduced-Calorie Cheese, 2 pcs.						2.5		
Sliced fresh nectarine, 1 pc.		10						
Hot herb tea, 1 cup							.5	
Lunch:								
Nutripoint Marinated Hawaiian Chicken, 4 oz.					3.5			
Nutripoint Potato Salad, ½ cup	9							
Nutripoint Cold Mixed-Vegetable Salad, ½ cup	17							
Fresh mango slices, ½ pc.		17.5						
No-calorie beverage							0	
Dinner:								
Nutripoint Scallop Kabobs w/Scallop Sauce, 2 pcs.					16.5			
Wild rice pilaf, ½ cup			6.5					
Tomato slices, ½ tomato	15							
Nutripoint Spinach Salad, 2 cups	65							
Nutripoint Lite Orange Vinaigrette Dressing, 2 tbs.							2.5	
Skim milk, 1 cup						9.5		
Sugar-Free Cherry Jell-O Gelatin (w/canned peaches), ½ cup		10.5						
Totals:	106	38	12	0	20	12	3	191
Goals:	55	15	10	5	5	10	0	100

NUTRIPOINT 1,000-1,200 CALORIE MENU								
Day: 13	Nutripoints							
Food Selection/Serving Size	Veg.	Fruit	Grain	Leg.	Meat	Milk	Other	
Breakfast:								
Nutripoint Oat Bran Muffin, 1 pc.			3.5					
Egg Beaters eggs w. Cheez, ½ cup						6		
Fresh kiwi slices, 1 kiwi		17						
Lunch:								
Nutripoint Navy Bean Soup, 1 cup French Market recipe w/navy beans				17				
Nutripoint Spinach Salad, 2 cups	65							
Nutripoint Lite Vinaigrette Dressing, 2 tbs.							-1.5	
Honeydew and cantaloupe melon slices, 1 cup		21.5						
No-calorie beverage							0	
Dinner:								
Nutripoint Chicken Primavera (Tyson's Diced Chicken Meat, 3 oz., and Nutripoint Fresh Pasta Salad, 1 cup)			9		4			
Nutripoint Tossed Salad, 2 cups	51.5							
Nutripoint Blue Cheese Dressing, 2 Tbls.							4	
Skim milk, 1 cup						9.5		
Fresh watermelon chunks, 1 cup		10.5						
Totals:	116.5	49	12.5	17	4	15.5	2.5	217
Goals:	55	15	10	5	5	10	0	100

NUTRIPOINT 1,000—1.200 CALORIE MENU								
Day: 14	Nutripoints							
Food Selection/Serving Size	Veg.	Fruit	Grain	Leg.	Meat	Milk	Other	
Breakfast:								
Shredded Wheat 'n Bran cereal, 2/3 cup			6					
Skim milk, 1 cup						9.5		
Fresh peach slices, 1 peach		11						
Lunch:								
Nutripoint Angel Hair Pasta w/Sunshine Sauce, 1½ cups			4.5					
Nutripoint Tossed Salad, 2 cups	51.5							
w/bean sprouts, 1 cup				9				
w/fresh peas, ¼ cup				3.5				
w/garbanzo beans (¼ cup)				2				
Nutripoint Lite Orange Vinaigrette Dressing, 2 Tbls.							2.5	
Nutripoint Rainbow Compote, ½ cup		18						
w/Nutripoint Banana Mint Sauce, 2 Tbls.						3		
Dinner:								
Baked sole w/lemon/Butter Buds, 6 oz.					6			
Baby Brussels sprouts, ½ cup	25							
Nutripoint Spinach Salad, 2 cups	65							
Nutripoint Lite Ranch Dressing, 2 Tbls.							2	
Nutripoint Bananas Flambé, 1/3 cup						2.5		
Totals:	141.5	29	10.5	14.5	6	15	4.5	221
Goals:	55	15	10	5	5	10	0	100

NUTRIPOINT RECIPES

MODIFYING YOUR FAVORITE RECIPES

Many of us have favorite recipes that we continue to make, even though we know they've got too much fat in them. But they're so good! And the family loves them! And you grew up having them every week, so they bring back memories. The excuses are endless.

We'd like you to pick out four favorite recipes and try modifying them to cut the fat *down,* not *out.* We all know general tips, such as bake, don't fry; use lemon juice and herbs instead of fat for seasoning; replace high-fat dairy products with low-fat ones; choose lean cuts of meat, well trimmed. These aren't new ideas, but sometimes it's hard to translate them into practical reality. Look at the two sample recipes on pages 204 and 205 to see how we do it—then work on some of your own. The text that appears in boldface represents a modification.

• Five-Cheese Casserole •

½ pound **lean** ground beef* } (vs. hamburger)
½ pound ground turkey }
1 onion, chopped
15 ounces tomato sauce
¾ teaspoon each dried basil and oregano
¼ teaspoon salt
½ cup **1-percent fat cottage cheese** (vs. 4%)
2 ounces **light cream cheese** (vs. regular: saves half the fat)
¼ cup **light sour cream** (vs. regular: saves half the fat)
½ cup **plain lowfat yogurt** (vs. sour cream)
1 tablespoon Parmesan cheese
8 ounces noodles, cooked
½ **cup** grated **part-skim mozzarella** cheese (vs. Swiss)
¼ **cup** grated **sharp cheddar** cheese (vs. ½ cup mild Cheddar: sharp is more flavorful, so less can be used)

DIRECTIONS Preheat oven to 350°F. Cook meat in **non-stick skillet** until browned (no fat needed for browning). **Pour off any excess fat and rinse meat with warm water.** Add onion and cook for 5 minutes. Stir in tomato sauce and seasonings. In a separate bowl blend together cottage cheese, cream cheese, sour cream, yogurt, and Parmesan cheese. Spray a 9 X 13-inch baking dish with **no-stick vegetable oil cooking spray** (instead of regular oil). Layer the baking dish with half the noodles, half the meat sauce, and all of the cheese mixture. Repeat with the rest of the noodles and sauce. Top with mozzarella and cheddar cheeses. Bake 30 minutes.

This recipe yields six very large servings. Before making our modifications, each serving contained 470 calories and 30 grams of fat. With our changes, each serving now has 317 calories and 10 grams of fat. It's amazing what a little creativity can do. Note that we didn't "save" by cutting down the total amount of food, but by making lower-calorie substitutions. And we didn't remove the things that make it wonderful, such as the bubbling cheese on top. Remember, healthy eating can also taste good.

SERVES: 6 SERVING SIZE: 1 heaping cup 5.5 Nutripoints

* Try adding broccoli or any other vegetable to increase portion size and decrease calories (broccoli has only 25 calories per half cup).

• Bran Muffins •

1 ½ cups **Whole Wheat Total** (or any other bran cereal)
1 ½ cup **orange juice** (vs. ½ cup apple juice), boiling
4 **egg whites** (vs. 3 eggs)
½ cup ½ -percent-fat buttermilk
4 ounces **orange juice concentrate** (vs. 4 ounces apple juice concentrate)
3 tablespoons safflower oil } (vs. ½ cup safflower oil)
1 large ripe **banana,** mashed }
½ cup **currants** (vs. ½ cup raisins)
2 **tablespoons** honey, brown sugar, or molasses (vs. ¾ cup)
½ teaspoon vanilla extract
1 cup **whole wheat flour** } (vs. 1 ½ cups white flour)
½ cup white flour }
1 ½ teaspoons baking soda
2 teaspoons baking powder
¾ teaspoon ground cinnamon
¾ teaspoon ground nutmeg
Zest of 1 orange, chopped fine

DIRECTIONS Preheat oven to 400°F. Combine Total in a large bowl with boiling orange juice. Let cool. Add the egg whites, milk, orange juice concentrate, oil, banana, currants, honey, and vanilla. Mix well. In a small bowl, combine flours, baking soda, baking powder, and spices. Add to wet mixture and mix very well.* Spray a 12-cup muffin tin with **nonstick spray.** Spoon batter into muffin cups. Bake for 20 minutes, or until done.

SERVES: 12 **SERVING SIZE: 1 muffin** **10.5 Nutripoints**

*Batter can be stored in refrigerator up to two weeks.

SOUPS

• Lentil Soup •

3 medium tomatoes, diced
2 cups dried lentils
3 medium onions, chopped
3 carrots, chopped
4 celery stalks, chopped
3 small potatoes, peeled and diced
4 sprigs parsley, chopped
1 can (28 oz.) tomatoes, with liquid
1 green pepper, chopped
3 cloves garlic, minced
2 bay leaves
2 tablespoons dried basil
1 teaspoon cayenne pepper
8 cups vegetable stock or chicken stock (low-sodium)
1 teaspoon salt
Freshly ground black pepper

DIRECTIONS In a large pot, combine all ingredients except the black pepper. Bring to a boil, cover, and simmer for 2 to 3 hours. Add black pepper to taste.

SERVES: 10 **SERVING SIZE: 1 ½ cups** **13.5 Nutripoints**

• French Market Soup •

¼ cup dried pinto beans
¼ cup dried lentils
¼ cup dried red beans
¼ cup dried split peas
¼ cup dried black beans
¼ cup dried black-eyed peas
¼ cup dried navy beans
¼ cup dried baby lima beans
¼ cup dried barley

DIRECTIONS Thoroughly mix dry beans in bowl. Split into two equal portions. Use one portion for this recipe and save other portion until you make the soup again. Soak beans overnight in 1 ½ quarts of water. Pour out soaking water and place the beans in a large Dutch oven with 1½ quarts of fresh water. Bring to a boil, reduce heat and simmer for 3 hours, and then add:

3 stalks celery, chopped
1 15-ounce can tomato sauce
1 medium onion, chopped
2 bay leaves
1 green bell pepper, seeded and chopped
¼ teaspoon dried thyme
1 14 ½-ounce can tomatoes
1 clove garlic
6 ounces lean turkey ham, cut into small pieces

DIRECTIONS Continue to cook 1 to 1½ hours. Just before serving, add black pepper to taste.

SERVES: 12 **SERVING SIZE: 1 cup** **17.0 Nutripoints**

• Hot and Sour Soup •

- 4 black Chinese mushrooms (use package directions for dried mushrooms), sliced
- ¼ pound boneless lean pork, cut into matchsticks (optional)
- 1 tablespoon dry sherry
- 4 cups chicken broth
- 1½ pound chicken breast, cut into matchsticks
- ¼ pound tofu, cut into half-inch cubes
- 2 tablespoons rice wine vinegar
- 1 tablespoon soy sauce
- 2 tablespoons cornstarch
- ¼ cup water
- ½ -¾ teaspoon white pepper
- ½ cup sliced bamboo shoots
- 1 teaspoon sesame oil
- 1 egg white, lightly beaten
- 2 scallions, chopped

DIRECTIONS Combine pork with sherry and let stand 10 minutes. Heat chicken broth to boil and add mushrooms, pork, chicken, and bamboo shoots. Stir, reduce heat, cover, and simmer for 5 minutes. Add tofu, vinegar, and soy sauce. Heat covered 1 minute. Blend cornstarch with cold water. Add to soup and cook until thickened. Add pepper and sesame oil. Slowly pour beaten egg white into soup while stirring. Sprinkle with scallions. Serve.

SERVES: 8 **SERVING SIZE: 1 cup** **4.0 Nutripoints**

• Wild Rice Soup •

- 2 teaspoons margarine
- ½ cup leeks, finely diced
- ½ onion, finely diced
- ½ cup carrots, finely diced
- ½ cup celery, finely diced
- 1 red pepper, seeded and finely diced
- 1 tablespoon flour
- 2½ cups chicken stock
- 1/3 cup wild rice
- 1–2 tablespoons dry sherry
- ⅛ teaspoon salt
- ½ cup evaporated skim milk
- 1 teaspoon chopped parsley

DIRECTIONS In a 2- to 3-quart saucepan, heat the margarine over medium heat. Add the leek, onion, carrots, celery, and red pepper. Cover pot and "sweat" the vegetables until translucent, about 7 minutes. Add the flour and stir well. Cook gently over low heat for approximately 3 minutes, stirring constantly. Add chicken stock gradually, making an increasingly thinner paste, until all stock has been added. Simmer 10 minutes. Add the wild rice, sherry, and salt. Simmer until rice grains have swollen and are tender, 30 to 40 minutes. Add evaporated skim milk and continue to cook on gentle heat. Garnish with parsley (you may want to add a dash more sherry just before serving).

SERVES: 8 **SERVING SIZE: 1 cup** **10.5 Nutripoints**

• Clear Spinach Soup •

3 cans low-sodium chicken broth
2 cups chopped fresh spinach
1 tomato, chopped
1 tablespoon low-calorie margarine
Juice of ½ lemon
Mrs. Dash (seasoning) and black pepper to taste

DIRECTIONS Bring broth to a boil. Add remaining ingredients and cook until spinach barely wilts. Serve immediately.

SERVES: 6 **SERVING SIZE: ½ cup** **23.5 Nutripoints**

• Chilled Blueberry Soup •

2 cups fresh or frozen blueberries (no added sugar)
¾ cup apple juice
½ cup orange juice
1 drop lemon extract
Dash of freshly grated nutmeg
Orange slices
Plain nonfat yogurt

DIRECTIONS Place first 4 ingredients in a saucepan. Bring to a boil over medium heat. Reduce heat and simmer 1 to 2 minutes. Add nutmeg. Pour soup into a blender and process until smooth. Chill. Garnish with orange slices and dollops of yogurt.

SERVES: 4 **SERVING SIZE: ¾ cup** **6.0 Nutripoints**

SANDWICHES

• Turkey Sandwich •

2 slices whole wheat bread
1 teaspoon low-cal. mayonnaise
2 teaspoons plain low-fat yogurt
1 ounce turkey, skinless light meat
¼ cup alfalfa sprouts
¼ tomato

DIRECTIONS Toast bread. Mix mayonnaise and yogurt in a small bowl. Spread mayonnaise mixture on toast. Assemble using remaining ingredients.

SERVES: 1 **SERVING SIZE: 1 sandwich** **4.0 Nutripoints**

• Cajun Chicken Sandwich •

5 skinless, boneless chicken breasts
10 slices whole grain bread, toasted
2 cups coarsely shredded lettuce

MARINADE: ¼ cup water
¼ cup Kikkoman teriyaki marinade
¼ cup red wine
1 ½ teaspoons dried thyme
1 ¼ teaspoons cayenne pepper
1 ¼ teaspoons black pepper
1 ¼ teaspoons white pepper
1 teaspoon garlic powder

SPREAD: ½ tablespoon plain nonfat yogurt
½ tablespoon light mayonnaise
1 tablespoon prepared horseradish

DIRECTIONS Combine marinade ingredients in a shallow glass casserole. Place chicken fillets in marinade, turning once to coat. Cover and refrigerate 2 to 4 hours. Remove chicken from marinade.

Combine yogurt, mayonnaise, and horseradish in a small bowl. Spread one side of each toasted bread slice with the mayonnaise mixture. Place shredded lettuce on half of the slices.

Grill marinated fillets over medium-hot coals approximately 4 minutes on each side, or until chicken is done. Add to sandwich and serve.

SERVES: 5 **SERVING SIZE: 1 sandwich** **5.5 Nutripoints**

• French Bread Pizza •

4 slices French bread
2 ounces part-skim mozzarella cheese
⅔ cup tomato sauce
¼ cup chopped onion
¼ cup chopped green pepper
¼ cup canned artichoke hearts, chopped
2 teaspoons grated Parmesan cheese

DIRECTIONS Preheat oven to 350°F. Slice French bread into pieces 1 inch thick. Spread with tomato sauce that has been mixed with chopped, steamed vegetables. Top with mozzarella and Parmesan cheeses. Bake until cheese melts.

SERVES: 2 **SERVING SIZE: 2 slices** **6.0 Nutripoints**

• Open-Face Pita Sandwich •

¼ cup julienned carrots
¼ cup julienned zucchini
¼ cup sliced mushrooms
¼ cup julienned onion
¼ cup julienned bell pepper
Salt, Mrs. Dash, Freshly ground black pepper
4 teaspoons mustard
2 pita breads
4 slices tomato
2 ounces shredded mozzarella cheese

DIRECTIONS Preheat oven to 375°F. Saute vegetables in water or steam until tender. Drain and season to taste. Spread a thin layer of mustard on top of whole, unsplit pita. Top with vegetables, tomato slices, and cheese. Bake until cheese melts.

SERVES: 2 **SERVING SIZE: 1 whole pita** **5.0 Nutripoints**

SALADS

• Tossed Salad •

1 cup romaine lettuce leaves, torn
½ cup fresh spinach leaves, torn
3 cherry tomatoes
⅛ cup purple cabbage, shredded
2 cucumber slices
1 mushroom, sliced

DIRECTIONS Wash vegetables. Combine ingredients and toss.

SERVES: 1 **SERVING SIZE: 2 cups** **51.5 Nutripoints**

• Spinach Salad •

1 ½ cups spinach leaves, chopped
2 fresh mushrooms, sliced
1 radish, sliced
¼ tomato, chopped

DIRECTIONS Wash vegetables. Combine ingredients and toss.

SERVES: 1 **SERVING SIZE: 2 cups** **65.0 Nutripoints**

• Black Bean Dip •

1 cup canned black bean soup
1 clove garlic, pressed
2 tablespoons Worcestershire sauce
1 tablespoon salsa (picante sauce)
½ tablespoon black pepper
2 teaspoons celery seed

DIRECTIONS Place all ingredients in food processor or blender and process until smooth. Add bean mixture to skillet and heat to reduce liquid volume. Remove from heat when mixture thickens. Refrigerate dip to allow mixture to continue to thicken. Serve with corn tortillas.

SERVES: 8 **SERVING SIZE: 2 tablespoons** **8.0 Nutripoints**

• Salad Greens with Balsamic Vinegar •

4 cups any combination of salad greens
(red leaf lettuce, spinach, Boston lettuce, endive)
1 cup fresh basil leaves
Balsamic vinegar to taste
Equal to taste (optional)
Freshly ground black pepper to taste

DIRECTIONS Wash and thoroughly dry the combination of leaves. Add just enough balsamic vinegar to satisfy your taste. You might like to try mixing a low-cal sweetener with the vinegar before adding it to the greens. Top with freshly ground pepper.

SERVES: 4 **SERVING SIZE: 1 cup** **42.0 Nutripoints**

• Slim Guacamole Dip •

- 1 ripe avocado, chopped and mashed
- 2 tablespoons fresh lime juice
- 2–3 tablespoons salsa (picante sauce)
- 1 ripe tomato, finely chopped
- 2 tablespoons plain low-fat yogurt
- ¼ small yellow onion, finely chopped
- ½ bell pepper, seeded and finely chopped
- Freshly ground black pepper to taste
- ¼ teaspoon ground cumin

DIRECTIONS Mix all ingredients and serve with tortilla chips.

SERVES: 8 **SERVING SIZE: ¼ cup** **7.5 Nutripoints**

• Coleslaw •

- 3 cups green cabbage, shredded
- 3 cups purple cabbage, shredded
- 1 large onion, sliced
- 2 carrots, shredded
- 1 green pepper, seeded and sliced

DRESSING:
- ¾ cup vinegar
- Low-cal sweetener or sugar to taste *
- ¼ teaspoon salt
- 1 teaspoon celery seed
- ¾ teaspoon dry mustard
- ¼ cup olive oil

DIRECTIONS Mix first 5 dressing ingredients together and bring to a boil. Add olive oil. Combine salad ingredients and toss with hot dressing. Chill.

SERVES: 8 **SERVING SIZE: 1 cup** **10.0 Nutripoints**

***If Equal used, do not add until salad is cool.**

• Tuna Salad •

1 6 ½ -ounce can water-packed tuna
1 stalk celery, diced
2 tablespoons fresh parsley, minced
⅛ cup onion, diced
¼ cup apple, diced
⅛ cup sweet pickle relish
½ cup grapes, cut in half
⅛ cup carrots, diced
¼ cup plain nonfat yogurt
⅛ cup light mayonnaise
1 tablespoon sesame seeds
¼ teaspoon dried dill
Freshly ground pepper to taste

DIRECTIONS Mix all ingredients together. Chill and serve.

SERVES: 4 **SERVING SIZE: ½ cup** **5.0 Nutripoints**

• Chicken Salad •

3 cups cooked, diced chicken breast (grilled chicken recommended)
1 ½ cups celery, diced
½ cup scallions, diced
¼ cup fresh parsley, minced
1 cup water chestnuts, diced
1 apple, diced
2 tablespoons whole-grain mustard
½ cup low-fat buttermilk
2 ½ tablespoons light mayonnaise
2 ½ tablespoons plain nonfat yogurt
1 ½ tablespoons lemon juice
Pinch of salt, freshly ground black pepper to taste

DIRECTIONS Mix first 6 ingredients and set aside. Mix remaining ingredients in a separate bowl and then add to chicken mixture.

SERVES: 15 **SERVING SIZE: ½ cup** **6.5 Nutripoints**

• Potato Salad •

- 6 ½ cups unpeeled new potatoes, boiled, cooled, and diced
- 2 hard-boiled egg whites, diced
- 1 bunch scallions, chopped
- ⅛ cup sweet pickle relish
- 1 tablespoon whole-grain mustard
- 2 ½ tablespoons light mayonnaise
- 1 ½ tablespoons orange juice concentrate
- ½ teaspoon rice wine vinegar
- 1 tablespoon low-fat buttermilk
- ¼ cup fresh parsley, minced
- Celery seed to taste
- Cayenne pepper to taste
- Freshly ground black pepper to taste
- Pinch of salt

DIRECTIONS Mix well, chill, and serve.

SERVES: 13 **SERVING SIZE: ½ cup** **9.0 Nutripoints**

• Cold Mixed-Vegetable Salad •

- 16 ounces frozen mixed vegetables (defrosted)
- 1 6-ounce can kidney beans (drained)
- 1 cup sliced water chestnuts (drained)
- ⅓ cup Bernstein's Low Calorie Italian salad dressing (or other low- cal dressing)
- ¼ cup apple juice concentrate
- 1 tablespoon rice wine vinegar
- Juice of ½ lemon
- 1–2 cloves garlic, pressed
- Freshly ground black pepper to taste

DIRECTIONS Combine vegetables and beans in a bowl. Mix remaining ingredients separately. Pour mixture over vegetables. Mix well and let marinate for at least 30 minutes. Serve as a salad, or use on top of fresh greens.

SERVES: 6 **SERVING SIZE: ½ cup** **17.0 Nutripoints**

VEGETABLE DISHES

• South-of-the-Border Vegetarian Chili •

2 15-ounce cans black beans, rinsed and drained
1 tablespoon cumin seed
1 ½ teaspoons dried oregano
1 ½ teaspoons dried basil
1 tablespoon olive oil
1 yellow onion, chopped
1 green pepper, chopped
1 yellow pepper, chopped
1 ½ cups carrots, sliced
2 cloves garlic, minced
2 teaspoons paprika
½ teaspoon cayenne pepper
2 tablespoons chili powder
¼ teaspoon Morton Lite Salt
1 ½ cups canned crushed tomatoes (salt-free), juice reserved
2 fresh jalapeno peppers, minced (remove seeds)
¼ cup plain nonfat yogurt
2 fresh tomatoes, chopped

DIRECTIONS In small nonstick skillet over medium heat, toast cumin seed, oregano, and basil, shaking pan occasionally until fragrant (5—10 minutes). Remove from heat.

In skillet over medium-high heat, heat oil until very hot. Add onion, peppers, carrots, garlic, toasted herbs, paprika, cayenne, chili powder, and Lite Salt. Saute 5—10 minutes. Add canned tomatoes, some tomato juice, and jalapeno pepper. Bring to a boil. Add beans; continue to simmer. Add fresh tomatoes; heat thoroughly.

Top with yogurt to serve.

SERVES: 8 **SERVING SIZE: ¾ cup** **13.0 Nutripoints**

• Vegetable Medley •

¼ cup julienned bell pepper
¼ cup julienned carrots
¼ cup julienned broccoli
Salt
Freshly ground pepper

DIRECTIONS Combine ingredients and steam or microwave until tender. Season to taste with McCormick's Salt Free Parsley Patch or Mrs. Dash.

SERVES: 1 **SERVING SIZE: ¾ cup** **48.5 Nutripoints**

• Vegetable Stir-Fry •

1 egg white
1 tablespoon sherry
1 tablespoon cornstarch
1 tablespoon peanut oil
¼ cup low-sodium soy sauce
1 cup sliced carrots
½ cup chopped scallions
1 clove garlic
1 small green pepper, thinly sliced
1 small red pepper, thinly sliced
1 cup zucchini, sliced
1 cup bok choy, shredded
1 cup fresh mushrooms, thinly sliced
1 cup broccoli, chopped
1 cup sliced water chestnuts
⅓ cup almonds, slivered

DIRECTIONS Combine egg white, sherry, and cornstarch; stir well.

Heat oil in a large skillet. Add soy sauce and carrots, stirring well. Stir-fry 2 minutes. Add scallions, garlic, and peppers; stir-fry an additional 2 to 3 minutes. Add zucchini, bok choy, mushrooms, broccoli, water chestnuts, and almonds; cook 2 to 3 minutes. Serve over hot rice.

SERVES: 6 **SERVING SIZE: ¾ cup** **13.5 Nutripoints**

• Marinated Asparagus •

32 fresh asparagus spears
1 ½ tablespoons Bernstein's Low Calorie Italian dressing
1 ½ tablespoons low-calorie vinaigrette dressing (or 3 T other low-calorie dressing)
1 pimiento, cut into four long strips

DIRECTIONS Wash and trim asparagus spears. Steam until tender (or microwave). Drain. Place in flat container. Add salad dressings and marinate in refrigerator until cold. To serve: wrap 8 spears of asparagus in one long piece of pimiento. Tie pimiento into a bow if possible.

SERVES: 4 **SERVING SIZE: 8 spears** **38.5 Nutripoints**

• Seasoned Turnip Greens •

¼ cup water
2 cups chopped turnip greens
¼ teaspoon ground black pepper
Tobasco to taste (optional)
1 ounce turkey ham (optional)
2 tablespoons Butter Buds, not reconstituted

DIRECTIONS Bring water to a boil. Add turnip greens, pepper, and Tobasco and turkey ham, if using. Cover and simmer until tender, adding water as needed. When tender, add Butter Buds and serve.

SERVES: 4 **SERVING SIZE: ½ cup** **67.0 Nutripoints**

• Home-Style Potatoes •

- 5 cups unpeeled new potatoes, cooked and diced
- 1 ½ tablespoons olive oil
- 1 ½ tablespoons water
- ¼ teaspoon paprika
- ½ teaspoon garlic powder
- ½ teaspoon ground black pepper
- Dash of cayenne pepper
- Pinch of salt
- Sprinkle of Parmesan cheese

DIRECTIONS Preheat oven to 425°F. Mix potatoes with oil, water, paprika, garlic powder, pepper, and salt. (Hands work best for mixing.) Spray a cookie sheet with a nonstick spray. Spread potato mixture on cookie sheet. Bake for at least 1 hour, or until done. Sprinkle lightly with Parmesan cheese.

SERVES: 9 **SERVING SIZE: ½ cup** **5.5 Nutripoints**

SEAFOOD DISHES

• Scallop Kabobs •

- 6 ounces scallops*
- ½ green pepper
- ½ yellow pepper
- 4 mushrooms
- 4 cherry tomatoes
- ¼ onion
- 4 skewers

DIRECTIONS Wash scallops. Cut vegetables into large pieces to be skewered. Skewer scallops and vegetables. Grill over open flame until done, about 5 minutes. (Indoor method: place under oven broiler until brown.)
Serve with Scallop Sauce (see page 253).

SERVES: 2 **SERVING SIZE: 2 skewers** **16.0 Nutripoints**

* You may substitute chunks of chicken, swordfish, fresh tuna, beef, or venison for scallops.

• Red Snapper Veracruz (w/wild rice) •

1 1 ½ -pound red snapper, dressed
3 ½ tablespoons fresh lime juice
Vegetable cooking spray
1 teaspoon olive oil
1 medium onion, thinly sliced
3 cloves garlic, minced
2 ½ cups peeled, chopped tomatoes (about 2 large tomatoes)
2 small fresh green chili peppers, seeded and halved, *or* 1–2 tablespoons canned green chili peppers
2 cups cooked wild rice
Fresh cilantro sprigs (optional)

DIRECTIONS Preheat oven to 400°F. Brush inside and outside of fish with lime juice. Place in a shallow roasting pan coated with vegetable oil spray, and set aside.

Coat a skillet with cooking spray; add oil, and place over medium heat until hot. Add onion and garlic; sauté 3 minutes. Add tomatoes and peppers; cook 5 minutes, stirring frequently.

Spoon sauce over fish; cover with foil and bake for 25 minutes. Place fish on bed of wild rice and garnish with fresh cilantro sprigs, if desired.

SERVES: 4 SERVING SIZE: 3 oz fish, ⅓ cup sauce, and ½ cup rice 13.5 Nutripoints

• Lettuce-Wrapped Salmon •

16 to 20 lettuce leaves
4 4-5 ounce salmon steaks
Juice of 1 lemon
Salt and pepper to taste

DIRECTIONS Place 4 or 5 lettuce leaves in steamer; cover and steam over boiling water 1 minute, or until barely wilted. Drain on paper towels. Repeat with remainder of leaves.

Spread out 4 or 5 of the steamed lettuce leaves, slightly overlapping. Place one salmon steak on leaves, season with lemon juice, salt, and pepper to taste. Wrap lettuce around fish to enclose completely. Repeat with remaining steaks.

Place fish packets in steamer. Cover and steam until done (7–10 minutes). Remove cooked fish. Roll into heated serving dish. Ladle Herb Sauce (see recipe below) over fish.

SERVES: 4 **SERVING SIZE: 1 4-5 oz. salmon steak** **10.5 Nutripoints**

• Herb Sauce •

1 cup parsley leaves
1 clove garlic
1 teaspoon dried (or fresh) tarragon leaves
1 teaspoon sugar
8 ounces plain low-fat yogurt
Salt and pepper to taste
1 tablespoon lemon juice
Other spices as desired (dill, capers, etc.)

DIRECTIONS Place parsley, garlic, tarragon, sugar, and ¼ cup of the yogurt in food processor; whirl to blend. Stir herb mixture into remaining ¾ cup yogurt. Add lemon juice, salt, and pepper. Spice as desired.

SERVES: 6 **SERVING SIZE: ¼ cup** **10.5 Nutripoints**

• Jambalaya* •

2 cups chopped onion
1 cup chopped celery
1 cup chopped green pepper
1 ½ teaspoons minced garlic
1 ½ teaspoons olive oil
2 ½ cups low-sodium chicken stock
Cayenne pepper to taste
2 teaspoons Kitchen Bouquet
1 ½ cups brown rice
½ cup wild rice
1 cup chopped scallions
½ cup chopped tomato

DIRECTIONS Sauté onion, celery, pepper, and garlic in olive oil to desired tenderness. Add chicken broth and cayenne, and bring to a boil. Add Kitchen Bouquet and rices. Return to boil. Cover and simmer for 10 minutes. Remove cover and stir. Continue cooking, uncovered, until rice is tender (approximately 20 minutes). Add more water if needed. Add scallions and chopped tomato. Serve. Freeze remainder of recipe in 1-cup servings.

SERVES: 12 **SERVING SIZE: 1 cup** **7.5 Nutripoints**

*** May add chicken or lean beef if desired.**

• Grilled Salmon with Yellow Bell Pepper Sauce •

- 2 large yellow bell peppers
- 3 tablespoons extra-virgin olive oil
- 3 cloves garlic, minced
- 2 shallots
- ⅛ teaspoon white peppercorns
- 1 tablespoon fresh thyme, chopped
- 3-4 ounces dry white wine
- 1 ½ tablespoons lemon juice
- 4 4-5 ounce salmon steaks*
- Red bell pepper strips
- Salt to taste
- 4 fresh oregano sprigs

DIRECTIONS Roast yellow bell peppers in a 400°F. oven or on grill until skins crack. Remove and let cool. Peel flesh and remove seeds and membranes. Reserve bell pepper flesh.

Heat olive oil in a saucepan and sauté garlic and shallots for approximately 1 minute. Add white peppercorns, thyme, salt, and wine. Lower heat to simmer; add lemon juice and cook until liquid is reduced by half.

Strain liquid into food processor. Add reserved bell pepper. Blend well.

Grill salmon steaks over hot coals until done, about 5 minutes per side.

Spoon bell pepper sauce onto each of 4 serving plates; top with salmon steaks. Garnish with red bell pepper strips and oregano.

SERVES: 4 **SERVING SIZE: 1 4-5 oz steak** **7.0 Nutripoints**

*Swordfish, halibut, or any firm-fleshed fish can be substituted.

• Crunchy Fish •

Lemon juice
3 fish fillets, about ½ -inch thick (3 ½ ounces each)
½ cup Nutri-Grain nuggets, Bran Buds, or Grape-Nuts cereal
1 tablespoon sesame seeds
1 tablespoon dried lemon peel
¼ cup flour
4 egg whites, beaten
Fresh parsley
Lemon slices

DIRECTIONS Preheat oven to 400°F. Rinse fish and pat dry. (You may wish to marinate fish in lemon juice 30 minutes before cooking.) Mix cereal, sesame seeds, and lemon peel in a shallow pan. Put flour and egg whites in separate shallow pans.

Thinly coat fish with flour, dip into egg whites, and then into cereal-seed mixture. Arrange fish on ungreased baking sheet; bake until done (5 minutes per ½ inch for fresh fish, and 10 minutes per ½ inch if frozen; fish turns opaque). Garnish with parsley and lemon.

SERVES: 3 **SERVING SIZE: 1 3 ½-ounce fillet** **6.5 Nutripoints**

MEAT AND POULTRY DISHES

• Aerobics Burger •

3 ounces lean ground round steak
1 whole wheat bun
¼ cup alfalfa sprouts
½ tomato
1 teaspoon mustard

DIRECTIONS Form beef into a patty. Grill beef over hot coals or under oven broiler to desired doneness. Remove excess grease by blotting with a paper towel. Assemble sandwich with remaining ingredients and serve.

SERVES: 1 **SERVING SIZE: 1 3-ounce burger** **5.0 Nutripoints**

• Beef Asada •

8 ounces lean beef flank steak
Salsa (picante sauce)
1 cup tomato, diced
4 whole wheat tortillas

STEAMED VEGETABLES:
1 cup onion, diced
1 cup green bell pepper, diced
1 cup yellow bell pepper, diced

SLIM GUACAMOLE DIP:
½ avocado, mashed
1 tablespoon lime juice
1-1 ½ tablespoons salsa (picante sauce)
½ tomato, diced
1 tablespoon plain nonfat yogurt
2 ½ tablespoons diced onion
¼ bell pepper, diced
¼ teaspoon freshly ground black pepper
⅛ teaspoon cumin seed

DIRECTIONS Marinate flank steak in salsa overnight. Grill until done, 5—7 minutes per side. Slice across grain into thin strips.

Steam (or microwave) vegetables until tender. Stir together the guacamole ingredients.

To serve, place the diced tomato and beef strips on the tortilla. Top with steamed vegetables and guacamole. Roll up tortillas and serve.

SERVES: 4 **SERVING SIZE: 1 filled tortilla** **7.0 Nutripoints**

• Chicken Enchiladas •

1 onion, chopped
2 cups frozen corn
2 cups mushrooms, sliced
1 can (10 ¾ -ounce) low-sodium cream of chicken (or low-sodium cream of mushroom) soup
1 cup plain yogurt
1 cup mozzarella cheese (divided use)
1 small can chopped green chili peppers
½ teaspoon cumin
½ teaspoon garlic powder
1 teaspoon chili powder
Black pepper to taste
1 cup cooked, diced chicken (try Tyson's frozen diced chicken)
10 corn tortillas

DIRECTIONS Preheat the oven to 350°F. Sauté onion, corn, and mushrooms (microwave works well). Add soup, yogurt, 1/2 cup cheese, chili peppers, and spices. Heat, but do not boil. Add chicken. Stir and heat 10 minutes. In a 9 X 13-inch pan, layer half of the mixture on 5 tortillas and then repeat. Top with remaining cheese. (You can make individual tortillas, if you prefer.) Bake for 20 minutes.

SERVES: 5 **SERVING SIZE: 2 tortillas** **5.0 Nutripoints**

• Chicken Stir-Fry •

1 egg white
1 tablespoon sherry
1 tablespoon cornstarch
12 ounces boneless chicken breast, skinned
1 tablespoon peanut oil
¼ cup soy sauce (low-sodium)
1 cup carrots, sliced
½ cup sliced scallions
1 clove garlic, minced
1 small green pepper, thinly sliced
1 small red pepper, thinly sliced
1 cup zucchini, sliced
1 cup bok choy, shredded
1 cup fresh mushrooms, thinly sliced
1 cup broccoli, chopped
1 cup water chestnuts
⅓ cup almonds, slivered

DIRECTIONS Combine egg white, sherry, and cornstarch; stir well. Cut chicken into bite-size pieces and add to sherry mixture, tossing gently to coat. Let stand 1 hour.

Heat oil in a large skillet. Remove chicken from marinade; sauté chicken in oil until lightly browned. Add soy sauce and carrots, stirring well. Cook 2 minutes. Add scallions, garlic, and peppers; stir-fry an additional 2 to 3 minutes. Add zucchini, bok choy, mushrooms, broccoli, water chestnuts, and almonds; cook 2 to 3 minutes. Serve over hot rice.

SERVES: 6 **SERVING SIZE: 1 cup** **8.5 Nutripoints**

• Lemon Chicken •

1 tablespoon grated lemon rind
½ cup lemon juice
⅛ cup water
⅛ cup corn oil
2 teaspoons soy sauce
1 clove garlic, minced
½ teaspoon Morton's Lite Salt
½ teaspoon ground black pepper
6 4-ounce chicken breasts, skin removed
½ cup flour
1 teaspoon paprika

DIRECTIONS Mix together lemon rind and juice, water, oil, soy sauce, garlic, Lite Salt, and pepper. Pour over chicken. Cover and refrigerate at least 3 hours, or overnight.

Preheat oven to 400° F. Drain chicken, reserving marinade. Combine flour with paprika and coat chicken. Shake off excess. Place in single layer with tops down in shallow pan and bake for 30 minutes.

Turn chicken. Pour marinade over chicken; bake 30 minutes longer, or until tender, basting occasionally.

SERVES: 6 SERVING SIZE: 1 4-ounce chicken breast 3.5 Nutripoints

• Low-Fat Fried Chicken •

⅓ cup flour
½ teaspoon salt
½ teaspoon paprika
¼ teaspoon cayenne pepper
¼ teaspoon onion powder or garlic powder
⅛ teaspoon black pepper
4 4-ounce pieces skinless, boneless chicken (3 oz cooked)
1 tablespoon olive oil
¾ cup water

DIRECTIONS Combine flour and spices in plastic bag or in bowl. Coat chicken in seasoned flour. Heat tablespoon oil in large nonstick skillet. Quickly add chicken. Brown over medium heat 5 to 10 minutes per side, until golden brown on all sides. Preheat oven to 350° F. Remove chicken from skillet and place on a cookie sheet which has been sprayed with nonstick vegetable spray. Bake until done (approximately 30 minutes).

SERVES: 4 SERVING SIZE: 3 oz cooked chicken 3.0 Nutripoints

PASTA AND GRAIN DISHES

• Angel Hair Pasta with Sunshine Sauce •

1 tablespoon olive oil
1 clove garlic, minced
2 14 ½ -ounce cans plum tomatoes, diced
2 cups fresh Roma tomatoes, diced
½ onion, chopped
1 yellow pepper, seeded and chopped
Pinch of salt
Freshly ground pepper
Italian seasoning to taste
1 package (or cube) low-sodium chicken broth
1 tablespoon sugar
4 tablespoons fresh parsley, chopped
1 tablespoon freshly grated Parmesan cheese
2 peeled, sliced, and slivered yellow onions
12—16 ounces angel hair pasta

DIRECTIONS Over low flame heat ½ tablespoon olive oil in saucepan. Add garlic and cook until soft. Add tomatoes, chopped onion, yellow pepper, salt, pepper, Italian seasoning, chicken broth, and sugar. Stir and cook uncovered over medium heat 15 minutes. Add parsley and cheese. Remove from heat. Keep warm.

Line cookie sheet with foil. Spread slivered onions on sheet and toss lightly with remaining ½ tablespoon olive oil. Place under broiler and cook until onions are wilted and slightly brown.

Cook pasta; drain and rinse. Top pasta with sauce. Sprinkle with onions. Serve.

SERVES: 6 SERVING SIZE: 1 ½ cups 10.0 Nutripoints

• Spinach Lasagna •

30 ounces frozen spinach
2 egg whites
8 large lasagna noodles
6 cups Nutripoint Tomato Sauce (see page 252) or use bottled sauce
1 ½ cups 1-percent-fat cottage cheese, partially drained
3 cups skim mozzarella cheese, sliced
¼ cup grated Parmesan cheese (Formagg brand)

DIRECTIONS This recipe requires one very large lasagna pan. Defrost frozen spinach and drain very well. Mix with egg white. Set aside. Cook lasagna noodles, drain, and rinse. Preheat oven to 350° F. Layer ingredients as follows:

1 ½ cups sauce
4 lasagna noodles
1 ½ cups sauce
¾ cup cottage cheese
1 ½ cups mozzarella cheese
1 ½ cups spinach
4 lasagna noodles
1 ½ cups sauce
¾ cup cottage cheese
1 ½ cups mozzarella cheese
1 ½ cups spinach
¼ cup Parmesan cheese
1 ½ cups sauce

Cover pan with foil. Bake about 1 hour. Remove from oven. Remove foil and let stand for 10 minutes. Serve. (This dish freezes well.)

SERVES: 12 **SERVING SIZE: 1 cup** **9.0 Nutripoints**

• Herbed Lentils and Wild Rice •

2 ¼ cups chicken or vegetable broth
¾ cup lentils
1 onion, chopped
1 cup mushrooms, sliced
1 red bell pepper, chopped
½ cup wild rice
½ cup dry white wine
½ teaspoon dried basil, crushed
½ teaspoon dried oregano, crushed
½ teaspoon dried thyme, crushed
¼ teaspoon salt
⅛ teaspoon garlic powder
¼ teaspoon freshly ground black pepper
1 cup shredded mozzarella cheese (divided use)
½ cup pimiento, chopped

DIRECTIONS Preheat oven to 350° F. Combine all the ingredients except ½ cup mozzarella cheese and pimiento. Pour mixture into an ungreased 1 ½-quart casserole with a tight-fitting lid. Cover and bake, stirring twice, 1 ½ to 2 hours, or until lentils and rice are done.

Uncover casserole; top with the remaining ½ cup mozzarella cheese and pimiento. Bake 5 minutes, or until cheese melts.

SERVES: 4 **SERVING SIZE: 1 cup** **6.5 Nutripoints**

• Fresh Pasta Salad •

1 cup fresh pasta
½ –1 tablespoon extra-virgin olive oil
¼ cup fresh basil, shredded
Squeeze of fresh lemon juice
12 cherry tomatoes, halved
⅛ teaspoon salt (optional)
Freshly ground black pepper

DIRECTIONS Cook pasta. Drain. Toss immediately with extra-virgin olive oil, basil, lemon juice, tomatoes, salt, and pepper.

SERVES: 8 **SERVING SIZE: ¼ cup** **4.5 Nutripoints**

FRUIT DISHES

• Fresh Fruit Slices •

¼ cantaloupe
¼ honeydew melon
½ cup sliced fresh strawberries

DIRECTIONS Slice melon pieces and arrange with strawberries.

SERVES: 2 **SERVING SIZE: 1 cup** **36.0 Nutripoints**

• Fruit Salad Plate •

2 bananas, sliced
2 kiwi fruit, sliced
1 ½ cups fresh pineapple chunks
2 ½ cups sliced fresh strawberries
2 cups chopped Bibb lettuce

DIRECTIONS Line 4 plates with the lettuce. Mix together the fruit; arrange on lettuce.

SERVES: 5 **SERVING SIZE: 1 cup** **14.5 Nutripoints**

• Rainbow Compote •

¼ cup fresh blueberries
¼ cup fresh raspberries
¼ cup sliced mango
¼ cup sliced fresh strawberries
4 sprigs fresh mint

DIRECTIONS Layer fruit in small glass bowls and garnish with mint. Serve.

SERVES: 2 **SERVING SIZE: ½ cup** **18.0 Nutripoints**

• Fresh Fruit Platter •

12 red grapes
¼ cantaloupe, cut into large chunks
1 cup fresh pineapple chunks
½ kiwi fruit, sliced
½ skinned orange, cut into chunks
1 cup fresh strawberries
⅛ papaya, sliced
⅛ mango, sliced
Leafy lettuce

DIRECTIONS Arrange fruit on platter lined with lettuce. Serve.

SERVES: 1 **SERVING SIZE: 2 ½ cups** **17.0 Nutripoints**

• Key Lime Mousse •

2 envelopes unflavored gelatin
¼ cup cold water
1 cup boiling water
1 cup fresh lime juice
1 tablespoon grated lime rind
½ cup sugar
3 cups nonfat yogurt cheese*

DIRECTIONS Dissolve gelatin in cold water. Add boiling water and stir until dissolved. Add lime juice, rind, and sugar. Stir well. Mix in yogurt cheese until smooth (food processor works well). Pour into a deep 9-inch pie pan, or pour into small individual serving-size containers. Chill until firm.

SERVES: 10 **SERVING SIZE: ½ cup** **5.5 Nutripoints**

• Fruit-Yogurt Pie •

1 envelope unflavored gelatin
⅓ cup cold water
2 8-ounce containers low-fat fruit yogurt
2 egg whites
⅓ cup sugar
1 ½ cups fresh berries
1 9-inch graham cracker pie crust

DIRECTIONS In a small saucepan over low heat, soften gelatin in water. Cook and stir until gelatin dissolves. Remove from heat. Stir in yogurt. Chill until partially set (the consistency of unbeaten egg whites).

In a large bowl, beat the egg whites until soft peaks form. Add sugar, 1 tablespoon at a time, beating until stiff peaks form. Stir fruit into yogurt mixture and fold mixture into beaten egg whites. Turn into graham cracker pie crust. Chill 3 to 4 hours, or until firm.

SERVES: 12 **SERVING SIZE: 1 small piece (1/12 of pie)** **0.5 Nutripoints**

*Make yogurt cheese by draining plain nonfat yogurt in cheesecloth or coffee filter for 8 to 10 hours. 2 cups yogurt yields 1 cup yogurt cheese.

• Poached Pears •

RASPBERRY
PUREE: 1 cup frozen raspberries
1–2 teaspoons cornstarch
2 tablespoons cold water

1 quart cranberry juice
1 cinnamon stick
6 black peppercorns
1 clove
2 pears, peeled with stems left on
8 ounces plain low-fat yogurt, mixed with vanilla and honey to taste

DIRECTIONS Heat raspberries in skillet. Strain to yield only liquid raspberry juice. Dissolve cornstarch in cold water and slowly add to raspberry juice. Stir well. Cook over medium heat until mixture thickens slightly.

Bring cranberry juice to a boil and add cinnamon stick, peppercorns, and clove. Simmer peeled pears in liquid for 5 minutes, covered, then chill.

Cut poached pears in half and then into ⅛-inch-thick slices, leaving them attached to the top of the pear. Spread 2 ounces yogurt on 4 plates. Fan pear slices on plate over the yogurt. Squeeze raspberry puree from a bottle into several horizontal lines on the yogurt surrounding the pear. Create pattern by running a knife vertically through the lines of raspberry puree from the bottom of the yogurt to the top.

SERVES: 4 **SERVING SIZE: ½ pear** **4.0 Nutripoints**

• Bananas Flambé •

4 small bananas
1 tablespoon orange juice
2 tablespoons reduced-calorie margarine
2 tablespoons brown sugar
¼ teaspoon ground cinnamon
¼ cup 151-proof (flames best) rum
1 quart low-fat frozen vanilla yogurt

DIRECTIONS Slice bananas in half lengthwise, then in half again. Toss with orange juice and set aside. Combine margarine with brown sugar in a large nonstick skillet. Cook over medium heat, stirring constantly until sugar melts. Add reserved bananas; cook 4 minutes. Sprinkle with cinnamon and remove from heat. Pour rum over banana mixture. Ignite; let flames die down. Serve immediately over frozen yogurt.

SERVES: 8 **SERVING SIZE: 2 banana slices + ½ c yogurt** **2.5 Nutripoints**

• Blackberry Freeze •

1 package frozen blackberries (no added sugar), semi-defrosted
1 ½ tablespoons orange juice concentrate
1 orange, sliced

DIRECTIONS Place first two ingredients into blender or food processor. Process until the mixture reaches the consistency of a sorbet. Garnish with fresh orange slices.

SERVES: 4 **SERVING SIZE: ¾ cup** **8.5 Nutripoints**

• Banana Gladje •

2 frozen bananas, cut into large pieces, semi-defrosted
3–4 tablespoons part-skim ricotta cheese (or 1 ounce Neufchâtel cheese)
⅛-¼ cup skim milk
Fresh mint

DIRECTIONS Place bananas into blender or food processor. Add remaining ingredients and process until smooth. Garnish with fresh mint.

SERVES: 3 **SERVING SIZE: ⅓ cup** **6.0 Nutripoints**

• Applesauce •

4 large apples
1 teaspoon cinnamon
½ teaspoon nutmeg
Pinch of cloves
Pinch of allspice
¼ cup water
2–4 packages favorite heat-stable low-cal sweetener
2 teaspoons honey

DIRECTIONS Core and peel apples. Add spices and water to a small saucepan; cover and simmer until apples are tender—approximately 25 minutes. Stir in sweetener and honey. Serve warm.

SERVES: 4 **SERVING SIZE: ½ cup** **3.0 Nutripoints**

BREAKFAST DISHES

• Bran Muffins •

- 1 ½ cups Whole Wheat Total (or other bran cereal)
- ½ cup orange juice, boiling
- 4 egg whites (or ¼ cup egg substitute)
- ½ cup ½ -percent-fat buttermilk
- 4 ounces orange juice concentrate
- 3 tablespoons safflower oil
- 1 large ripe banana, mashed
- ½ cup currants
- 2 tablespoons honey, brown sugar, or molasses
- ½ teaspoon vanilla extract
- 1 cup whole wheat flour
- ½ cup white flour
- 1 ½ teaspoons baking soda
- 2 teaspoons baking powder
- ¾ teaspoon cinnamon
- ¾ teaspoon nutmeg
- Zest of 1 orange, chopped finely

DIRECTIONS Preheat oven to 400° F. Combine cereal in a large bowl with boiling orange juice. Let cool. Add the egg whites, buttermilk, orange juice concentrate, oil, banana, currants, honey, and vanilla. Mix well. In a small bowl, combine flours, baking soda, baking powder, and spices. Add to cereal mixture and mix very well.* Spray a muffin tin with nonstick spray. Spoon into muffin cups. Bake for 20 minutes, or until done.

SERVES: 12 **SERVING SIZE: 1 muffin** **10.0 Nutripoints**

* **Batter can be stored in refrigerator up to 2 weeks.**

• Oat Bran Muffins •

1 ¼ cups oat bran cereal
1 cup whole wheat flour
¼ cup dried apricots, coarsely chopped
1 tablespoon baking powder
½ cup skim milk
½ cup orange juice
¼ cup molasses (or honey)
2 tablespoons vegetable oil
3 egg whites

DIRECTIONS Preheat oven to 425°F. Spray bottom and sides of 12 medium-size muffin cups with nonstick spray (or line with paper baking cups). Combine dry ingredients. Add milk, juice, egg whites, molasses, and oil. Mix just until dry mixture is moistened. Fill prepared muffin cups ¾ full. Bake for 15 minutes.

SERVES: 12 **SERVING SIZE: 1 muffin** **3.5 Nutripoints**

• French Toast •

1 egg yolk
2 egg whites
1/16 teaspoon salt
½ teaspoon vanilla extract
2 teaspoons brown sugar
Cinnamon to taste
3 slices cinnamon bread

DIRECTIONS Combine first six ingredients and beat well. Pour mixture into baking dish and add bread. Turn bread to coat with mixture. Spray nonstick skillet with nonstick spray. Add bread and cook over medium heat until golden brown on both sides.

SERVES: 2 **SERVING SIZE: 1 ½ pieces toast** **0.5 Nutripoints**

Serving suggestions

1. Serve with frozen fruit which has been heated in the microwave and sweetened to taste.
2. Top with vanilla-flavored low-fat yogurt.

• Garden Scrambled Eggs •

⅛ green pepper, diced
onion, diced
2 fresh mushrooms, diced
2 egg whites
1 egg yolk
⅛ cup low-fat cottage cheese

DIRECTIONS Place first 3 ingredients in a microwave-safe container, cover, and microwave on medium setting until vegetables are tender, or spray a nonstick skillet with a non-stick spray and lightly sauté vegetables. Whip egg whites with yolk and cottage cheese. Scramble eggs in skillet with cooked vegetables until done.

SERVES: 1 **SERVING SIZE: ¾ cup** **5.5 nutripoints**

• Fruited Cinnamon Cereal •

¾ cup cooked old-fashioned oatmeal
¼ apple, shredded
1 tablespoon raisins or chopped dried apricots
Cinnamon to taste

DIRECTIONS Mix all ingredients together and serve.

SERVES: 1 **SERVING SIZE: 1 cup** **5.0 nutripoints**

• Whole Grain Pancakes •

2 cups whole wheat flour
½ teaspoon baking soda
½ teaspoon Morton Lite Salt
2 egg whites
1 egg yolk
1 tablespoon oil
1 ¾ cups orange juice

DIRECTIONS Sift flour, baking soda, and Lite Salt together in a bowl.

Blend eggs, oil, and orange juice in a bowl. Add dry ingredients. Mix just until blended.

Heat nonstick skillet and spray with nonstick vegetable spray. Drop batter onto skillet to make small pancakes. Cook over medium heat until bubbles burst and bottoms are golden brown, about 2 minutes. Flip pancakes and brown other side.

SERVES: 6 **SERVING SIZE: 4 pancakes** **5.5 Nutripoints**

• Hot Blueberry Topping •

1 16-ounce package frozen, unsweetened blueberries (or 2 pints fresh blueberries)
1 tablespoon honey
Favorite heat-stable low-cal sweetener, to taste
4 teaspoons cornstarch
4 teaspoons cold water
2 teaspoons orange juice

DIRECTIONS Heat fruit in large pan (or in microwave). Add honey and sweetener. Dissolve cornstarch in cold water and slowly add to hot fruit mixture. Stir well. Mixture will look cloudy at this point. Add orange juice. Bring to a boil, which will clear mixture. Serve hot.

SERVES: 3—4 **SERVING SIZE: ½ cup** **2.5 Nutripoints**

• Hot Peach Topping •

1 16-ounce package frozen, unsweetened peaches (or 4 cups sliced fresh peaches)
1 tablespoon honey
Favorite heat-stable low-cal sweetener, to taste
4 teaspoons cornstarch
4 teaspoons cold water
2 teaspoons orange juice
Cinnamon to taste

DIRECTIONS Heat fruit in large pan (or in microwave). Add honey and other sweetener. Dissolve cornstarch in cold water and slowly add to hot fruit mixture. Stir well. Mixture will look cloudy at this point. Add orange juice and cinnamon.

Bring to a boil, which will clear mixture. Serve hot.

SERVES: 3—4 **SERVING SIZE: ½ cup** **7.0 Nutripoints**

• Hot Red Raspberry Topping •

1 16-ounce package frozen, unsweetened raspberries (or 2 pints fresh raspberries)
1 tablespoon honey
Favorite heat-stable low-cal sweetener, to taste
4 teaspoons cornstarch
4 teaspoons cold water
2 teaspoons orange juice
Cinnamon to taste

DIRECTIONS Follow directions for Hot Peach Topping. Add cinnamon to taste.

SERVES: 3—4 **SERVING SIZE: ½ cup** **9.0 Nutripoints**

• Honey Cream Cheese •

8 ounces low-fat cream cheese (Neufchâtel)
1 tablespoon honey
1 package favorite low-cal sweetener
1 tablespoon milk

DIRECTIONS Place ingredients in food processor. Mix until smooth.

SERVES: 8–16 **SERVING SIZE: 1—2 tablespoons** **5.5 Nutripoints**

DRESSINGS AND SAUCES

• Lite Spicy Mustard Dressing •

½ cup of Dijon mustard
2 cloves garlic, minced
Juice of 2 lemons
2 packages favorite low-cal sweetener
⅛ cup water (or plain nonfat yogurt, if desired)

DIRECTIONS Mix all ingredients. Refrigerate and serve.

SERVES: 16 **SERVING SIZE: 1 tablespoon** **0.5 Nutripoints**

• Lite Zero Salad Dressing •

½ cup tomato juice or V8 (may add low-sodium canned tomatoes pureed in food processor to thicken)
2 tablespoons fresh lemon juice
1 tablespoon finely chopped onion (or dehydrated onion)
¼ cup fresh finely chopped parsley
½ cup canned tomatoes (no added salt), chopped

DIRECTIONS Combine ingredients in jar with tight lid and shake well, or whiz in a blender.

SERVES: 10 **SERVING SIZE: 2 tablespoons** **1.0 Nutripoint**

• Balsamic Vinegar Dressing •

4 tablespoons low-fat buttermilk
1 tablespoon rice wine vinegar
1 tablespoon balsamic vinegar
1 teaspoon sugar
Freshly ground black pepper and Morton Lite Salt to taste

DIRECTIONS Mix ingredients well and serve.

SERVES: 6 **SERVING SIZE: 1 tablespoon** **0.0 Nutripoints**

• Blue Cheese Dressing •

½ cup low-fat cottage cheese
¼ cup low-fat buttermilk
1 tablespoon white vinegar
1 ½ tablespoons blue cheese salad dressing mix

DIRECTIONS Blend all ingredients until smooth. Refrigerate for 1 hour to develop full flavor.

SERVES: 8 **SERVING SIZE: 2 tablespoons** **8.0 Nutripoints**

• Lite 16-Island Dressing •

1 cup plain nonfat yogurt
1 tablespoon Dijon mustard
2 tablespoons olive oil
½ teaspoon horseradish
1 tablespoon fresh lemon juice
1 teaspoon minced chives (or scallions)
2 tablespoons tomato paste or crushed tomatoes
1 tablespoon chopped fresh parsley
1 teaspoon dried basil*
Freshly ground black pepper to taste
Morton's Lite Salt to taste

DIRECTIONS Combine all ingredients and mix until smooth.

SERVES: 12 **SERVING SIZE: 2 tablespoons** **2.5 Nutripoints**

• Honey Yogurt Dressing •

1 cup plain nonfat yogurt
1 ⅔ tablespoons honey

DIRECTIONS Mix well in a blender or food processor.

SERVES: 16 **SERVING SIZE: 1 tablespoon** **2.0 Nutripoints**

• Lite Mayonnaise Mix •

¾ cup plain nonfat yogurt
¼ cup light mayonnaise

DIRECTIONS Mix ingredients until smooth.

SERVES: 16 **SERVING SIZE: 1 tablespoon** **1.5 Nutripoints**

• New Way Sour Cream •

1 cup low-fat cottage cheese
2 tablespoons fresh lemon juice
1 tablespoon skim milk

DIRECTIONS Mix all ingredients in a food processor and whiz until smooth.

SERVES: 8 **SERVING SIZE: 2 tablespoons** **6.5 Nutripoints**

• Lite Caper Dressing •

¼ cup light mayonnaise
⅔ cup plain low-fat yogurt
3 tablespoons red wine vinegar
2 ½ –3 tablespoons capers, rinsed and minced
2 tablespoons minced fresh chives
2 tablespoons chopped fresh parsley
2 tablespoons minced shallots
1 clove garlic, minced
1 tablespoon fresh chopped basil
2 tablespoons Dijon mustard

DIRECTIONS Combine all ingredients. Mix until smooth.

SERVES: 12 **SERVING SIZE: 2 tablespoons** **2.0 Nutripoints**

• Lite Vinaigrette Dressing •

2 large cloves garlic, crushed
2 tablespoons olive oil
4 tablespoons mild vinegar (cider vinegar recommended)
1–2 tablespoons lemon juice
2 tablespoons water
½ teaspoon dry mustard
¼ teaspoon freshly ground black pepper
1 teaspoon sugar or low-cal sweetener to taste
¼ teaspoon salt

DIRECTIONS Combine ingredients and mix well.

SERVES: 3 **SERVING SIZE: 2 tablespoons** **1.5 Nutripoints**

Variations

1. Substitute any fruit vinegar for cider vinegar.
2. Add 4 diced artichoke hearts, a bit more dry mustard, and 1 tablespoon balsamic vinegar.

• Lite Orange Vinaigrette Dressing •

½ cup orange juice concentrate
¼ cup olive oil
¼ cup apple cider vinegar
2 teaspoons Dijon mustard
2 egg whites, beaten
Herbs as desired

DIRECTIONS Slowly add oil to orange juice while using a hand beater. Add vinegar and mustard; beat again. Fold in egg whites and herbs and serve.

SERVES: 8 **SERVING SIZE: 2 tablespoons** **2.5 Nutripoints**

• Lite Ranch Dressing •

1 cup low-fat buttermilk
¾ cup plain low-fat yogurt
¼ cup light mayonnaise
2 tablespoons chopped fresh parsley
2 ½ teaspoons minced fresh dill, or ¾ teaspoon dried
2 teaspoons chopped fresh basil, or ¾ teaspoon dried
½ teaspoon Worcestershire sauce
1–2 cloves garlic, pressed
¾ teaspoon onion powder

DIRECTIONS Blend all ingredients. Chill at least 8 hours before serving.

SERVES: 16 **SERVING SIZE: 2 tablespoons** **3.5 Nutripoints**

• Juniper Berry Marinade and Sauce (For Venison, Quail, or Chicken) •

MARINADE:

½ cup olive oil
2–3 stalks celery, diced
Salt and freshly ground pepper to taste
6 juniper berries, crushed
Juice of 6 lemons
1 carrot, diced

SAUCE:

2 tablespoons cornstarch
Cold water
1 cup warm low-sodium beef broth
1 teaspoon margarine
6 juniper berries, crushed
Dash of salt
Freshly ground pepper and other spices to taste

DIRECTIONS Stir together marinade ingredients. Place meat of your choice in a large nonmetallic bowl and pour marinade over it. Set aside in refrigerator for 4 to 8 hours, turning the meat occasionally.

Mix cornstarch with small amount of cold water to form a paste; add slowly to beef broth. Place over medium heat and reduce until thick. Add margarine and crushed berries. Add salt, pepper, and spices to taste.

Marinate meat; grill meat; ladle ¼ cup sauce on top, Serve hot.

SERVES: 4 **SERVING SIZE: ¼ cup** **0.0 Nutripoints**

• Hawaiian Marinade for Chicken or Fish •

½ cup low-sodium soy sauce
½ cup pineapple juice
½ cup water
1 teaspoon minced garlic
½ tablespoon dry mustard
¼ cup sugar
⅛ cup vegetable oil (or olive oil)
1 kiwi fruit, peeled and mashed
1 cup fresh pineapple, cut into large chunks

DIRECTIONS Mix together all the ingredients. Place skinless chicken breasts or fish in a shallow nonmetallic container and pour marinade over all. Set aside in the refrigerator for about 2 hours. Remove chicken or fish from marinade and grill. Meanwhile, simmer marinade in a saucepan until reduced and thickened. Ladle 1 ounce on top of chicken or fish, making sure that each plate gets a few chunks of fresh pineapple.

SERVES: 6
SERVING SIZE: Marinade for 6 4-ounce chicken breasts or 6 4-ounce fish fillets **4.0 Nutripoints**

• Tomato Sauce •

1 carrot
2 stalks celery
1 red or green bell pepper, halved and seeded
1 ½ medium onions
2 cloves garlic
2 large tomatoes, skins removed
½ medium zucchini
Small amount of olive oil
6 cups crushed tomatoes

SPICES: 1 tablespoon Italian seasoning
2 teaspoons basil
2 teaspoons sugar
1 tablespoon fennel seed, crushed
1 bay leaf
⅛ cup chopped fresh parsley
2 teaspoons oregano
2 teaspoons salt
2 teaspoons chili powder

DIRECTIONS Using a food processor, chop the vegetables into small pieces. Heat olive oil in large saucepan and sauté vegetables until tender (about 10 to 12 minutes). Add the crushed tomatoes and the spices and let simmer about 2 hours.

SERVES: 12 cups **SERVING SIZE: 1 cup** **19.0 Nutripoints**

• Mango Sauce •

1 shallot, minced
½ tablespoon margarine
1 15-ounce can mangoes (no sugar), puréed
2 tablespoons cornstarch
Sherry to taste
1 fresh mango, peeled and mashed

DIRECTIONS Sauté shallot in margarine. Add puréed mango. Combine cornstarch with a small amount of cold water and add to puréed mixture. Bring to a boil. Add sherry to taste. Stir in fresh mango. Pour small amount of sauce over baked chicken breasts.

SERVES: 8 **SERVING SIZE: ¼ cup** **1.0 Nutripoint**

• Scallop Sauce •

⅛ cup diced onion
½ tablespoon minced garlic (or shallots)
½ tablespoon olive oil
1 ½ tablespoons sherry
½ cup ½-percent-fat milk
4 teaspoons low-sodium chicken bouillon
1 tablespoon fresh lemon juice
¼ teaspoon tarragon
½ teaspoon dill
½ teaspoon basil
Pinch of salt
Freshly ground pepper to taste
¼ cup fresh tomato, peeled and diced
3 fresh mushrooms, sliced
1–2 tablespoons cornstarch
½ cup cold water

DIRECTIONS Sauté onion and garlic in olive oil. Add sherry, milk, bouillon, lemon juice, and spices. Steam tomato and mushrooms and add to mixture. Dissolve cornstarch in cold water and add to mixture to thicken. Serve over broiled or baked scallops.

SERVES: 6 **SERVING SIZE: ¼ cup** **1.0 Nutripoints**

• Banana Mint Sauce •

1 frozen banana
1 cup low-fat plain yogurt
Fresh mint leaves

DIRECTIONS Peel and break banana into pieces and freeze. Combine frozen banana, yogurt, and mint. Mix all ingredients in a food processor until smooth. Spoon over seasonal fruit.

SERVES: 16 **SERVING SIZE: 2–4 tablespoons** **6.5 Nutripoints**

FRUIT DRINKS

• Strawberry Smoothie •

½ cup low-fat milk
½ cup strawberries
2 packages favorite low-cal sweetener
3–4 ice cubes

DIRECTIONS Mix ingredients in blender until smooth.

SERVES: 1 **SERVING SIZE: 1-1½ cups** **13.5 nutripoints**

• Sunrise Cooler •

3 cups freshly squeezed orange juice
1 cup frozen strawberries
2 cups sparkling mineral water
Ice cubes as desired

DIRECTIONS Purée frozen strawberries in food processor. Mix with orange juice and freeze until just firm. Before serving add mineral water and pour over ice cubes.

SERVES: 8 **SERVING SIZE: ½ cup** **15.5 Nutripoints**

PART VII

NUTRIPOINT LISTS

THE LISTS THAT FOLLOW CONTAIN NUTRIPOINT RATINGS FOR MORE than 3,600 foods. The lists are in three parts:

The Nutrigroup Ratings lists show the rating of every food within its Nutrigroup, highest to lowest. There are six basic Nutrigroups:

1. Vegetables
2. Fruits
3. Grains
4. Legumes/nuts/seeds
5. Milk/dairy
6. Meat/fish/poultry

There are five types of foods on the Nutrigroup Ratings lists:

1. Nutripoint recipes
2. Basic foods
3. Generic foods
4. Brand-name foods
5. Fast foods

There are also five Other Group lists:

1. Fats/oils
2. Sugar
3. Alcohol
4. Condiments
5. Miscellaneous

The following are notes and explanations concerning various aspects of the lists.

Nutripoint Recipes These are easily identified because they always include the words *Nutripoint Recipe.* Two examples of such entries from the lists include "Red Snapper, Veracruz, Nutripoint" and "Dressing, Lite, Blue Cheese, Nutripoint Recipe." These are recipes we've created for dishes that are high in Nutripoints, and, of course, delicious. You'll find the recipes for them in the recipe section (page 201). (You'll also find these foods featured on the Nutripoint fourteen-day menus, beginning on page 185.)

Basic Foods These are just what you would think: apples, whole wheat flour, milk, chicken breast, and so on. They're foods that are unprocessed.

Generic Foods You'll notice that some of the foods on the list are neither brand names nor basic foods such as grapes. These foods are what we call *generic foods.* They have ratings based on USDA nutritional information. Some of these are foods that have had some processing, such as canned pumpkin or tomato sauce; others are what are known as *home recipes,* such as coleslaw. Home recipes are standard recipes that most people would use at home to prepare certain foods. Of course, your recipe for tuna noodle casserole might well differ from the USDA home recipe version, but to assume a certain standard is the only way to evaluate these foods.

Brand-Name Foods These are foods that have been processed by a particular manufacturer who also provided the nutritional information used as the basis of analysis of these foods. These foods include everything from Birds Eye frozen whole leaf spinach to Gatorade.

Fast Foods These are foods that are served by fast-food restaurants. We've included most of the major fast-food chains, from Arby's to McDonald's, and we've tried to include the most popular items on their menus, from salads, to burgers, to pizzas.

You'll notice that there are three columns for the food ratings. The *Nutripoints* column, obviously, is the rating of the food.

The *Food Name* column, of course, identifies the food.

The *Serving Size* column shows the amount of food that is rated. The measurements include cups, pieces, fluid ounces, ounces by weight, tablespoons, and teaspoons. Various explanations concerning serving sizes appear in the text.

Next to a food name you'll sometimes find an asterisk (*), a dagger (†), or a double dagger (††). An asterisk means that the food is fortified, a dagger indicates that it contains too much cholesterol, and a double dagger warns the reader to exercise caution when eating a food because it may contain contaminants.

Fortification You'll notice, particularly in the grain Nutrigroup, that many of the foods have an asterisk (*). This means that these foods derive at least 50 percent of their nutritional value from fortification. There are further discussions of this topic in the text (see page 152), but I'll simply reiterate here that some controversy exists about the value of fortification. Often, nutrients have been removed through processing and then replaced artificially. While these foods do contain large amounts of certain nutrients, they're not "natural" in that they aren't as nature formulated them. In general, the fortified foods at the top of the list are far preferable to fortified foods lower on the list because the top foods (cereals usually) begin with a whole food and then fortify it. The foods lower down sometimes have sugar as a primary ingredient, with vitamins and minerals added to that.

My basic suggestion concerning fortified foods is that if you choose them, check the labels to be sure that the food is based on a real, basic food. One of the best tip-offs to a fortified food with little value is if the label contains any of the various terms for sugar (see page 84) listed among its first few ingredients.

Cholesterol Some foods, particularly those in the meat/ poultry/fish Nutrigroup, have a dagger (†) indicating cholesterol. Again, this has been discussed more fully in the text (see pages 145-146), but briefly, the notation means that these foods have a content of cholesterol per calorie of 1 milligram or more. This is a high concentration of cholesterol and, whatever the ranking of the food, I suggest that you avoid foods with the cholesterol mark.

Caution Some shellfish have a double dagger (††), which indicates the possibility of contamination. While many of these foods are high in Nutripoints, care must be taken when eating them.

NUTRIGROUP RATINGS

VEGETABLE GROUP

Nutripoints	Serving Size		Food Name—Vegetables
79.0	1	cup	Turnip Greens, Chopped, Cooked
75.0	2	cups	Spinach, Raw, Chopped
72.5	1	cup	Bok Choy, Raw, Shredded
67.0	1	cup	Turnip Greens, Seasoned, Nutripoint Recipe
65.0	2	cups	Salad, Spinach, Nutripoint Recipe
61.5	1	cup	Mustard Greens, Cooked
57.0	1	cup	Spinach, Whole Leaf, Fzn, Birds Eye
56.5	1	cup	Beet Greens, Cooked
54.5	1	cup	Parsley, Fresh
53.5	1	cup	Spinach, Fresh, Cooked
53.0	1	cup	Broccoli, Raw
52.5	20	pieces	Watercress
51.5	2	cups	Salad, Tossed, Nutripoint Recipe
48.5	1	cup	Vegetable Medley, Nutripoint Recipe
48.0	1	cup	Mustard Greens, Fzn, Cooked
47.5	2	cups	Lettuce, Romaine
46.0	1/2	cup	Broccoli Spears, Fzn, Birds Eye
44.5	3	wt oz	Turnip Greens, Allen's
44.5	1	cup	Dandelion Greens, Raw
44.0	8	stalks	Asparagus, Fresh
42.5	2	whole	Peppers, Sweet, Red, Raw
42.5	3/4	cup	Spinach, Frozen, Cooked
42.5	1	cup	Collard Greens, Raw, Chopped
42.0	1	cup	Swiss Chard, Cooked
42.0	1	cup	Collard Greens, Fresh, Cooked
42.0	1	cup	Salad, Greens, Balsamic Vinegar, Nutripoint Recipe
41.5	1	cup	Broccoli, Cauliflower and Red Peppers, Fzn, Birds Eye
41.5	1 1/2	cups	Spinach, Chopped, Fzn, 365 Organic, Whole Foods
40.5	1	cup	Cauliflower, Raw
40.0	3/4	cup	Dandelion Greens, Cooked
40.0	1/2	cup	Collard Greens, Frozen, Cooked
40.0	1/2	cup	Brussels Sprouts, Cooked

Nutripoints	Serving Size		Food Name—Vegetables
39.5	1	cup	Cress, Garden, Cooked
39.0	1	cup	Cabbage, Common, Raw, Shredded
39.0	1	cup	Broccoli, Organic, Fzn, Cascadian Farm
38.5	8	stalks	Asparagus, Marinated, Nutripoint Recipe
38.5	1	cup	Broccoli, Cooked
38.5	1	cup	Kale, Chopped, Cooked
37.5	2	whole	Green Pepper, Raw
37.0	1	cup	Cauliflower, Cooked
36.0	1	cup	Broccoli, Carrots, and Cauliflower, Fzn, Pictsweet
35.5	1	cup	Chicory Greens, Raw
35.5	3/4	cup	Spinach, Early Garden, Canned, Del Monte
35.5	1	whole	Carrots, Raw
34.0	2	cups	Lettuce, Butterhead/Boston/Bibb, chopped
33.0	1	cup	Broccoli, Cauliflower and Carrots, Fzn, Green Giant
33.0	1	cup	Salad, Tossed, No Dressing
32.5	1	cup	Mushrooms, Fresh
32.5	8	stalks	Asparagus, Canned
31.5	1	cup	Cabbage, Common, Chopped, Cooked
31.0	1/2	cup	Broccoli, Baby Carrots, & Water Chestnuts, Fzn, Birds Eye
31.0	1/2	cup	Okra, Cooked
30.5	1	cup	Broccoli, Cauliflower and Carrots, Fzn, Birds Eye
30.5	10	pieces	Lettuce, Loose leaf
30.0	1	whole	Tomato, Fresh
30.0	1/2	cup	Carrots, Sliced, Cooked
30.0	6	fl oz	Juice, V8 , Essential Antioxidants
29.5	1	cup	Spinach, Leaf, No Salt Added, Canned, Del Monte
29.5	1	cup	Cabbage, Red, Raw, Shredded
29.0	1	cup	Radishes, Raw
29.0	6	pieces	Gummies, Juice Plus+® , Veggie
29.0	1	serving	Wendy's Side Salad
28.5	6	fl oz	Juice, V8 Vegetable, No Salt Added
28.0	½	cup	Peas and Carrots, Frozen, Cooked
27.0	8	fl oz	Juice, V8 , Bone Health
27.0	½	cup	Brussels Sprouts, Frozen, Cooked
27.0	8	stalks	Asparagus, Frozen, Cooked
26.5	½	cup	Squash, Butternut, Baked
26.0	6	fl oz	Juice, V8 Vegetable, Spicy
26.0	1	cup	Okra, Raw
26.0	6	fl oz	Juice, Tomato, Low Sodium
25.5	½	cup	Pumpkin, Canned
25.0	½	cup	Brussels Sprouts, Baby, Fzn, Seabrook Farms
25.0	½	cup	Peas and Carrots, Canned
24.5	1	cup	Squash, Summer, Cooked

Nutripoints	Serving Size		Food Name—Vegetables
24.5	1	cup	Cabbage, Savoy, Raw, Shredded
24.5	1/2	cup	Broccoli, Sweet Peas, and Carrots, Fzn, Green Giant
24.5	6	fl oz	Juice, V8 Vegetable
24.5	2	cups	Kohlrabi, Raw
24.5	6	fl oz	Juice, Tomato
24.5	1	cup	Beans, Green Cooked
24.0	10	pieces	Scallions
23.5	1	cup	Soup, Spinach, Clear, Nutripoint Recipe
23.5	1 1/2	cups	Broccoli Florets, Fzn, 365 Organic , Whole Foods
23.0	1	cup	Cauliflower, Fzn, Birds Eye
23.0	1/2	cup	Squash, Winter, Cooked, Fzn, Birds Eye
23.0	1/2	cup	Tomatoes, Canned
22.0	1/2	cup	Vegetables, Mixed, Canned
21.5	1	cup	Salad, Tossed, w/Tomato
21.0	1/2	cup	Mixed Vegetables, Fzn, Veg-All
20.0	8	stalks	Celery, Raw
20.0	1	whole	Cucumber, Raw
20.0	1/2	cup	Spinach, Cut Leaf, In Butter, Fzn, Green Giant
20.0	1/4	cup	Tomato Paste, Canned
19.5	1	cup	Turnips, Cooked
19.0	1/2	cup	Sauce, Tomato, Nutripoint Recipe
19.0	1	cup	Mushrooms, Cooked
18.5	1	cup	Lettuce and Tomato
18.5	1/2	cup	Mixed Vegetables, Natural Pack, Canned, Libby's
18.0	1/2	cup	Kelp
18.0	1/2	cup	Turnips, Raw
18.0	1/2	cup	Rutabagas, Cooked
18.0	10	pieces	Lettuce, Iceberg
18.0	1/2	cup	Vegetables, Custom Cuisine w/Dijon, Fzn, Birds Eye
18.0	1/2	cup	Vegetables, Mixed, Frozen, Cooked
18.0	1/2	cup	Vegetables, Mixed, Fzn, Birds Eye
17.5	1/2	cup	Pumpkin, Cooked
17.5	2	cups	Alfalfa Sprouts, Raw
17.5	1/2	cup	Sauce, Tomato, Canned
17.0	3/4	cup	Broccoli, Carrots, and Red Peppers, Fzn, Birds Eye
17.0	1/2	cup	Bamboo Shoots, Raw
17.0	1	cup	Sauerkraut, Canned
17.0	1/2	cup	Salad, Mixed Vegetable, Nutripoint Recipe
17.0	1/2	cup	Eggplant, Cooked
17.0	1/2	cup	Broccoli, Corn and Red Peppers, Fzn, Birds Eye
16.5	1/2	serving	Wendy's Garden Salad (take out)
16.5	1	cup	Bamboo Shoots, Canned
16.0	1/2	cup	Squash, Winter, Baked

Nutripoints	Serving Size		Food Name—Vegetables
16.0	6	fl oz	Juice, Just Carrot, Naked Juice
16.0	2	whole	Leeks, Raw
16.0	1	cup	Zucchini, Raw
16.0	1	cup	Mixed Vegetables, Organic, Fzn, Cascadian Farm
15.5	1	cup	Beans, Green, Cut, Fzn, Birds Eye (Large Portion)
15.5	1/2	cup	Sauce, Tomato, Thick & Zesty, Contadina
15.0	1	cup	Zucchini, Cooked
15.0	6	fl oz	Juice, Carrot
14.5	1	cup	Asparagus, 50-Percent Less Salt, Canned, Green Giant
14.0	1	cup	Tomatoes, Peeled, Del Monte
14.0	1/2	cup	Asparagus, Cuts, Canned, Green Giant
13.5	1/2	cup	Vegetable Stir Fry, Nutripoint Recipe
13.5	1/2	cup	Beans, Yellow Snap, Cooked
13.5	1	Tbls	Wendy's Crushed Red Peppers
13.5	1	cup	Beans, Green, Cut, No Salt Added, Canned, Del Monte
13.0	1	cup	Soup, Vegetable, No Salt, Health Valley
13.0	1	cup	Alfalfa Sprouts, Arrowhead Mills
13.0	1	cup	Mushrooms, Canned, Green Giant
13.0	1/2	cup	Broccoli, Caul. & Carrots w/Cheese Sauce, Fzn, Birds Eye
13.0	1/2	cup	Broccoli, Caul. & Carrots w/Cheese Sauce, Green Giant
13.0	1	cup	Beans, Green, Whole, Canned, Del Monte
12.5	1	cup	Vegetarian Stew
12.5	1/4	cup	Tomato Paste, Contadina
12.5	1	cup	Soup, Vegetable, Health Valley
12.5	1/2	cup	Beans, Green, Cut, Fzn, Birds Eye (small portion)
12.5	1	whole	Artichoke, Cooked
12.0	1/2	piece	Sweet Potato/Yam, Baked
12.0	1/2	cup	Soup, Tomato, No Salt, Health Valley
12.0	1/2	cup	Brussels Sprouts w/Butter, Fzn, Green Giant
12.0	3/4	cup	Juice, Tomato, Campbell's
12.0	1	cup	Soup, Vegetable
11.5	2/3	cup	Mixed Vegetables, Fzn, 365 Organic , Whole Foods
11.5	1/2	cup	Parsnips, Raw
11.5	1/2	cup	Squash, Acorn, Baked
11.5	1/2	cup	Soup, Tomato, Health Valley
11.0	1	cup	Soup, Chunky 5 Bean Vegetable, Health Valley
11.0	1/2	cup	Beets, Cooked
10.5	1/2	cup	Sauce, Tomato, Del Monte
10.0	1/2	cup	Coleslaw, Bavarian, Nutripoint Recipe
9.5	1/2	cup	Sauce, Spaghetti, Pritikin
9.0	1/2	cup	Sauce, Tomato, Hunts
9.0	1/2	cup	Potato Salad, Nutripoint Recipe
8.5	1/2	cup	Onion, Raw

Nutripoints	Serving Size		Food Name—Vegetables
8.5	1/4	cup	Shallots, Raw
8.5	1/2	potato	Potato, Baked
8.5	1	serving	Carl's Jr. Garden Salad to Go
8.5	1/2	cup	Parsnips, Cooked
8.0	1/2	cup	Corn, Frozen, Cooked
8.0	1	cup	Beans, Green 50-Percent Less Salt, Canned, Green Giant
8.0	1/2	yam	Sweet Potato/Yam, Canned
8.0	1/2	cup	Celeriac, Raw
7.5	1/2	cup	Mixed Vegetables, w/Butter, Fzn, Green Giant
7.5	1/2	cup	Succotash, Cooked
7.5	1	cup	Leeks, Cooked
7.5	1/2	cup	Beets, Canned, Cooked
7.0	1/2	cup	Vegetables, Pasta Primavera Style, Fzn, Birds Eye
7.0	1/2	cup	Succotash, Frozen, Cooked
7.0	8	fl oz	Juice, V8 Splash
7.0	1	cup	Soup, Healthy Request, Vegetable, Campbell's
7.0	1/2	cup	Tomatoes, Stewed, Hunts
7.0	1	piece	Corn, Little Ears, Fzn, Birds Eye
6.5	1	cup	Soup, Tomato w/ Vegetables, Progresso
6.5	1	cup	Soup, Vegetable, Pritikin
6.0	1/2	cup	Corn, Golden, Family Style, No Salt, Canned, Del Monte
6.0	1/2	cup	Broccoli Spears, w/Butter Sauce, Fzn, Green Giant
6.0	1/2	cup	Cauliflower, Cheese Sauce, Fzn, Green Giant
6.0	1/2	cup	Corn, Sweet, Fzn, Birds Eye
6.0	1/4	serving	Wendy's Chef Salad (take out)
6.0	1/2	piece	Corn On Cob, Fresh, Cooked
5.5	1	burger	Hamburger, Garden Veggie Patties, Morningstar Farms
5.5	1/2	cup	Potatoes, Homestyle, Nutripoint Recipe
5.5	1/4	cup	Flour, Potato
5.5	1	cup	Water Chestnuts, Canned
5.0	1	cup	Soup, Broccoli, Creamy Organic, Imagine Foods
5.0	1	cup	Soup, Chunky Vegetable, Campbell's
5.0	2/3	cup	Broc/Caul/Carrots/97% Fat-Free Sauce, Fzn, Green Giant
5.0	1	cup	Soup, Minestrone
5.0	1/2	cup	Corn w/Red and Green Peppers, Canned
4.5	1	cup	Beans, Green, Kitchen Cut, Canned, Green Giant
4.5	8	wt oz	Soup, Vegetarian Vegetable, Campbell's
4.5	1/2	cup	Corn, Creamed, Canned
4.5	1	cup	Soup, Vegetable Beef
4.5	1	cup	Soup, Garden Vegetable, Healthy Choice
4.5	1/2	portion	Vegetables, Spring, Cheese Sauce, Fzn, Budget Gourmet
4.5	1/4	Potato	Wendy's Hot Stuffed Potato
4.5	1/2	Cup	Corn, Canned

Nutripoints	Serving Size		Food Name—Vegetables
4.0	1/2	cup	Salad, Spinach, w/Egg/Bacon/Tomato
4.0	1/2	piece	Carl's Jr. Chef Salad (take-Out)
4.0	1/2	piece	Sweet Potatoes, Candied
4.0	1/2	cup	Sauce, Spaghetti, Meatless, Aunt Millie's
4.0	1/2	cup	Sauce, Spaghetti, No Salt Added, Prego
4.0	1/4	portion	Eggplant Rollettes, Fzn, Celentano
3.5	1	cup	Beans, Green, French Style Cut, Canned, Green Giant
3.5	1/2	cup	Sauce, Spaghetti, w/Pepperoni/Sausage, Aunt Millie's
3.5	1	cup	Soup, Minestrone, Campbell's
3.5	1/2	cup	Poi
3.5	1	cup	Soup, Chunky Minestrone, Campbell's
3.5	1/2	cup	Beets, Pickled, Canned
3.0	1/2	portion	Spinach, Au Gratin, Fzn, Budget Gourmet
3.0	1/2	cup	Sauce, Spaghetti, w/Mushrooms, Homestyle, Ragu
3.0	1/2	piece	Carl's Jr. Lite Potato
3.0	1/4	portion	Eggplant Parmigiana, Fzn, Celentano
3.0	1/2	cup	Coleslaw
3.0	1/2	cup	Corn, 50% Less Salt, Canned, Green Giant
3.0	1	cup	Soup, Vegetable, 1/3 Less Salt, Campbell's
3.0	2	whole	Pickles, Kosher Crunchy Dills, Half/Salt Vlasic
3.0	1/2	cup	Beans, Green, French Cut, In Butter, Green Giant
3.0	1/4	cup	Artichoke Hearts, Marinated
3.0	1/2	cup	Vegetables, Italian Style, Fzn, Birds Eye
2.5	1/2	cup	Kentucky Fried Chicken, Corn
2.5	1/2	cup	Soup, Tomato Minestrone, Couscous, Nile Spice Foods
2.5	1/2	cup	Corn, Whole Kernel, Canned, Green Giant
2.5	1/2	serving	Moroccan Stew, Organic, Fzn, Moosewood
2.5	1	cup	Carl's Jr. Lumber Jack Mix Vegetable Soup
2.5	2	cups	Popcorn, Gourmet, O. Redenbacher
2.5	1/2	cup	Soup, Vegetable Parmesan, Couscous, Nile Spice Foods
2.5	1	cup	Soup, Tomato
2.5	1/2	cup	Vegetables, Japanese Style, Fzn, Birds Eye
2.5	1	whole	Pickles, Sweet 'n Sour, Claussen
2.5	1/4	cup	Potatoes, Au Gratin
2.0	1	cup	Soup, Vegetable, Campbell's
2.0	1/4	cup	Potatoes, Scalloped
2.0	1/4	cup	Wendy's Deluxe Three Bean Salad
2.0	20	chips	Potato Chips, Lay's Light, Nonfat
2.0	1/2	cup	Soup, Squash, Creamy Organic, Imagine Foods
2.0	1/2	cup	Corn, Whole Kernel, Canned, Del Monte
2.0	1	cup	Soup Mix, Country Vegetable, Lipton

- - -

2.0	1/4	serving	Carl's Jr. Broccoli and Cheese Potato

Nutripoints	Serving Size		Food Name—Vegetables
2.0	1/4	cup	Potatoes, Mashed, From Flakes
2.0	1/2	portion	Cauliflower, Cheddar Cheese Sauce, Fzn, Budget Gourmet
2.0	1/2	portion	Broccoli w/Cheddar Cheese Sauce, Fzn, Stouffer's
1.5	1/4	potato	Wendy's Hot Stuffed Potato w/Broccoli & Cheese
1.5	1/4	serving	Carl's Jr. Taco Salad to Go
1.5	1/2	cup	Corn, Niblets, In Butter, Fzn, Green Giant
1.5	1/2	cup	Goulash
1.5	1/2	cup	Kentucky Fried Chicken , Cole Slaw
1.5	12	chips	Potato Chips, Baked Lay's
1.5	1/4	serving	Taco Bell Tostada Red Sauce
1.5	1/2	portion	Cabbage Roll, Frozen Dinner
1.5	1/4	cup	Taco Salad
1.5	1/4	serving	Taco Bell Tostada Green Sauce
1.5	1/4	portion	Potato, Baked, Broccoli & Cheese, Fzn, Weight Watchers
1.5	17	chips	Potato Chips, Ruffles Light, Nonfat
1.5	1/2	portion	Potatoes, Cheddared, w/Broccoli, Fzn, Budget Gourmet
1.5	1/4	cup	Broccoli, Fried, w/Breading
1.5	1/4	portion	Potato, Baked, Chicken Divan, Fzn, Weight Watchers
1.5	1	cup	Gazpacho
1.0	1	portion	Ratatouille, Frozen Dinner
1.0	1/2	cup	Soup, Cream of Asparagus
1.0	1/4	serving	Tostada
1.0	1/4	cup	Potatoes, Mashed, Home Recipe
1.0	1/4	cup	Okra, Fried w/Breading
1.0	9	chips	Potato Chips, Light, Ruffles
1.0	20	chips	Potato Chips, Lay's Light, BBQ, Nonfat
1.0	16	chips	Potato Chips, Pringles Fat Free
1.0	1	serving	McDonald's Side Salad
1.0	1/2	cup	Soup, Tomato, Low Sodium, w/Pieces, Campbell's
1.0	1/4	cup	Wendy's California Coleslaw
1.0	1/2	cup	Carl's Jr. Cream of Broccoli Soup
1.0	1/4	serving	Carl's Jr. Sour Cream & Chive Potato
1.0	2	Tbls	Catsup
1.0	4	pieces	French Fries (18 pc=.5 c)
0.5	1	cup	Broth, Vegetable Organic, Imagine Foods
0.5	1/2	cup	Soup Mix, Green Pea, Cup-A-Soup, Lipton
0.5	1/4	serving	Wendy's Spring Mix Salad
0.5	1	cup	Soup, Tomato, Campbell's
0.5	2	Tbls	Catsup, Tomato, Del Monte
0.5	1/2	cup	Sauce, Spaghetti, w/Mushrooms, Prego
0.5	1/4	serving	Taco Bell Taco Salad w/Salsa w/o Shell
0.5	2	whole	Pickles, Kosher Dill Spears, Vlasic
0.5	11	chips	Tortilla Chips, Doritos, Light, Lowfat, Nacho Cheese

Nutripoints	Serving Size		Food Name—Vegetables
0.5	1/3	serving	Wendy's Caesar Side Salad
0.5	1/4	serving	Carl's Jr. Cheese Potato
0.5	1/2	cup	Vegetables, San Francisco Style, Fzn, Birds Eye
0.5	2	Tbls	Catsup, Low Sodium/Sugar
0.5	1	cup	Soup, Tomato, 1/3 Less Salt, Campbell's
0.5	1/4	serving	Carl's Jr. Fiesta Potato
0.5	1/2	serving	McDonald's Garden Salad
0.5	1/2	cup	Sauce, Spaghetti, Prego
0.5	1/4	cup	Potatoes, Hash Browned
0.5	1/2	cup	Soup, Potato
0.5	1/2	portion	Potatoes, Scalloped, Fzn, Stouffer's
0.5	1/2	portion	Soufflé, Corn, Fzn, Stouffer's
0.5	1/2	cup	Potatoes, Golden Crinkles, Ore-Ida
0.0	1/4	serving	Taco Bell Taco Salad w/o Shell
0.0	8	chips	Potato Chips, Unsalted, Lay's
0.0	1/2	cup	Corn, Cream Style, Golden Sweet, Canned, Del Monte
0.0	1/4	cup	Potatoes, Instant Mashed, Hungry Jack
0.0	1/2	cup	Sauce, Spaghetti, Plain, Extra Thick & Zesty, Ragu
0.0	1/2	cup	Soup, Tomato w/Milk, 1/3 Less Salt, Campbell's
0.0	5	chips	Potato Chips
0.0	1/4	cup	Potato Sticks, Shoestring
0.0	1/4	serving	Taco Bell Taco Salad w/Salsa w/Shell
0.0	8	chips	Potato Chips, Lay's
0.0	1/2	cup	Sauce, Spaghetti, w/Meat, Ragu
0.0	1/4	serving	Wendy's Hot Stuffed Potato w/Sour Cream & Chives
0.0	1/2	cup	Sauce, Spaghetti, Plain, Ragu
0.0	9	chips	Potato Chips, Ruffles
0.0	2	pieces	Onion Rings, Fried
-0.5	1/4	cup	Potatoes, Tater Tots, Ore-Ida
-0.5	1/4	serving	Wendy's Hot Stuffed Potato w/Bacon & Cheese
-0.5	1/2	cup	Corn, Cream Style, Canned, Green Giant
-0.5	1/4	serving	Corn, Fried w/Breading
-0.5	1/4	cup	Potatoes, Au Gratin, Betty Crocker
-0.5	3	Tbls	Sauce, Traditional Pizza Quick, Ragu
-0.5	1/2	cup	Soup, Cream of Celery
-0.5	1/2	cup	Sauce, Spaghetti, Extra Thick & Zesty, w/Meat, Ragu
-0.5	2	cup	Popcorn, Gourmet, Microwave, O. Redenbacher
-0.5	1/4	cup	Potatoes, Instant Mashed, Betty Crocker
-0.5	1/4	serving	McDonald's Regular French Fries
-0.5	1/4	cup	Sauce, Spaghetti, Garden Tomato w/Mushroom, Prego
-0.5	1/4	serving	McDonald's Chef Salad
-0.5	1/4	cup	Sauce, Spaghetti, Extra Chunky Mushroom/Onion, Prego
-0.5	1	cup	Jack In the Box Side Salad

Nutripoints	Serving Size		Food Name—Vegetables
-0.5	1/4	cup	Cauliflower, Fried w/Breading
-0.5	1/3	serving	Corn, Sweet, Butter Sauce, Fzn, Budget Gourmet
-0.5	1/2	portion	Potatoes, Au Gratin, Fzn, Stouffer's
-0.5	1/4	serving	Jack In the Box Mexican Chicken Salad
-0.5	1/4	serving	Carl's Jr. Bacon and Cheese Potato
-0.5	1/4	cup	Wendy's Old Fashioned Corn Relish
-1.0	1/2	cup	Soup, Tomato w/Milk, Campbell's
-1.0	1/2	cup	Potato Chips, Light, Pringle's
-1.0	1	piece	Carl's Jr. Onion Rings
-1.0	1/4	cup	Sauce, Spaghetti, Meat Flavor, Prego
-1.0	0.25	cup	Potato Salad, Home Recipe
-1.0	5	chips	Potato Chips, Wise
-1.0	17	chips	Corn Chips, Fritos
-1.0	1	serving	Carl's Jr. Fried Zucchini
-1.0	1	cup	Soup, Creamy Natural Broccoli, Campbell's
-1.0	1/4	cup	Mushrooms, Fried w/Breading
-1.0	1/4	cup	Squash, Fried, w/Breading
-1.0	8	slices	Pickles, Bread 'n Butter, Cucumber Slices, Heinz
-1.0	1/4	cup	Soup, Cream of Mushroom
-1.0	1/2	cup	Soup, Creamy Natural Broccoli w/Milk, Campbell's
-1.0	1/4	cup	Soup, Mushroom, Cream Of, Campbell's
-1.0	1/4	serving	Jack In the Box Taco Salad
-1.5	2	pieces	Carl's Jr. Hash Browns Nuggets
-1.5	1/2	cup	Salad, Chef, w/Ham/Cheese, w/o Dressing
-1.5	1	cup	Soup, Onion
-1.5	1/4	cup	Wendy's Red Bliss Potato Salad
-1.5	1/2	cup	Potato Chips, Sour Cream 'n Onion, Pringle's
-1.5	1	cup	Soup, Tomato Rice, Old Fashioned, Campbell's
-1.5	1/2	cup	Potato Chips, Pringle's
-2.0	1	serving	Jack In the Box Hash Browns
-2.0	1/2	serving	McDonald's Hashbrown Potatoes
-2.0	1/4	serving	Wendy's Hot Stuffed Potato w/Cheese
-2.0	1	cup	Soup, Cream of Mushroom, 1/3 Less Salt, Campbell's
-2.0	1/4	cup	Rhubarb, Cooked, w/Sugar
-2.5	1/4	serving	Jack In the Box Chef Salad
-2.5	1/4	serving	Pie, Rhubarb, Homemade
-2.5	2	Tbls	Relish, Hot Dog, Vlasic
-2.5	1/2	cup	Soup, Creamy Natural Potato w/Milk, Campbell's
-2.5	1	cup	Soup Mix, Cream of Mushroom, Cup-A-Soup, Lipton
-2.5	1	cup	Soup Mix, Tomato, Cup-A-Soup, Lipton
-2.5	1/2	cup	Kentucky Fried Chicken, Mashed Potatoes
-2.5	1	whole	Pickles, Sweet Gherkins, Heinz
-3.0	1/2	cup	Soufflé, Spinach

Nutripoints	Serving Size		Food Name—Vegetables
-3.0	1	cup	Soup, Cream of Celery, Campbell's
-3.5	2	Tbls	Relish, Sweet, Heinz
-3.5	1	cup	Soup, French Onion, Campbell's
-3.5	2	whole	Pickles, Dill
-4.0	2	whole	Pickles, Kosher, Claussen
-4.0	1/2	cup	Soup, Creamy Natural Potato, Campbell's
-4.5	1	cup	Soup, Cream of Mushroom, Campbell's
-5.0	1	whole	Pickles, Sweet
-5.5	1	cup	Soup Mix, Onion, Lipton
-6.0	2	Tbls	Pickle Relish

FRUIT GROUP

Nutripoints	Serving Size		Food Name—Fruits
34.0	6	pieces	Gummies, Juice Plus+®, Fruit
29.0	1/4	melon	Melon, Cantaloupe
26.5	8	fl oz	Fruit Drink, Fuze White Tea (*)
24.5	16	fl oz	Juice, V8 Splash, Diet, All Flavors
24.5	16	fl oz	Sports Drink, Motion Potion (*)
22.5	6	fl oz	Juice, Blue Machine, Naked Juice (*)
22.0	16	wt oz	Juice, Kombucha Organic (*)
22.0	16	wt oz	Juice, Synergy Organic Elixir (*)
22.0	8	fl oz	ViaViente Nutritional Drink (*)
22.0	8	fl oz	Fruit Drink, Fuze Green Tea (*)
22.0	8	fl oz	Juice, Orange, Light 'n Healthy, Tropicana
21.0	1	whole	Guava
20.5	1/2	fruit	Papaya
20.0	1	cup	Fruit Slices, Fresh, Nutripoint Recipe
19.0	1	cup	Strawberries, Fresh
19.0	3/4	cup	Currants, Black
18.0	1/2	cup	Fruit, Rainbow Compote, Nutripoint Recipe
18.0	8	fl oz	Fruit Drink, Fuze Replenish (*)
17.5	1/2	fruit	Mango
17.5	8	fl oz	Juice, Orange Light, Minute Maid
17.0	1	whole	Kiwi Fruit
17.0	1	cup	Strawberries, Frozen, Unsweetened
16.5	1/2	cup	Fruit Platter, Fresh, Nutripoint Recipe
16.5	1	cup	Strawberries, Organic, Fzn, Cascadian Farm
16.0	6	whole	Litchi, Fresh
15.5	1/2	cup	Fruit Drink, Sunrise Cooler, Nutripoint Recipe
15.5	1/2	cup	Mandarin Oranges, Canned, Unsweetened
15.0	6	fl oz	Juice, Orange w/C, E, Zinc, Minute Maid
15.0	8	fl oz	Fruit Drink, Fuze Refresh (*)
15.0	10.5	fl oz	Smoothie, Slim-Fast Optima (*)
14.5	3	wt oz	Currants, Red, Raw
14.5	1/2	cup	Fruit Salad Plate, Nutripoint Recipe
14.0	1/4	melon	Melon, Honeydew
14.0	1/2	cup	Plums, Canned, Unsweetened
13.5	1	whole	Orange, Fresh
13.5	3	whole	Apricot, Fresh
13.0	1	cup	Fruit Drink, Strawberry Smoothie, Nutripoint Recipe
13.0	1	whole	Tangerine
13.0	1/2	fruit	Grapefruit, Fresh
13.0	1/2	cup	Blackberries, Fresh

Nutripoints	Serving Size		Food Name—Fruits
13.0	1	cup	Berries, Fresh, Nutripoint Recipe
13.0	6	fl oz	Juice, Orange, Healthy Heart, Tropicana
13.0	1/2	cup	Fruit Salad, Fresh
13.0	6	fl oz	Juice, Just Apple, Naked Juice
13.0	6	fl oz	Juice, Red Machine, Naked Juice
12.5	6	fl oz	Juice, Orange, Immunity Defense, Tropicana
12.5	1	cup	Juice, Cranberry, Low Cal
12.5	1	whole	Carambola (starfruit)
12.5	8	fl oz	Vitamin Water, Stress-B Lemon-Lime, Glaceau(*)
12.5	8	fl oz	Juice, Cranapple, Low Cal, Ocean Spray
12.5	1/2	cup	Raspberries, Fresh
12.0	3	wt oz	Elderberry, Raw
12.0	6	fl oz	Juice, Orange, Kids+, Minute Maid
12.0	6	fl oz	Juice, Just Grapefruit, Naked Juice
12.0	6	fl oz	Juice, Orange, Healthy Kids, Tropicana
11.5	8	fl oz	Juice, V8 Splash, Mango Peach
11.5	6	fl oz	Juice, Orange, Fresh Squeezed
11.5	6	fl oz	Juice, Tropical Blend, Vruit
11.5	6	fl oz	Juice, Orange, Home Squeezed + Calc. & D, Minute Maid
11.5	6	fl oz	Juice, Just Fresh O-J, Naked Juice
11.5	6	fl oz	Juice, Orange, Heartwise, Minute Maid
11.0	1	whole	Peach, Fresh
11.0	6	fl oz	Juice, Orange, Tropicana
11.0	6	fl oz	Juice, Just O-J, Naked Juice
11.0	8	fl oz	Fruit Drink, Fuze Vitaboost (*)
11.0	6	fl oz	Juice, Orange, Low Acid, Tropicana
11.0	1/4	melon	Melon, Casaba
11.0	6	fl oz	Juice, Green, Machine, Naked Juice
11.0	6	fl oz	Juice, Orange Tangerine, Minute Maid
11.0	6	pieces	Apricots, Dried
11.0	6	fl oz	Juice, Grapefruit, Unsweetened
11.0	8	fl oz	Juice, V8 Splash, Tropical Blend
11.0	6	fl oz	Juice, Orange, Calcium Fortified, Minute Maid
11.0	1/2	cup	Apricots, Canned, Unsweetened
11.0	1	cup	Gelatin, Holiday Dessert
11.0	6	fl oz	Juice, Orange, Frozen, Reconstituted
11.0	6	fl oz	Fruit Drink, Snapple-A-Day Meal Replacement (*)
10.5	6	fl oz	Juice, Orange, w/Calcium, Citrus Hill
10.5	1	cup	Watermelon
10.5	1/2	cup	Peaches, Canned, Unsweetened
10.5	1/2	portion	Apples, Glazed, Raspberry Sauce, Fzn, Budget Gourmet
10.5	8	fl oz	Juice, Cranberry, Low Cal, Ocean Spray
10.0	6	fl oz	Juice, Orange-Grapefruit, Unsweetened, Canned

Nutripoints	Serving Size		Food Name—Fruits
10.0	6	fl oz	Juice, Orange, Fzn, Minute Maid
10.0	1	whole	Prickly pear
10.0	6	whole	Kumquats
10.0	1/2	cup	Fruit Cocktail, Canned, Unsweetened
10.0	1	whole	Nectarine, Fresh
10.0	1	cup	Cranberry, Raw
10.0	3	wt oz	Bilberry, Raw
10.0	5	whole	Loquat, Fresh
9.5	6	fl oz	Juice, Orange-Pineapple
9.5	6	fl oz	Juice, Orange, Home Squeezed, Minute Maid
9.5	6	fl oz	Juice, Orange, Low Acid, Minute Maid
9.5	8	fl oz	Juice, V8 Splash Smoothies, All Flavors
9.5	8	fl oz	Fruit Drink, Fuze Focus (*)
9.0	1/2	cup	Boysenberries, Frozen
9.0	1/2	cup	Topping, Red Raspberry, Hot, Nutripoint Recipe
9.0	2	whole	Passion Fruit, Purple, Fresh
9.0	6	fl oz	Juice, Orange Passion, Minute Maid
8.5	1/2	serving	Wendy's Fresh Fruit Bowl
8.5	3/4	cup	Blackberry Freeze, Nutripoint Recipe
8.5	1/2	cup	Strawberries, Halved, Light Syrup, Fzn, Birds Eye
8.0	6	pieces	Apricots, Dried, Sun-Maid
8.0	6	fl oz	Juice, Grapefruit, Ocean Spray
8.0	1/2	cup	Pineapple, Fresh
7.5	6	pieces	Apricots, Dried, Del Monte
7.5	1/2	cup	Cherries, Sour, Canned, Unsweetened
7.5	1/2	cup	Blackberries, Frozen, Unsweetened
7.5	10	pieces	Cherries, Sour, Raw
7.5	1/2	fruit	Banana
7.5	4	fl oz	Juice, Verry Pro-Berry, Naked Juice
7.5	1	whole	Persimmon
7.0	6	fl oz	Juice, Cranberry Cocktail, Ocean Spray
7.0	6	fl oz	Juice, Mighty Mango, Naked Juice (*)
7.0	1/2	cup	Topping, Peach, Hot, Nutripoint Recipe
7.0	6	fl oz	Juice, Grapefruit, Sweetened
7.0	6	fl oz	Juice, Tropical Orange, Tropicana
7.0	1/2	cup	Blueberries, Fresh
6.5	1/2	cup	Prunes, Cooked, Unsweetened
6.5	1/2	cup	Frozen Dessert, Peach, Vitari Soft Serve
6.5	8	fl oz	Juice, SoBe Synergy
6.5	8	fl oz	Fruit Drink, SoBe Elixir 3C, Orange Carrot (*)
6.5	1	cup	Peaches, Canned In Juice
6.5	1	bar	Snack Bar, Think! Bar (*)
6.5	1/2	cup	Strawberries, Frozen, Sweetened

Nutripoints	Serving Size		Food Name—Fruits
6.5	1/2	cup	Peaches, Light Yellow Cling, Fruit Juice, Canned, Libby's
6.5	8	fl oz	Fruit Drink, Fuze Lemon AID (*)
6.0	3	prunes	Prunes, Whole, Sunsweet
6.0	1/3	cup	Banana Gladje, Nutripoint Recipe
6.0	2	whole	Plum, Fresh
6.0	1	whole	Quince
6.0	1/2	fruit	Plantain, Fresh
6.0	4	fl oz	Juice, Protein Zone, Naked Juice
6.0	3/4	cup	Soup, Blueberry, Chilled, Nutripoint Recipe
6.0	6	fl oz	Juice, Grapefruit, Pink, Ocean Spray
6.0	8	fl oz	Vitamin Water, Essential Orange-Orange, Glaceau (*)
6.0	4	prunes	Prunes, Dried
6.0	6	fl oz	Juice, Pineapple, Unsweetened, Canned
5.5	1/2	cup	Cherries, Sweet, Canned, Water
5.5	1/2	cup	Plantain, Cooked
5.5	6	fl oz	Juice, Grape, Unsweetened, Fzn, Welch's
5.5	6	fl oz	Juice, Grape, Unsweetened
5.5	16	fl oz	Fruit Drink, SoBe Lean (*)
5.5	8	fl oz	Vitamin Water, Formula 50 Grape, Glaceau (*)
5.5	10	whole	Cherries, Sweet, Fresh
5.0	8	fl oz	Fruit Drink, Fuze Energize (*)
5.0	6	fl oz	Juice, Pineapple, Dole
5.0	1/4	cup	Strawberries, Fzn, Heavy Syrup, Birds Eye
5.0	4	fl oz	Juice, Prune, Canned
5.0	2	figs	Figs, Dried
5.0	1/2	cup	Mandarin Oranges, Canned
5.0	1/2	cup	Fruit Cocktail, Hot, Nutripoint Recipe
5.0	1	wt oz	Prunes, Pitted, Bite Size, Sunsweet
5.0	4	pieces	Peaches, Dried, Sun-Maid
5.0	2	pieces	Peaches, Dried, Sulfured, Uncooked
4.5	4	fl oz	Apricot Nectar, Canned
4.5	1/2	cup	Blueberries, Frozen, Unsweetened
4.5	1/4	cup	Currants, Zante
4.5	1/2	cup	Frozen Dessert, Orange, Vitari Soft Serve
4.5	1/4	cup	Prunes, Canned, Heavy Syrup
4.5	1	whole	Pear, Fresh
4.5	8	fl oz	Fruit Drink, Hawaiian Punch, Low Cal
4.5	1	bar	Snack Bar, SnackWells (*)
4.5	6	fl oz	Juice, Apple, Fzn, Seneca
4.5	6	fl oz	Juice, Kiwi, Sweetened, Kiwi Island
4.5	1/4	cup	Raspberries, Frozen, Sweetened
4.5	1/4	cup	Guacamole
4.5	2	figs	Figs, Mission, Sun-Maid

Nutripoints	Serving Size		Food Name—Fruits
4.5	20	grapes	Grapes, Raw
4.5	1	whole	Apple, Fresh
4.0	1/2	cup	Pineapple, Chunks, In Juice, Canned, Del Monte
4.0	1/2	cup	Pineapple, Sliced, In Juice, Canned, Del Monte
4.0	2	figs	Figs, Calimyrna, Sun-Maid
4.0	1/4	fruit	Avocado, Florida
4.0	1	whole	Figs, Fresh
4.0	8	fl oz	Fruit Shake, Melaleuca Sustain
4.0	8	fl oz	Sports Drink, Bodyfuel
4.0	1/2	serving	Pear, Poached, Nutripoint Recipe
4.0	1/2	cup	Pineapple, Sliced, In Juice, Canned, Dole
4.0	1/4	cup	Raisins
4.0	4	fl oz	Juice, Prune, Sunsweet
4.0	1/4	cup	Prunes, Cooked, w/Sugar
4.0	6	fl oz	Peach Nectar, Canned
4.0	1/2	cup	Peaches, Yellow Cling, Light Syrup, Canned, Del Monte
4.0	6	fl oz	Papaya Nectar, Canned
4.0	5	dates	Dates
3.5	1	whole	Pomegranate
3.5	6	fl oz	Fruit Drink, Citrus Punch, Sunny Delite
3.5	2	wt oz	Mixed Fruits, Dried, Sun-Maid
3.5	1/2	cup	Applesauce, No Sugar
3.5	6	fl oz	Juice, Cranberry, Sweetened
3.5	1	wt oz	Fruit Bits, Dried, Sun-Maid
3.5	6	fl oz	Juice, Mango Nectar, Kern's
3.5	6	fl oz	Juice, Strawberry/Banana Nectar, Kern's
3.5	6	fl oz	Juice, Grape, Red, Welch's
3.5	6	fl oz	Juice, Grape, Purple, Welch's
3.5	1/2	cup	Pears, Canned No Sugar
3.5	1/4	cup	Currants, Zante, Sun-Maid
3.5	1/2	cup	Frozen Dessert, Wild Berry, Vitari Soft Serve
3.0	6	fl oz	Fruit Drink, Guava, Ocean Spray
3.0	1/2	cup	Frozen Dessert, Strawberry, Vitari Soft Serve
3.0	1/2	cup	Applesauce, Nutripoint Recipe
3.0	1/2	cup	Applesauce, Natural Style, Mott's
3.0	8	fl oz	Sports Drink, LowOz
3.0	6	fl oz	Juice, Guava Nectar, Kern's
3.0	2	Tbls	Raisins, California Golden, Sun-Maid
3.0	2	pieces	Pears, Dried
3.0	2	Tbls	Raisins, Thompson Seedless, Natural, Sun-Maid
2.5	1/2	cup	Apricots, Canned In Heavy Syrup
2.5	6	fl oz	Fruit Drink, Crangrape, Ocean Spray
2.5	6	fl oz	Juice, Apple

Nutripoints	Serving Size		Food Name—Fruits
2.5	1/2	cup	Fruit Cocktail, Light Syrup, Del Monte
2.5	2	wt oz	Apples, Dried, Chunks, Sun-Maid
2.5	1	bar	Snack Bar, Melaleuca Fruit & Fiber Bar
2.5	1/2	cup	Topping, Blueberry, Hot, Nutripoint Recipe
2.5	1/2	cup	Fruit Cocktail, Light Syrup, Libby's
2.5	6	fl oz	Pear Nectar, Canned
2.5	6	fl oz	Juice, Apple, Mott's
2.0	1/4	fruit	Avocado, California
2.0	1/2	cup	Applesauce, Unsweetened, Musselman
2.0	6	fl oz	Juice, Grape, Sweetened, Fzn, Welch's
2.0	6	fl oz	Juice, Grape, White, Welch's
2.0	6	fl oz	Juice, Mango-Mango, Ocean Spray
2.0	2	tablets	Thins, Juice Plus+® Fiber Snack
2.0	1/2	cup	Cherries, Sweet, Frozen, Sweetened
2.0	1/2	cup	Pineapple, Sliced, Canned, Light Syrup, Dole
2.0	1	wt oz	Fruit Leather
2.0	2	Tbls	Apple Butter
1.5	8	fl oz	Sports Drink, Exceed
1.5	1/2	cup	Pears, Bartlett, Light Syrup, Canned, Del Monte
1.5	6	fl oz	Juice, Apple, From Concentrate, Tree Top
1.5	6	fl oz	Juice, Cranapple, Ocean Spray
1.5	6	fl oz	Fruit Drink, Fruit Juicy Red, Hawaiian Punch
1.5	6	fl oz	Fruit Drink, Grape, Hi-C
1.0	1	bar	Frozen Dessert, Fruit Bar

1.0	6	fl oz	Juice, Apple, From Concentrate, Fzn, Tree Top
1.0	1/2	cup	Pineapple, Canned, Heavy Syrup
1.0	1/2	cup	Frozen Dessert, Strawberry, Chunky, Frozfruit
1.0	1	Tbls	Taco Bell Guacamole
1.0	1	cup	Gelatin, Cherry, Sugar-Free, Jell-O
1.0	8	fl oz	Sports Drink, Recharge
1.0	1/2	cup	Fruit Cocktail, Canned, Heavy Syrup
1.0	6	fl oz	Juice, Apple, Lucky Leaf
1.0	1/2	cup	Cherries, Sour, Canned, Heavy Syrup
0.5	1	bar	Frozen Dessert, Fudgesicle
0.5	2	Tbls	Jelly, Grape, Imitation, Smucker's
0.0	8	fl oz	Fruit Drink, SoBe Elixir 3C, Pomegranate Cranberry (*)
0.0	1/2	cup	Cherries, Sweet, Canned, Heavy Syrup
0.0	6	fl oz	Juice, Cranberry Cocktail, Fzn, Welch's
0.0	1/2	cup	Peaches, Canned, Heavy Syrup
0.0	4	olives	Olives, Ripe, Lindsay
0.0	6	fl oz	Fruit Drink, Grape, Fzn, Welchade
0.0	1	Tbls	Jelly, Fruit Butters, All Flavors

Nutripoints	Serving Size		Food Name—Fruits
0.0	1/2	cup	Plums, Canned, Heavy Syrup
-0.5	1/2	portion	Apples, Escalloped, Fzn, Stouffer's
-0.5	1	bar	Frozen Dessert, Pineapple, Frozfruit
-0.5	1/2	cup	Applesauce, w/Sugar
-0.5	2	Tbls	Jam, Low Cal
-0.5	1	slice	Luncheon Meat, Olive Loaf
-1.0	1	piece	Raspberry, Peccavi, Nutripoint Recipe
-1.0	1	wt oz	Raisins, Carob-Covered
-1.0	1/2	piece	Pie, Raspberry
-1.0	1/2	piece	Pie, Banana Cream
-1.0	1/4	piece	Pie, Mincemeat
-1.0	1/2	cup	Pears, Canned, Heavy Syrup
-1.0	1/4	piece	Burger King Apple Pie
-1.0	1/4	cup	Apple Crisp
-1.5	1/2	cup	Pie Filling, Apple, Lite, Thank You
-1.5	6	fl oz	Fruit Drink, Sugar Added
-1.5	1/2	piece	Pie, Blackberry
-1.5	1/2	piece	Pie, Strawberry
-1.5	1/2	cup	Frozen Dessert, Banana, Creamy, Frozfruit
-1.5	1	wt oz	Raisins, Chocolate-Covered
-1.5	6	fl oz	Fruit Drink, Cranicot, Ocean Spray
-1.5	1/4	serving	Banana Split
-1.5	6	fl oz	Fruit Drink, Hawaiian Punch
-2.0	1/2	piece	Pie, Apple, Fzn, Weight Watchers
-2.0	1	piece	Fruit Leather, With Sugar
-2.0	1/4	piece	Pie, Apple
-2.0	1/2	piece	Pie, Peach
-2.0	1/2	piece	Pie, Blueberry
-2.0	1/2	piece	Pie, Berry
-2.0	1/4	piece	McDonald's Apple Pie
-2.0	1/4	piece	Pie, Fruit
-2.0	1	Tbls	Coconut
-2.0	1/4	piece	Pie, Cherry, Hostess
-2.0	1/4	piece	Pie, Blueberry, Hostess
-2.0	8	olives	Olives, Black
-2.0	1	piece	Coconut, Chocolate-Covered
-2.0	1/4	piece	Pie, Cherry, Natural Juice, Mrs. Smith's
-2.0	8	fl oz	Fruit Drink, Five Alive, Minute Maid
-2.0	1/2	cup	Salad, Waldorf
-2.5	1/2	cup	Sherbet, Orange
-2.5	1/4	piece	Pie, Apple, Natural Juice, Mrs. Smith's
-2.5	1/4	piece	Jack In the Box Hot Apple Turnover
-2.5	17	pieces	Gummy Bear, Fruit Juice

Nutripoints	Serving Size		Food Name—Fruits
-2.5	1/4	piece	Pie, Peach, Mrs. Smith's
-2.5	1/2	serving	Mousse, Raspberry, Fzn, Weight Watchers
-3.0	2	Tbls	Sauce, Cranberry, Canned, Sweetened
-3.0	1/2	piece	Pie, Pumpkin, Homemade
-3.0	1	piece	Frozen Dessert, Banana, Pudding Pops, Jello
-3.0	1	Tbls	Jam, Preserves, All Flavors
-3.0	8	pieces	Olives, Medium, Mammoth Queen, S&W
-3.0	1/2	cup	Pie Filling, Apple, Thank You
-3.0	1	cup	Fruit Drink, Limeade
-3.5	1/4	cup	Berries, Fresh, w/Zabaglione Sauce
-3.5	1/4	piece	Pie, Cherry, w/Cream Cheese & Sour Cream
-3.5	1/2	piece	Pie, Coconut Cream
-3.5	1	Tbls	Coconut, Shredded Premium, Baker's
-3.5	1	wt oz	Coconut, Raw
-3.5	2	pieces	Cherries, Chocolate Covered
-3.5	1	Tbls	Topping, Strawberry, Smucker's
-4.0	1	Tbls	Coconut, Dried, Sweetened, Shredded
-4.0	8	pieces	Olives, Green
-4.0	1/2	bar	Candy Bar, Coconut Almond Joy
-4.0	1/2	cup	Pie Filling, Cherry, Thank You
-4.0	1/4	piece	Pie, Lemon Meringue
-4.0	1/2	cup	Gelatin, Strawberry-Banana, Royal
-4.5	6	fl oz	Fruit Drink, Lemonade
-4.5	1/4	cup	Sauce, Cranberry, Whole Berry, Ocean Spray
-4.5	8	fl oz	Energy Drink, AMP, Pepsi
-5.0	6	fl oz	Lemonade, Minute Maid
-5.0	1/2	piece	Pie, Cherry
-5.0	1/2	cup	Gelatin, Cherry Flavor, Jell-O
-5.0	1	Tbls	Preserves, All Varieties, Kraft
-5.5	6	fl oz	Fruit Drink, Punch, Capri Sun
-5.5	6	fl oz	Fruit Drink, Orange, Capri Sun
-5.5	2	Tbls	Jelly, Cranberry
-5.5	2	Tbls	Jelly, Blackberry Spread, Smucker's
-5.5	1	Tbls	Jam, Grape, Welch's
-5.5	1	Tbls	Jelly, Grape, Welch's
-5.5	1	Tbls	Preserves, Strawberry, Welch's
-6.0	1	Tbls	Jam, Strawberry, Smucker's
-6.0	1	Tbls	Jelly, Grape, Concord, Smucker's
-6.0	1	Tbls	Marmalade, Orange, Smucker's
-6.0	1	Tbls	Preserves, Raspberry, Smucker's

GRAINS

Nutripoints	Serving Size		Food Name—Grains
64.5	1	cup	Cereal, Whole Grain Total, General Mills (*)
57.5	1	cup	Cereal, Total Corn Flakes, General Mills (*)
56.0	1	cup	Cereal, Product 19, Kellogg's (*)
55.5	3/4	cup	Cereal, Total Brown Sugar & Oat, General Mills (*)
48.5	1	cup	Cereal, Multi-Grain Cheerios, General Mills (*)
43.5	1/2	cup	Cereal, All Bran Extra Fiber, Kellogg's
43.5	3/4	cup	Cereal, Total Protein, General Mills (*)
40.5	1/3	cup	Cereal, All-Bran (*)
40.5	1/2	cup	Cereal, Total Raisin Bran, General Mills (*)
36.5	3/4	cup	Cereal, Just Right w/Fruit and Nuts, Kellogg's (*)
31.5	1/2	cup	Cereal, Fiber One, General Mills (*)
31.0	1/2	cup	Cereal, 100% Bran, Nabisco (*)
29.5	1	bar	Snack Bar, Pounds Off Bar (*)
28.5	2/3	cup	Cereal, Fruitful Bran, Kellogg's (*)
27.5	1	wt oz	Bran, Wheat, Toasted, Kretschmer
26.5	1/2	cup	Bran, Wheat
26.5	1	cup	Cereal, Smart Start, Kellogg's (*)
25.0	1	bar	Snack Bar, Tiger's Sports Bar (*)
23.5	1/2	cup	Cereal, 100% Bran With Oat Bran, Nabisco (*)
23.0	1	bar	Snack Bar, Energia (*)
23.0	3/4	cup	Cereal, Heart to Heart, Kashi (*)
22.5	1	bar	Snack Bar, Power Bar, All Flavors (*)
21.0	2/3	cup	Cereal, 40+bran Flakes, Kellogg's (*)
21.0	2/3	cup	Cereal, Bran Flakes, Kellogg's (*)
21.0	1	serving	Energy Bites, Power Bar (*)
20.0	8	fl oz	BrainSustain Drink (Rice) (*)
19.5	1	cup	Cereal, Empower, Health Valley (*)
18.5	3/4	cup	Cereal, Kellogg's Complete Wheat Bran Flakes (*)
18.0	1	cup	Cereal, Corn Flakes, Kellogg's (*)
18.0	7/8	cup	Cereal, Grape-Nut Flakes, Post (*)
17.5	2/3	cup	Cereal, Natural Bran Flakes, Post (*)
17.0	1/2	cup	Cereal, Oat Squares, Quaker (*)
16.5	1	bar	Candy Bar, Slim-Fast (*)
15.5	1/2	cup	Cereal, Fruit & Fiber w/Raisins, Peaches, Almonds, Post (*)
15.5	1/2	cup	Cereal, Fruit & Fiber w/Dates, Raisins, Walnuts, Post (*)
15.5	3/4	cup	Cereal, Raisin Bran, Kellogg's (*)
15.5	3/4	cup	Cereal, Bran Chex, General Mills (*)
15.5	2	waffles	Waffles, Honey Oat, Heart to Heart, Kashi (*)
14.5	3/4	cup	Cereal, Benefit, General Mills (*)
14.5	1	bar	Snack Bar, ZonePerfect (*)

Nutripoints	Serving Size		Food Name—Grains
14.0	1	cup	Cereal, Special K, Kellogg's (*)
14.0	1/2	cup	Cereal, Cracklin' Oat Bran, Kellogg's (*)
13.5	1	serving	Cereal, Heart to Heart Hot Oatmeal, Kashi (*)
13.5	1/4	cup	Cereal, Grape-Nuts, Post (*)
13.5	2	pieces	Candy Bar, Ideal Green Apple, Thompson Foods (*)
13.0	2/3	cup	Cereal, Wheat Chex, General Mills (*)
13.0	1 1/4	cups	Cereal, Cheerios, General Mills (*)
13.0	1/2	cup	Cereal, Raspberry Fruit Wheats, Nabisco (*)
13.0	1	cup	Cereal, Cheerios, Multi-Grain, General Mills (*)
13.0	1	cup	Cereal, Fruit Loops, Kellogg's (*)
13.0	1/2	cup	Cereal, Blueberry Fruit Wheats, Nabisco (*)
12.5	1	bar	Meal Bar, Glucerna (*)
12.5	1/2	cup	Cereal, Mueslix, Bran Muesli, Kellogg's (*)
12.5	1	cup	Cereal, Trix, Reduced Sugar, General Mills (*)
12.5	1	cup	Cereal, Cocoa Puffs, Reduced Sugar, General Mills (*)
12.5	1/2	cup	Cereal, Frosted Mini-Wheats, Kellogg's (*)
12.0	1/2	cup	Cereal, Oat Bran Prepared w/Low-Fat Milk, Nabisco (*)
12.0	1/4	cup	Wheat Germ, Kretschmer
12.0	1	cup	Cereal, Wheaties, General Mills (*)
11.5	1/2	cup	Cereal, Frosted Wheat Squares, Nabisco (*)
11.5	1	cup	Cereal, Rice Krispies, Kellogg's (*)
11.5	1	cup	Cereal, Slender, Health Valley (*)
11.5	1	cup	Cereal, Multi-Bran Chex, General Mills (*)
11.5	1	cup	Cereal, Team Flakes, Nabisco (*)
11.0	2/3	cup	Cereal, Life, Cinnamon, Quaker (*)
10.5	2	slices	Bread, Hunger Filler Whole Grain, Natural Ovens Bakery
10.5	1	muffin	Muffin, Nutripoint Recipe
10.5	1/4	cup	Wheat Germ
10.5	2	waffles	Waffles, Whole Grain Wheat/Oat Bran, Aunt Jemima
10.5	1	cup	Soup, Wild Rice, Nutripoint Recipe
10.5	1	cup	Cereal, Lucky Charms, General Mills (*)
10.5	1	cup	Cereal, Sun Flakes, Ralston (*)
10.5	1	cup	Cereal, Heart Wise, Health Valley (*)
10.0	1/2	cup	Cereal, Mueslix, 5 Grain Muesli, Kellogg's (*)
10.0	1/3	cup	Cereal, Oatbake, Kellogg's (*)
10.0	1 1/2	cups	Cereal, Kix, General Mills (*)
10.0	1/2	cup	Cereal, Raisin Nut Bran, General Mills (*)
10.0	3/4	cup	Cereal, Honey Nut Cheerios, General Mills (*)
10.0	1/3	cup	Cereal, Horizon Trail Mix, Post (*)
10.0	1	cup	Cereal, Corn Chex, General Mills (*)
10.0	1	cup	Cereal, Benefit w/Raisins, General Mills (*)
10.0	1	cup	Cereal, Crispix, Kellogg's (*)
10.0	1 1/2	cups	Pasta, Angel Hair, w/Sunshine Sauce, Nutripoint Recipe

Nutripoints	Serving Size		Food Name—Grains
9.5	1/2	cup	Cereal, Oatmeal Crisp Raisin, General Mills (*)
9.5	1	bar	Breakfast Bar, Slim-Fast Optima (*)
9.5	2/3	cup	Cereal, Life, Quaker (*)
9.5	1	cup	Cereal, Apple Jacks, Kellogg's (*)
9.5	1/2	cup	Cereal, Oats, Instant w/Bran, Lowfat Milk, 3-Minute Brand
9.0	8	crackers	Cracker, Snackbread, High Fiber Ryvita
9.0	1	cup	Lasagna, Spinach, Nutripoint Recipe
9.0	1 1/8	cups	Cereal, Rice Chex, General Mills (*)
9.0	1 1/4	cups	Cereal, Toasties Corn Flakes, Post (*)
9.0	2	wt oz	Bran, Rice
9.0	3/4	cup	Cereal, Golden Grahams, General Mills (*)
9.0	1/3	cup	Bran, Oat, Arrowhead Mills
9.0	3/4	cup	Cereal, Cap'n Crunch, Peanut Butter, Quaker (*)
8.5	1	cup	Cereal, Alpha-Bits, Post (*)
8.5	1	bar	Snack Bar, Clif ZBar (*)
8.5	3/4	cup	Cereal, Cap'n Crunch, Quaker (*)
8.5	1	cup	Cereal, Multi-Grains/Raisins/Oats, Healthy Choice
8.5	1 1/4	cups	Cereal, Quaker Oat Bran
8.5	3	small	Pancakes, Whole Wheat, Aunt Jemima (from mix)
8.5	1 1/3	cups	Cereal, Honey-Comb, Ralston (*)
8.5	1/4	cup	Cereal, Hot, High Fiber, Ralston
8.5	1	bar	Meal Bar, Slim-Fast Optima (*)
8.0	1	wt oz	Wheat Germ, Kretschmer, Honey Crunch
8.0	7/8	cup	Cereal, Golden Crisp, Post (*)
8.0	3	small	Pancakes, Lite Buttermilk, Aunt Jemima (from mix)
8.0	1	cup	Cereal, Trix, General Mills (*)
8.0	3/4	cup	Cereal, Apple Cinnamon Cheerios, General Mills (*)
8.0	1	cup	Cereal, Corn Pops, Kellogg's (*)
7.5	3	crackers	Cracker, Crispbread Fiber Plus, Wasa
7.5	3/4	cup	Cereal, Cinnamon Toast Crunch, General Mills (*)
7.5	1	cup	Cereal, Malt O Meal, w/Water, Cooked (*)
7.5	1	cup	Jambalaya, Nutripoint Recipe
7.5	1/2	cup	Cereal, C.W. Post, w/Raisins, Post (*)
7.5	7/8	cup	Cereal, Fruity Pebbles, Post (*)
7.5	7/8	cup	Cereal, Cocoa Pebbles, Post (*)
7.0	2/3	cup	Cereal, Honeybunches of Oats w/Almonds, Post (*)
7.0	3/4	cup	Cereal, Cocoa Krispies, Kellogg's (*)
7.0	3	pancakes	Pancakes, Lite, Buttermilk, Aunt Jemima
7.0	3/4	cup	Cereal, Frosted Flakes, Kellogg's (*)
7.0	1/2	cup	Cereal, Oat Bran, Quaker
6.5	1/2	cup	Cereal, Oat Bran, Instant, w/Skim Milk, 3-Minute Brand
6.5	2/3	cup	Cereal, Honey Nut Chex, General Mills
6.5	1	cup	Cereal, Cocoa Puffs, General Mills (*)

Nutripoints	Serving Size		Food Name—Grains
6.5	2	slices	Bread, Health Max, Natural Ovens Bakery
6.5	3	slices	Bread, Hi-Fiber, Wonder
6.5	4	wt oz	Pilaf, Vegetarian Amaranth, Health Valley
6.0	1	whole	Muffin, English, Whole Wheat
6.0	1	cup	Cereal, Basic 4, General Mills (*)
6.0	1/4	cup	Cereal, Hot, High Fiber, w/Milk, Ralston
6.0	1	wt oz	Cereal, Oat Bran, Instant, w/Water, 3 Minute Brand
6.0	1	piece	Pizza, French Bread, Nutripoint Recipe
6.0	1/4	cup	Flour, Whole Wheat
6.0	3	small	Pancakes, Buckwheat, Aunt Jemima (from mix)
6.0	1	bar	Snack Bar, FIBAR (all flavors) (*)
6.0	1	bar	Snack Bar, Nutra Blast (*)
6.0	2/3	cup	Cereal, Atkins, All Flavors
6.0	3	slices	Bread, Less, Mrs. Baird's
6.0	1	wt oz	Spicer's Cheddar Cheese Wheat Snacks
6.0	2	slices	Bread, Whole Wheat, Stone-Ground, the Sourdough
6.0	2	slices	Bread, Whole Wheat
6.0	1	wt oz	Cereal, Shredded Wheat 'n Bran, Nabisco
5.5	1	cup	Cereal, Puffed Wheat, Quaker
5.5	4	pancakes	Pancake, Whole Wheat, Orange, Nutripoint Recipe
5.5	3	slices	Bread, Light Bran & Oat, Oatmeal Goodness
5.5	1	cup	Cereal, Oat Bran, Instant, w/Whole Milk, 3-Minute Brand
5.5	3	slices	Bread, Oat Bran N' Honey, Light, Roman Meal
5.5	1	cup	Cereal, Instant Oatmeal w/Peaches and Cream, Quaker
5.5	1	wt oz	Quinoa, Dry, Arrowhead Mills
5.5	1	bagel	Bagel, Whole Grain, Natural Ovens Bakery
5.5	1/2	cup	Cereal, Oatmeal, Dry
5.5	1/2	cup	Rice, Wild, Cooked w/o Salt
5.5	1/4	cup	Flour, Whole Wheat, Gold Medal
5.5	3	slices	Bread, Diet 40 Cal/Slice
5.0	2	slices	Bread, Wheat, Fresh Horizons
5.0	2	slices	Bread, Mixed Grain
5.0	1	bar	Candy Bar, Tiger's Milk Nutrition (*)
5.0	1/2	piece	Sandwich, Open Face Pita, Nutripoint Recipe
5.0	2	Tbls	McDonald's Croutons
5.0	1	wt oz	Amaranth, Dry, Arrowhead Mills
5.0	1	piece	Cereal, Shredded Wheat (large Biscuit), Nabisco
5.0	6	crackers	Cracker, Rykrisp, Ralston
5.0	1	cup	Cereal, Oatmeal, Fruited Cinnamon, Nutripoint Recipe
5.0	1	serving	Subway Veggie Delight Sandwich (6")
5.0	1	piece	Muffin, Raisin Oat Bran, Health Valley
5.0	2	slices	Bread, Sprouted Wheat
5.0	2	slices	Bread, 5 Bran, Home Pride

Nutripoints	Serving Size		Food Name—Grains
5.0	2/3	cup	Cereal, Shredded Wheat, Spoon Size, Nabisco
4.5	1	bar	Breakfast Bar, Chocolate, Carnation
4.5	1	bar	Snack Bar, Ensure (*)
4.5	2/3	cup	Rice, Whole Grain Brown, Uncle Ben's
4.5	2	slices	Bread, Whole Wheat, Thin, Pepperidge Farm
4.5	1/2	cup	Cereal, Malt-O Meal, Quick, w/Whole Milk
4.5	1	cup	Cereal, Cream of Wheat, Quick, Nabisco
4.5	1/2	cup	Pasta Salad, Fresh, Nutripoint Recipe
4.5	1	piece	Tortilla, Whole Wheat
4.5	2	cups	Cereal, Puffed Wheat
4.5	2	slices	Bread, Wheat, Lite 35, Earth Grains
4.5	2	slices	Bread, Whole Wheat, Stone-Ground, Country Hearth
4.5	3	cakes	Rye Cakes, Quaker
4.5	1	cup	Soup, Healthy Classics, Garlic & Pasta, Progresso
4.5	3	cakes	Wheat Cakes, Quaker
4.5	1/2	cup	Cereal, Instant Cream of Wheat, w/Low-Fat Milk, Nabisco
4.5	1	piece	Roll, Whole Wheat
4.5	1	whole	Muffin, English, w/Raisins
4.5	2	wt oz	Wheat, Whole Grain, Dry, Arrowhead Mills
4.5	1/2	cup	Cereal, Whole Wheat, Cooked
4.5	1/2	cup	Rice, Wild, Sherry, Frozen, Green Giant
4.5	2	slices	Bread, Cracked Wheat
4.5	1	bar	Breakfast Bar, Honey Nut, Carnation
4.5	1/2	cup	Ravioli
4.5	1	whole	Muffin, English, Roman Meal
4.5	1	wt oz	Cereal, H-O Super Bran
4.5	2	slices	Bread, Triticale
4.5	2	slices	Bread, Roman Meal
4.5	3/4	cup	Cereal, Oats, Old Fashioned, Quaker
4.5	2	slices	Bread, Pumpernickel
4.0	1/2	cup	Pasta Accents, Cheddar Cheese, Green Giant
4.0	1/2	cup	Rice, Brown, Cooked w/o Salt
4.0	2	slices	Bread, Whole Rye
4.0	1	whole	Muffin, English
4.0	2	slices	Bread, Wheat Germ
4.0	1	serving	Pizza, Four Cheese, Fzn, South Beach Diet
4.0	1/2	serving	Lasagna, Low Cal Frozen Meal
4.0	1/4	cup	Flour, Rye, Whole Grain
4.0	3	crackers	Cracker, Crispbread Golden Rye, Wasa
4.0	1	serving	Pizza Deluxe, Fzn, South Beach Diet
4.0	1/2	cup	Rotini Cheddar, Garden Gourmet, Green Giant
4.0	2	pieces	Cereal, Whole Wheat, Weetabix
4.0	2	pieces	Tortilla, Corn

Nutripoints	Serving Size		Food Name—Grains
4.0	1	serving	Pasta e Fagioli, Organic, Fzn, Moosewood
4.0	1	wt oz	Cereal, Oats, Steel-Cut, Arrowhead Mills
4.0	1/2	cup	Spaghetti, w/Sauce
4.0	1	serving	Rice, Wild & Long Grain, Veg. & Herb, Uncle Ben's
4.0	1/2	cup	Spaghetti, Hi-Protein
4.0	1	piece	Bread, Pita, Whole Wheat
4.0	1	wt oz	Cereal, 7 Grain, Stone-Buhr
4.0	1	piece	Granola Bar, Chewy Fruit & Nut, Jack La Lanne
4.0	1/4	cup	Flour, Ezekiel, Arrowhead Mills
4.0	1/2	cup	Noodles, Whole Wheat
4.0	1	whole	Muffin, English, Pepperidge Farm
4.0	2	slices	Bread, 100% Whole Wheat, Wonder
4.0	10	pieces	Cookies, Animal, Oat Bran, Health Valley
4.0	1/4	cup	Barley, Uncooked
4.0	1/2	cup	Macaroni & Spaghetti, Enriched, Prince
4.0	2	slices	Bread, Raisin
4.0	1	waffle	Waffles
4.0	2	slices	Bread, Wheat Berry, Honey, Earth Grains
4.0	1	whole	Bagel, Whole Wheat
4.0	1/2	cup	Rice, Spanish
3.5	1/4	cup	Flour, Triticale, Whole, Arrowhead Mills
3.5	1/2	cup	Rice, Brown, Natural Long Grain, Mahatma
3.5	2	slices	Bread, Protogen Protein, Thomas'
3.5	2	slices	Bread, Bran'nola, Oroweat
3.5	1	slice	Pizza Hut Fit 'N Delicious Pizza (ave. all varieties)
3.5	2	slices	Bread, Wheat, Stone-Ground, Earth Grains
3.5	2	slices	Bread, 100% Whole Wheat, Home Pride
3.5	1/2	cup	Pasta Accents, Garlic Seasoning, Green Giant
3.5	1/4	cup	Flour, Whole Wheat, Pillsbury
3.5	1	whole	Bagel, Pumpernickel
3.5	1	wt oz	Macaroni, Dry (2 wt oz=1 c cooked)
3.5	1	portion	Spaghetti, w/Meatball Dinner, Frozen, Morton
3.5	1/2	cup	Macaroni, Cooked, No Salt (2 oz dry = 1 c cooked)
3.5	1/2	cup	Pilaf, Breakfast, 7 Whole Grains & Sesame, Kashi
3.5	2	slices	Bread, Bran
3.5	2	slices	Bread, Sandwich, Salt-Free, Earth Grains
3.5	1/4	cup	Flour, Whole Buckwheat
3.5	1	piece	Biscuit (mix), Multigrain, Arrowhead Mills
3.5	1/4	cup	Cereal, Alpen
3.5	1	bar	Snack Bar, Nutri-Grain, Kellogg's (all flavors)
3.5	1	whole	Muffin, English, Cracked Wheat
3.5	2	slices	Bread, Original Bran'nola, Arnold
3.5	2	slices	Bread, Honey Wheat Berry, Arnold

Nutripoints	Serving Size		Food Name—Grains
3.5	1	muffin	Muffin, Oat Bran, Nutripoint Recipe
3.5	1/4	cup	Corn Meal, Yellow Enriched, Aunt Jemima
3.5	1	slices	Pizza Hut Veggie Lover's Thin 'N Crispy Pizza
3.5	1/2	cup	Linguine, Spinach High-Protein, Buitoni
3.5	1/2	cup	Rice, Brown, Instant, Minute
3.5	1	roll	Roll, Rye
3.5	6	pieces	Breadsticks
3.5	1/2	serving	Subway Gardenburger Sandwich (6")
3.5	1 1/2	waffles	Waffles, Common Sense Oat Bran, Eggo
3.5	2	slices	Bread, Honey Nut and Oat Bran, Roman Meal
3.5	1 1/4	wt oz	Cereal, Instant Oatmeal w/Apples and Cinnamon, Quaker
3.5	3	crackers	Cracker, Crispbread Hearty Rye, Wasa
3.5	2	slices	Bread, Oatmeal and Bran, Oatmeal Goodness
3.5	1/2	cup	Macaroni, Cooked, All Shapes, Mueller's
3.5	1	muffin	Muffin, Bran, w/Raisin & Nuts
3.5	2	slices	Bread, Oatmeal and Sunflower Seeds, Oatmeal Goodness
3.5	2	slices	Bread, Low-Sodium
3.5	1/4	cup	Corn Meal, Dry
3.5	1	muffin	Muffin, Extra Crisp, Arnold
3.5	2	pancakes	Pancake Mix, Complete Buttermilk, Aunt Jemima
3.5	1/2	piece	Pizza Hut Supreme Hand Tossed Pizza
3.5	1	piece	Bread, Pita
3.5	1/2	cup	Noodles, Spinach
3.5	1	muffin	Fruit and Nut Muffins
3.0	1/2	cup	Macaroni, Superoni, Prince
3.0	1/2	cup	Spaghetti, Cooked (1 c = 2 wt oz dry)
3.0	2	slices	Bread, Wheat Berry, Home Pride
3.0	1	bar	Snack Bar, GOLEAN Crunchy, Kashi
3.0	4	pieces	Cracker, Crispbread Dark Rye, Ryvita
3.0	1/2	cup	Rice, Brown Pilaf, w/Vegetables & Herbs, Pritikin
3.0	2	slices	Bread, Wheat and Oatmeal, Oatmeal Goodness
3.0	2	slices	Bread, 7 Grain, Home Pride
3.0	2	cup	Cereal, Puffed, 7 Whole Grains and Sesame, Kashi
3.0	2	biscuits	Biscuit, Extra Rich Buttermilk, Hungry Jack
3.0	2	slices	Bread, Oat Bran, Honey, Earth Grains
3.0	1/4	cup	Flour, All-Purpose Enriched, Pillsbury
3.0	6	crackers	Cracker, Seasoned, Rykrisp
3.0	1/2	piece	Pizza Hut Pepperoni Pan Pizza
3.0	1	roll	Roll, Cracked Wheat
3.0	2	wt oz	Linguine, Buitoni, (2 oz dry = 3/4 c cooked)
3.0	2	slices	Bread, Honey Wheat Berry, Pepperidge Farm
3.0	1/2	cup	Rice, White, Regular, w/Added Salt
3.0	2	slices	Bread, Grape-Nuts, Oroweat

Nutripoints	Serving Size		Food Name—Grains
3.0	1/2	piece	Bun, Submarine/Hoagie
3.0	1	wt oz	Rotini, Rainbow, Creamette
3.0	1/2	cup	Cereal, Oats, Quick, Prepared w/Low-Fat Milk, Quaker
3.0	2	slices	Bread, Sprouted Wheat, Pepperidge Farm
3.0	1/2	cup	Pilaf, Couscous, Casbah
3.0	1/4	cup	Flour, White, All-Purpose Plain, Martha
3.0	2/3	cup	Rice, White, Instant, Cooked
3.0	3	cakes	Rice Cakes, Plain, Lightly Salted, Quaker
3.0	3	cakes	Rice Cakes, Plain, Salt-Free, Quaker
3.0	3	cakes	Rice Cakes, Sesame, Lt. Salted, Quaker
3.0	8	fl oz	Rice Milk, Rice Dream Original, 1% Fat
3.0	1	cup	Soup, Chicken w/Rice, Healthy Choice
3.0	1/4	cup	Flour, All-Purpose, Gold Medal
3.0	2	slices	Bread, Rye, Family, Pepperidge Farm
3.0	8	pieces	Cracker, Whole Wheat
3.0	1/2	cup	Spaghetti, San Giorgio
3.0	1/2	cup	Rice, White, Regular, Cooked, w/o Salt
3.0	3	cookies	Cookies, Fruit Chunks, Health Valley
3.0	2	slices	Bread, White, Butter-Top, Home Pride
3.0	1	muffin	Muffin, Bran
3.0	1/4	cup	Flour, White
3.0	1	whole	Muffin, English, Health Nut, Oroweat
3.0	1	slice	Bread, Health Nut, Oroweat
3.0	2	slices	Bread, White, Brick Oven, Arnold
3.0	3	cups	Popcorn, Light, Orville Redenbacher's
3.0	1/2	portion	Cavatelli, Frozen, Celentano
3.0	1/2	cup	Spaghetti, Ronzoni
3.0	2	slices	Bread, French
3.0	1	cup	Grits, Cooked
3.0	2	slices	Bread, Rye, Light, Earth Grains
3.0	2	slices	Bread, Bran'nola Rice Bran, Oroweat
3.0	2	slices	Bread, Old-Fashioned Buttermilk, Country Hearth
3.0	1/4	cup	Bulgur, Dry
3.0	1	wt oz	Noodles, Egg, Cholesterol Free, No Yolks
3.0	1/2	cup	Macaroni Ribbons, Spinach, Creamette, Borden
3.0	1	piece	Pizza Hut Cheese Thin 'n Crispy Pizza
3.0	2	slices	Bread, Oatmeal, Pepperidge Farm
2.5	1/2	piece	Pizza Hut Cheese Pan Pizza
2.5	1/2	portion	Spaghetti, Meat Sauce, Frozen, Weight Watchers
2.5	2	wt oz	Linguine, San Georgio (2 oz dry = 3/4 c cooked)
2.5	2	slices	Bread, Italian
2.5	3	crackers	Cracker, Norwegian Crispbread, Thick Style, Kavli
2.5	1/2	cup	Lasagna

Nutripoints	Serving Size		Food Name—Grains
2.5	1/2	portion	Pasta Primavera, Frozen, Weight Watchers
2.5	6	crackers	Cracker, Crispbread Dark, Finn
2.5	2	slices	Bread, Rye, Jewish, Real Unseeded, Levy's
2.5	1	cup	Cereal, Puffed Rice, Quaker
2.5	1/2	cup	Macaroni, Elbow, Creamette, Borden
2.5	1/2	cup	Spaghetti, Creamette, Borden
2.5	1/4	cup	Cracker Meal, Keebler
2.5	2	slices	Bread, Sourdough
2.5	1/2	portion	Lasagna, Primavera, Frozen, Celentano
2.5	1/2	roll	Roll, French, Brown 'n Serve, Pepperidge Farm
2.5	2	rolls	Roll, Sourdough, French Extra, Earth Grains
2.5	1/2	portion	Spaghetti, Low Cal, Frozen Dinner
2.5	2	crackers	Cracker, Crispbread Breakfast, Wasa
2.5	1/4	cup	Flour, Soybean
2.5	1	whole	Muffin, English, Regular, Thomas'
2.5	1	wt oz	Noodles, Egg, Veggie, Hodgson Mill
2.5	1	wt oz	Spaghetti Substitute, Spinach, Deboles
2.5	2	slices	Bread, Whole Wheat, Brick Oven, Arnold
2.5	1	wt oz	Noodles, Spaghetti, Whole Wheat, Hodgson Mill
2.5	2	slices	Bread, Oatnut, Oroweat
2.5	2	pancakes	Pancake Mix, Original Complete, Aunt Jemima
2.5	3	pieces	Cookies, Fat-Free, Health Valley (all flavors)
2.5	3	cakes	Corn Cakes, Quaker
2.5	10	crackers	Cracker, Fat Free, Premium Saltine, Nabisco
2.5	2	slices	Bread, Honey Wheat Berry, Oroweat
2.5	1/4	cup	Flour, Rye, Medium, Pillsbury
2.5	1	roll	Roll, Diet
2.5	1/2	cup	Rice, Minute Rice
2.5	1	roll	Roll, French or Vienna
2.5	1	roll	Roll, Sourdough
2.5	1	cup	Farina, Cooked
2.5	8	crackers	Cracker, Crispbread Light Natural, Krispen
2.5	2	slices	Bread, Bran'nola Multi-Bran, Oroweat
2.5	1/2	cup	Rice, Brown, Quick, Vegetable Herb, Arrowhead Mills
2.5	1/2	cup	Rice, Converted, Uncle Ben's
2.5	1	cracker	Cracker, Matzo
2.5	3/4	cup	Cereal, Cream of Rice, Cooked
2.5	2	slices	Bread, White
2.5	2	wt oz	Linguine, Thin, Ronzoni (2 oz dry = 3/4 c cooked)
2.5	2	slices	Bread, White, Wonder
2.5	1/2	cup	Fettuccini, Garden Gourmet, Frozen, Green Giant
2.5	1	piece	Muffin Mix, Oat Bran, Wheat Free, Arrowhead Mills
2.5	6	pieces	Breadsticks, Plain, Keebler

Nutripoints	Serving Size		Food Name—Grains
2.5	1/4	cup	Cereal, Familia, w/Fruit & Nuts
2.0	1/2	cup	Rice, Ext Long Grain Enriched, Carolina
2.0	1/2	cup	Rice, Long Grain Enriched, Mahatma
2.0	1/2	cup	Cereal, Seven in the Morning, Kashi
2.0	2	cups	Bread, Family Style Distinctive, Pepperidge Farm
2.0	1/2	cup	Rice, Pilaf
2.0	2	rolls	Kentucky Fried Chicken, Roll
2.0	1	whole	Muffin, English, Honey Wheat, Thomas'
2.0	1/2	piece	Pizza Hut Hand Tossed Cheese Pizza
2.0	1	wt oz	Noodles, Egg, Whole Wheat, Hodgson Mill
2.0	1	wt oz	Noodles, Spinach, Whole Wheat, Hodgson Mill
2.0	1/2	cup	Noodles, Egg, Cooked, Mueller's
2.0	2	cups	Cereal, Puffed Rice
2.0	1	wt oz	Ramen, Natural Whole Wheat, Westbrae
2.0	1/2	piece	Pizza Hut Super Supreme Pan Pizza
2.0	1	roll	Roll, Frankfurter, Wonder
2.0	1	bun	Bun, White, Hamburger
2.0	2	whole	Bagel, Plain, Lender's
2.0	1	roll	Roll, Hard
2.0	1	whole	Bagel, Raisin 'n Honey, Lender's
2.0	1/2	cup	Spaghetti, w/Meat Sauce
2.0	1	piece	Bagel
2.0	1/2	piece	Pizza Hut Supreme Pan Pizza
2.0	1/2	cup	Pilaf, Kashi
2.0	1	piece	Muffin Mix, Bran, Original Wheat, Arrowhead Mills
2.0	1/2	cup	Bread Crumbs
2.0	6	crackers	Cracker, Melba Toast, White, Old London
2.0	1/2	portion	Lasagna, Zucchini, Lean Cuisine, Stouffer's
2.0	1/2	piece	Pizza Hut Supreme Thin 'n Crispy Pizza
2.0	1	roll	Roll, White
2.0	12	crackers	Cracker, 5-grain, Harvest Crisps, Nabisco
2.0	1	tart	Tarts, Fat-Free, Health Valley (all flavors)
2.0	1/2	cup	Ramen, Natural Mushroom, Westbrae
2.0	6	pieces	Breadsticks, Onion, Keebler
2.0	1	piece	Tortilla, Flour
2.0	4	crackers	Cracker, Crispbread Lite Rye, Wasa
2.0	2	biscuits	Biscuit, Butter, Pillsbury
2.5	2	slices	Bread, Pumpernickel, Arnold
2.0	1/2	piece	Pizza Hut Super Supreme Hand Tossed Pizza
2.0	1/2	piece	Pizza Hut Super Supreme Thin 'n Crispy Pizza
2.0	1/2	portion	Pizza, Cheese, French Bread, Lean Cuisine, Stouffer's
2.0	2	slices	Bread, Oatmeal
2.0	1	piece	Cornbread, Southern, Nutripoint Recipe

Nutripoints	Serving Size		Food Name—Grains
2.0	1/2	cup	Croutons
2.0	1	wt oz	Ramen, Natural Spinach, Westbrae
2.0	1/2	portion	Ravioli, Mini, Frozen, Celentano
2.0	1/2	bar	Candy Bar, Fruit Nut, Concentrated, Pemmican
2.0	2	cups	Popcorn, Air Popped
2.0	1	cup	Cereal, Oatmeal, Cooked, Prepared w/Water
2.0	1/4	piece	Pizza Hut Supreme Personal Pan Pizza
2.0	2	pieces	Waffles, Blueberry, Aunt Jemima
2.0	2	slices	Bread, Potato
2.0	1	portion	Linguini, Seafood, Frozen, Weight Watchers
2.0	1	bar	Breakfast Bar
1.5	1/4	cup	Cereal, Orangeola w/Bananas/Hawaiian Fruit, Health Valley
1.5	1/4	piece	Pizza Hut Pepperoni Personal Pan Pizza
1.5	2	pieces	Biscuit, Country Style, Pillsbury
1.5	1/2	cup	Rice, Rice A Roni, Spanish
1.5	2	slices	Bread, Gluten
1.5	1	piece	Domino's Large 16" Cheese Pizza
1.5	1	roll	Roll, Sweet, w/Fruit
1.5	1/2	cup	Bread Crumbs, Plain, Progresso
1.5	1	cup	Wendy's Pasta Deli Salad
1.5	2	cups	Cereal, Puffed, Kashi
1.5	1	bun	Bun, Hot Dog, Arnold
1.5	1.25	wt oz	Cereal, Instant Oatmeal w/Maple and Brown Sugar, Quaker
1.5	1/2	portion	Rice, Fried, w/Chicken, Frozen, Chun King
1.5	2	pieces	Cracker, Honey Graham, Health Valley
1.5	1/2	portion	Lasagna, Frozen, Celentano
1.5	1/4	cup	Granola, Maple Nut, Arrowhead Mills
1.5	1/2	cup	Spaghetti, w/Meatballs
1.5	4	crackers	Cracker, Rice Cake
1.5	1 1/2	waffles	Waffles, Nutri-Grain, Frozen, Eggo
1.5	10	crackers	Cracker, Low Salt, Saltine, Nabisco
1.5	10	crackers	Cracker, Saltine, Nabisco
1.5	10	crackers	Cracker, Whole Wheat, Saltine, Nabisco
1.5	1	fl oz	Pretzel, Fat Free, Mr. Salty, Nabisco
1.5	1/2	portion	Fettucini, w/Meat Sauce, Slim, Frozen, Budget Gourmet
1.5	1	roll	Roll, Frankfurter, Side-Sliced, Pepperidge Farm
1.5	1/2	piece	Pizza Hut Pepperoni Hand Tossed Pizza
1.5	1	piece	Pizza, Cheese, Frozen, Weight Watchers
1.5	1/2	piece	Pizza Hut Pepperoni Thin 'n Crispy Pizza
1.5	1/2	cup	Egg Noodles, Cooked (1.125 C=2 wt oz Dry)
1.5	6	pieces	Biscuit, Uneeda
1.5	1/2	portion	Lasagna, w/Bread, Frozen, Morton

Nutripoints	Serving Size		Food Name—Grains
1.5	1/2	cup	Pretzels, Keebler
1.5	2	pieces	Roll, Dinner, Wheat Loaf, Pipin' Hot
1.5	1/2	piece	Domino's Large 16" Sausage/Mushroom Pizza
1.5	6	pieces	Breadsticks, Sesame, Keebler
1.5	1/4	cup	Granola, No Sugar
1.5	1/2	piece	Pizza, Combo, Deluxe, Frozen, Weight Watchers
1.5	1/3	portion	Lasagna, Three Cheese, Frozen, Budget Gourmet
1.5	1/2	portion	Pasta Shells & Beef, Frozen, Budget Gourmet
1.5	2	rolls	Roll, Dinner, White Loaf, Pipin' Hot
1.0	11	crackers	Cracker, Wheat Vegetable, Stone ground, Hain
1.0	1/2	serving	Beef & Broccoli, Uncle Ben's Pasta Bowl
1.0	1/2	piece	Domino's Large 16" Veggie Pizza
1.0	6	pieces	Breadsticks, Garlic, Keebler
1.0	1/2	cup	Stuffing Mix, Herb Seasoned, Pepperidge Farm
1.0	1/2	piece	Domino's Large 16" Ham Pizza
1.0	10	crackers	Cracker, Saltine, Low Sodium
1.0	2	waffles	Waffles, Original, Aunt Jemima
1.0	4	crackers	Cracker, Melba Toast
1.0	1	whole	McDonald's English Muffin w/Butter
1.0	1	piece	Pizza, w/Cheese
1.0	1/2	portion	Pasta Casino, Frozen, Stouffer's
1.0	4	crackers	Cracker, Oat Bran Krisp, Ralston
1.0	1	wt oz	Pretzels, Twists, Rold Gold
1.0	1/2	portion	Lasagna, Meat Sauce, Frozen, Weight Watchers
1.0	10	crackers	Cracker, Melba Toast, Garlic, Keebler
1.0	10	crackers	Cracker, Melba Toast, Onion, Keebler
1.0	10	crackers	Cracker, Melba Toast, Plain, Keebler
1.0	4	crackers	Cracker, Amaranth Graham, Health Valley
1.0	1/2	piece	Pizza, French Bread Pepperoni, Stouffer
1.0	1/2	piece	Pizza, Sausage, Frozen, Weight Watchers
1.0	1/2	portion	Lasagna, Italian Cheese, Frozen, Weight Watchers
1.0	50	crackers	Crackers, Oyster, Small
1.0	1/2	cup	Croutons, Cheddar and Romano Cheese, Pepperidge Farm
1.0	6	crackers	Cracker, Low Salt, Triscuit, Nabisco
1.0	6	crackers	Cracker, Wheat 'n Bran, Triscuit, Nabisco
1.0	1	serving	Pasta, Penne & Ricotta, Weight Watchers
1.0	1	biscuit	Biscuit, Buttermilk, From Mix
1.0	1	pancake	Pancake, Cornmeal
1.0	2	crackers	Cracker, Sea Toast, Keebler
1.0	1/2	cup	Fettuccini, Cooked (1 C=2 wt oz Dry)
1.0	1/2	portion	Rice, Fried, w/Pork, Frozen, Chun King
1.0	8	crackers	Cracker, Saltine
1.0	2	cups	Popcorn, Original Lite

Nutripoints	Serving Size		Food Name—Grains
1.0	1	piece	Cornbread
1.0	1/2	serving	Penne Pasta, Spicy Puttanesca, Organic, Fzn, Moosewood
1.0	1	piece	Cake, Elfin Loaves, Blueberry, Frozen, Keebler
1.0	1/2	piece	Pizza, Pepperoni, Frozen, Weight Watchers
1.0	1 1/2	waffles	Waffles, Homestyle, Frozen, Eggo
1.0	2	waffles	Waffles, Organic Gorilla Banana, Nature's Path
1.0	1/4	cup	Granola, Heartland
1.0	1	pancakes	Pancake, Buckwheat
1.0	1	piece	Pizza, Cheese, Deluxe, Frozen, Totino's
1.0	2	biscuits	Biscuit, Buttermilk, Big Country, Pillsbury
1.0	5	pieces	Nachos, Cheese/Hot Peppers
1.0	1	biscuit	Biscuit
1.0	1	serving	Lasagna Florentine, Weight Watchers Smart Ones
1.0	1/4	cup	Noodles & Cheese Dinner, Deboles
1.0	6	crackers	Cracker, 7 Grain Vegetable, Stoned Wheat, Health Valley
1.0	1	whole	Carl's Jr. English Muffin w/Margarine
1.0	15	chips	Tortilla Chips, Light Nacho Cheese, Doritos
1.0	1/4	cup	Noodles, Chow Mein
1.0	1/4	cup	Cereal, 100% Natural, Quaker
1.0	1/4	cup	Pasta & Sauce, Marinara, Hain
1.0	1/2	piece	Domino's Large 16" Pepperoni Pizza
1.0	50	crackers	Crackers, Oyster, Small, Keebler
1.0	1	muffin	Muffin, Oatmeal
0.5	1/2	portion	Pasta Oriental, Frozen, Stouffer's
0.5	1	tart	Pop-Tarts, Frosted Strawberry, Kellogg's
0.5	20	crackers	Crackers, Cheese Nips
0.5	1/2	portion	Lasagna, Meat Sauce, Frozen, Stouffer's
0.5	1/4	cup	Cereal, Country Morning
0.5	1/2	cup	Pasta Salad, Italian, Cool Side, Lipton
0.5	1	pancake	Pancake, Whole Wheat
0.5	1	pancake	Pancake, Plain
0.5	10	crackers	Cracker, Saltine, Premium
0.5	1	pancake	Pancake, w/Fruit
0.5	1/2	piece	Pizza, French Bread Deluxe, Frozen, Weight Watchers
0.5	1/2	piece	Pizza, Cheese, Frozen, Tree Tavern
0.5	1	muffin	Muffin, Cornbread
0.5	1/2	serving	Lasagna, Vegetable, 365 Organic, Whole Foods
0.5	2	cups	Popcorn, Natural Salt Free, Orville Redenbacher's
0.5	10	pieces	Pretzels, 3 Ring
0.5	1/2	portion	Spaghetti, Beef & Mushroom Sauce, Stouffer's
0.5	1	bar	Granola Bar, Chewy Chocolate Chip, Quaker
0.5	10	crackers	Cracker, Rice, Small
0.5	1/2	piece	Domino's Large 16" Deluxe Pizza

Nutripoints	Serving Size		Food Name—Grains
0.5	1	tart	Pop-Tarts, Blueberry, Kellogg's
0.5	10	crackers	Cracker, Melba Toast, Sesame, Keebler
0.5	1/2	portion	Lasagna, Vegetable, Single Serving, Frozen, Stouffer's
0.5	1/2	piece	Pizza, French Bread, Cheese, Frozen, Stouffer's
0.5	1/2	piece	Pizza, French Bread, Vegetable Deluxe, Frozen, Stouffer's
0.5	1/2	piece	Pizza, Cheese, French Bread, Frozen, Weight Watchers
0.5	1/4	serving	Del Taco Macho Nachos
0.5	50	pieces	Pretzels, Sticks
0.5	1/2	serving	Pizza, Mushroom & Spinach, Linda McCartney
0.5	1	piece	Cake, Elfin Loaves, Apple Cinnamon, Frozen, Keebler
0.5	1	piece	Cake, Elfin Loaves, Banana, Frozen, Keebler
0.5	10	crackers	Cracker, Soda
0.5	1/2	portion	Linguini, w/Shrimp, Frozen, Budget Gourmet
0.5	12	crackers	Crackers, Oat Thins, Nabisco
0.5	1	bar	Candy Bar, Rice Krispies, Kellogg's
0.5	10	crackers	Cracker, Low Salt, Ritz
0.5	10	crackers	Cracker, Whole Wheat, Ritz
0.5	22	crackers	Crackers, Teddy Grahams, Nabisco
0.5	1	tart	Pop-Tarts, Kellogg's Lowfat
0.5	1/4	portion	Lasagna, Italian Sausage, Frozen, Budget Gourmet
0.5	1	piece	Pizza, 9 Slice, Frozen, Celentano
0.5	1/2	portion	Rigatoni, Baked, w/Meat Sauce/Cheese, Frozen, Stouffer's
0.5	1/2	serving	Lasagna, Vegetarian, Boca
0.5	1/2	serving	Pasta, Farfalle & Spinach Pesto, Organic, Fzn, Moosewood
0.5	15	chips	Tortilla Chips
0.5	2	biscuits	Biscuit, Flaky, Hungry Jack
0.5	1 1/2	pieces	French Toast, Nutripoint Recipe
0.5	1	serving	Portabello Mushroom, Uncle Ben's Pasta Bowl
0.5	4	wt oz	Pizza, Cheese, Chef Boy-Ar-Dee
0.5	4	crackers	Cracker, Graham, Honey Maid
0.5	1	tart	Pop-Tarts, Frosted Cherry w/Smucker's Fruit, Kellogg's
0.5	1	serving	Pasta Shells, Stuffed, Fzn, Healthy Choice
0.5	1	piece	Pizza, Thick Crust, Frozen, Celentano
0.5	1/2	cup	Rice, Chicken Rice-A-Roni
0.5	1	muffin	Muffin
0.5	7	crackers	Cracker, Oat Bran Graham, Health Valley
0.5	1/2	cup	Bread, Stuffing
0.5	26	crackers	Crackers, Oyster, Large, Keebler
0.5	1/2	piece	Domino's Large 16" Double Cheese/Pepperoni Pizza
0.5	1	piece	Pizza, Party Cheese, Frozen, Totino's
0.0	1/2	portion	Lasagna, w/Meat Sauce, Slim Frozen, Budget Gourmet
0.0	1/2	portion	Lasagna, Single Serving, Frozen, Stouffer's
0.0	1/2	cup	Rice, Rice A Roni

Nutripoints	Serving Size		Food Name—Grains
0.0	1/2	portion	Pasta Alfredo, w/Broccoli, Frozen, Budget Gourmet
0.0	1	roll	Roll, Sweet, w/Fruit, Frosted
0.0	1/2	piece	Pizza, Pepperoni, French Bread, Frozen, Weight Watchers
0.0	15	crackers	Crackers, TLC 7 Grain, Kashi
0.0	2	crackers	Cracker, Graham, Plain
0.0	1/4	cup	Macaroni & Cheese
0.0	2	Tbls	McDonald's Chow Mein Noodles
0.0	1/2	serving	Pasta, Broccoli and Parmesan, Organic, Fzn, Moosewood
0.0	1/2	cup	Macaroni & Cheese Dinner, Deluxe, Kraft
0.0	1/4	cup	Cereal, 100% Natural, Raisin & Date, Quaker
0.0	1	piece	Bun, Cinnamon
0.0	2	cookies	Cookies, Commodore, Keebler
0.0	1	roll	Roll, Sweet, w/Fruit & Nuts, Frosted
0.0	1/2	portion	Ravioli, Frozen, Celentano
0.0	2	waffles	Waffles, Buttermilk, Jumbo, Downyflake
0.0	1/2	portion	Pasta & Cheese, Baked, Frozen, Celentano
0.0	1/2	portion	Spaghetti, w/Meat Sauce, Frozen, Stouffer's
0.0	1	cup	Popcorn, Caramel
0.0	1/4	serving	Taco Bell Nachos Bellgrande
0.0	1/2	piece	Pizza, French Bread, Pepperoni/Mushroom, Fzn, Stouffer's
0.0	1	piece	Pizza, Cheese, Frozen, Celeste
0.0	1	piece	Pizza, Cheese, Round Family Style, Elios
0.0	11	chips	Corn Chips, Pringles
0.0	1	serving	Macaroni & Cheese, Weight Watchers 99% Fat Free
0.0	1/4	cup	Granola
0.0	3/4	cup	Cereal, Kashi Medley
0.0	6	crackers	Cracker, Harvest Wheat, Keebler
0.0	1/2	cup	Macaroni Salad
0.0	1	wt oz	Pizza, Combos
0.0	1/2	cup	Shells & Cheese Dinner, Velveeta
0.0	1	serving	Carl's Jr. Hot Cakes w/Margarine
0.0	1/2	portion	Macaroni & Cheese, Frozen, Budget Gourmet
0.0	1/2	portion	Rice, Oriental, Vegetables, Frozen, Budget Gourmet
0.0	2	cups	Popcorn, Cooked w/Oil
0.0	1/2	piece	Pizza, Pepperoni, Frozen, Elio's
0.0	1/2	cup	Noodles, Egg, Ronzoni
0.0	1	piece	Bread, Garlic
0.0	1	muffin	Muffin, Blueberry
0.0	1	piece	Gingerbread
0.0	1	wt oz	Wendy's Taco Chips
0.0	1	burger	Hamburger, Vegetarian, Fzn, Gardenburger
-0.5	1/2	piece	Cake, Upside Down, Pineapple
-0.5	1	piece	Cake, White

Nutripoints	Serving Size		Food Name—Grains
-0.5	1/2	piece	Carl's Jr. Danish (all Varieties)
-0.5	16	crackers	Cracker, Wheat Thins
-0.5	1	slice	Bread, Banana
-0.5	1/4	cup	Graham Crumbs, Keebler
-0.5	1	piece	Cake, Carrot, Frozen, Weight Watchers
-0.5	6	crackers	Cracker, Triscuit
-0.5	4	wt oz	Pizza, Pepperoni, Chef Boy-Ar-Dee
-0.5	1	bar	Granola Bar
-0.5	15	chips	Tortilla Chips, Nacho Cheese, Doritos
-0.5	1/2	cup	Stuffing Mix, American New England, Stove Top
-0.5	1	wt oz	Crackers, Wheat Thins, Multi-Grain, Kraft
-0.5	3	crackers	Cracker, Cheese & Peanut Butter, Keebler
-0.5	1/2	serving	Taco Bell Nachos
-0.5	1/2	biscuit	McDonald's Biscuit w/Biscuit Spread
-0.5	1	serving	Pizza, Veggie Supreme, Morningstar Farms
-0.5	1/2	portion	Linguini, Clam Sauce, Frozen, Stouffer's
-0.5	18	chips	Tortilla Chips, Doritos
-0.5	1/2	portion	Linguini, w/Scallops & Clams, Slim Fzn, Budget Gourmet
-0.5	1	cracker	Cracker, Petite Butter Crescents, Pepperidge Farm
-0.5	1	wt oz	Corn Chips
-0.5	1/2	serving	McDonald's Hotcakes w/Butter & Syrup
-0.5	1/2	serving	Jack In the Box Pancake Platter
-0.5	1	muffin	Muffin, w/Fruit And/Or Nuts
-0.5	1/4	piece	Taco Bell Mexican Pizza
-0.5	1/2	slice	Pizza, Thai Recipe Chicken, California Pizza Kitchen
-0.5	1	piece	Tamales, In Chili Sauce, Old El Paso
-1.0	1/2	piece	Wendy's Apple Danish
-1.0	4	crackers	Cracker, Toast & Peanut Butter, Keebler
-1.0	1	wt oz	Crackers, Wheat Thins, Kraft
-1.0	1/2	piece	Pizza, w/Sausage
-1.0	8	crackers	Cracker, Ritz
-1.0	1/2	portion	Pasta Mexicali, Frozen, Stouffer's
-1.0	7.5	wt oz	Spaghetti, w/Meatballs/Tomato Sauce, Chef Boyardee
-1.0	1/2	portion	Fettuccini, Chicken, Frozen, Weight Watchers
-1.0	1	bar	Candy Bar, Ultra, Wild Cherry, Excel
-1.0	1/2	piece	Taco Bell Meximelt
-1.0	1	cookie	Cookies, Sugar
-1.0	1	muffin	Muffin Mix, Corn, Betty Crocker
-1.0	1	muffin	Muffin Mix, Bran Date, Jiffy
-1.0	1	roll	Roll, Sweet, Cinnamon Bun, Frosted
-1.0	1	muffin	Carl's Jr. Bran Muffin
-1.0	1	piece	Fruitcake
-1.0	1	piece	Snack Cake, Lights, Hostess

Nutripoints	Serving Size		Food Name—Grains
-1.0	4	crackers	Cracker, Hearty Wheat, Pepperidge Farm
-1.0	1/2	piece	Shortcake, Sponge Type w/Fruit
-1.0	1	muffin	Muffin Mix, Corn, Jiffy
-1.0	1	muffin	Muffin Mix, Corn, Old Fashioned, Fzn, Pepperidge Farm
-1.0	1/4	serving	Burger King French Toast Sticks
-1.0	2	pancakes	Pancake & Waffle Mix, Extra Light, Hungry Jack
-1.0	1	pancake	Pancake & Waffle Mix, Blue Corn
-1.0	1	bar	Granola Bar, Chewy Honey & Oats, Quaker
-1.0	1/4	cup	Pudding, Rice
-1.0	45	crackers	Cracker, Original Tiny Goldfish, Pepperidge Farm
-1.0	2	wt oz	Candy Bar, Club Sandwich, Hoffman's
-1.0	1/4	cup	Pasta Salad, Home Recipe
-1.0	2	pieces	Hush Puppies
-1.5	2	pancakes	Pancake & Waffle Mix, Buttermilk, Hungry Jack
-1.5	10	crackers	Crackers, Animal, Barnum's
-1.5	1/2	slice	Pizza, BBQ Chicken, California Pizza Kitchen
-1.5	1	whole	Doughnut, Whole Wheat
-1.5	1	wt oz	Corn Puffs, Cheese, Cheez Doodles, Borden
-1.5	7	cookies	Cookies, Nilla Wafers
-1.5	1	slice	Bread, Date, Pillsbury
-1.5	1/2	cup	Stuffing
-1.5	1/2	piece	Egg Roll
-1.5	4	cookies	Cookies, Lemon Creme, Keebler
-1.5	1	bar	Granola Bar, w/Roasted Almonds, Nature Valley
-1.5	1	muffin	Muffin Mix, Blueberry, Wild, Betty Crocker
-1.5	1/2	cup	Stuffing Mix, Cornbread, w/Butter, Stove Top
-1.5	2	cookies	Cookies, Oatmeal
-1.5	1	roll	Roll, Sweet, Apple, Frozen, Weight Watchers
-1.5	1	bar	Granola Bar, Chewy, Low-Fat, Quaker (all flavors)
-1.5	1	cake	Snack Cake, 97% Fat-Free, Hostess (all flavors)
-1.5	10	crackers	Crackers, Animal
-1.5	1	muffin	Muffin Mix, Blueberry, Wild, Duncan Hines
-1.5	1	piece	Turnover, Fruit
-1.5	2	cookies	Cookies, O.F. Oatmeal, Keebler
-1.5	1	serving	Carl's Jr. French Toast Dips
-1.5	1/2	portion	Macaroni & Cheese, Casserole, Frozen, Morton
-1.5	2	cookies	Cookies, Chocolate Fudge Sandwich, Keebler
-1.5	1/2	piece	Tamale
-1.5	1/4	cup	Pasta & Sauce, Swiss, Creamy, Hain
-1.5	2	cookies	Cookies, O.F. Sugar, Keebler
-1.5	2	pieces	Cookies, Keebies, Keebler
-1.5	1/2	piece	Wendy's Cinnamon w/Raisin Danish
-1.5	2	cookies	Cookies, French Vanilla Creme, Keebler

Nutripoints	Serving Size		Food Name—Grains
-1.5	25	pieces	Cheese Puffs, Cheetos
-1.5	1	piece	Cake, Angel Food, Duncan Hines
-1.5	2	cookies	Cookies, Pitter Patter, Keebler
-1.5	1/2	piece	Wendy's Cheese Danish
-1.5	1/4	portion	Pasta Carbonara, Frozen, Stouffer's
-1.5	1/2	slice	Pizza, Five Cheese & Tomato, California Pizza Kitchen
-1.5	5	cookies	Cookies, Vanilla Wafers, Keebler
-1.5	1/2	biscuit	Wendy's Buttermilk Biscuit
-1.5	1	wt oz	Wendy's Cheddar Chips
-1.5	1/2	muffin	Carl's Jr. Blueberry Muffin
-1.5	1	bar	Granola Bar, Chewy Fruit, Quaker
-1.5	1/2	piece	Danish, Apple, Pillsbury
-1.5	1/2	portion	Macaroni & Cheese, Frozen, Stouffer's
-2.0	2	cookies	Cookies, O.F. Double Fudge, Keebler
-2.0	1/2	piece	Taco Bell Cinnamon Crispas
-2.0	1	bar	Granola Bar, Oats 'n Honey, Nature Valley
-2.0	2	cookies	Cookies, Homeplate, Keebler
-2.0	2	cookies	Cookies, Molasses
-2.0	1/2	portion	Fettuccini Primavera, Frozen, Stouffer's
-2.0	2	cookies	Cookies, Applesauce
-2.0	1	piece	Cake, Banana, w/Frosting
-2.0	1	piece	Cake, Crumb
-2.0	1	piece	Cake, Crumb, Hostess
-2.0	1	piece	Wendy's French Toast
-2.0	1	bar	Snack Bar, GOLEAN, Kashi
-2.0	1/2	piece	Cake, Coffee
-2.0	2	cookies	Cookies, O.F. Chocolate Chip, Keebler
-2.0	1	slice	Bread, Carrot, Nut, Pillsbury
-2.0	1/2	piece	Pizza, w/Pepperoni
-2.0	1	piece	Cake, Chocolate, Frozen, Weight Watchers
-2.0	1	cookie	McDonald's McDonaldland Cookies
-2.0	4	cookies	Cookies, Buttercup, Keebler
-2.0	1/2	piece	Chocolate Éclair
-2.0	1	piece	Cake, German Chocolate, Frozen, Weight Watchers
-2.0	1	piece	Cake, Banana, Sara Lee
-2.0	1/2	cup	Pudding, Bread
-2.0	1/4	bar	Dairy Queen Fudge Nut Bar
-2.0	1/2	piece	Turnover, Blueberry, Frozen, Pepperidge Farm
-2.0	1	piece	Doughnut, Cake w/o Frosting
-2.0	1/2	cup	Egg Noodles, Creamette, Borden
-2.0	2	pieces	Fig Newton
-2.0	1	piece	Shortcake, Strawberry, Frozen, Weight Watchers
-2.0	1	piece	Doughnut, Powdered Strawberry Filled, Krispy Kreme

Nutripoints	Serving Size		Food Name—Grains
-2.0	2	cookies	Cookies, Macaroon
-2.0	1	piece	Snack Cake, Light, Apple 'n Spice, Pepperidge Farm
-2.0	1/2	piece	Cake, Sponge, w/Whipped Cream and Fruit
-2.0	1	piece	Snack Cake, Ding Dong, Hostess
-2.5	1	piece	Snack Cake, Drake's Devil Dogs
-2.5	1	whole	Doughnut, Glazed
-2.5	1/2	piece	Danish Pastry
-2.5	1	piece	Pie Crust Mix, Betty Crocker
-2.5	1	roll	Roll, Sweet, Cinnamon, w/Icing, Pillsbury
-2.5	1	whole	Croissant
-2.5	1/2	piece	Cake, Carrot, w/Cream Cheese Frosting
-2.5	1/2	piece	Doughnut, Chocolate, w/ Chocolate Icing
-2.5	1	piece	Cake, Black Forest, Frozen, Weight Watchers
-2.5	1	cookie	McDonald's Chocolaty Chip Cookies
-2.5	1	piece	Doughnut, Original Glazed, Krispy Kreme
-2.5	1	piece	Cake, Angel Food, Plain
-2.5	2	cookies	Cookies, Oatmeal Cremes Sandwich, Keebler
-2.5	1	piece	Pie Crust, Pet Ritz
-2.5	1/2	roll	Roll, Sweet
-2.5	1	piece	Doughnut, Cake w/Frosting
-2.5	3	pieces	Shortbread, Lorna Doone
-2.5	1 1/4	wt oz	Candy Bar, Crunchy Nut, Kudos
-2.5	1	piece	Doughnut, Traditional Cake, Krispy Kreme
-2.5	2	cookies	Cookies, Sandwich, Chocolate/Vanilla
-2.5	1	piece	Cake, Pound, Blueberry Topping, Frozen, Weight Watchers
-2.5	1	piece	French Toast
-2.5	2	cookies	Cookies, Oreo
-3.0	1/2	piece	Doughnut, Old Fashioned, Glazed, Earth Grains
-3.0	1	piece	Twinkies, Hostess
-3.0	1	piece	Brownie, Walnut, Betty Crocker
-3.0	1	cookie	Cookies, O.F. Granola, Large, Pepperidge Farm
-3.0	1	wt oz	Candy, Cracker Jacks
-3.0	1	piece	Pie Crust
-3.0	1/2	piece	Doughnut, Jelly
-3.0	1/2	piece	Doughnut, Chocolate Creme Filled
-3.0	1/2	piece	Doughnut, Custard Filled
-3.0	1	piece	Snack Cake, Drake's Ring Ding Jr.
-3.0	1	piece	Doughnut, Chocolate Iced Kreme Filled, Krispy Kreme
-3.0	1/2	piece	Doughnut, Devil's Food, Earth Grains
-3.0	1/2	piece	Cake, German Chocolate
-3.0	6	cookies	Cookies, Vanilla Wafer
-3.0	3	cookies	Cookies, Oatmeal Raisin, Pepperidge Farm
-3.0	1/2	piece	Cake, Torte

Nutripoints	Serving Size		Food Name—Grains
-3.0	2	cookies	Cookies, Chips Deluxe, Keebler
-3.0	1/2	piece	Cake, Bundt Pound Supreme, Pillsbury
-3.0	1/2	cookie	Carl's Jr. Chocolate Chip Cookie 2.5 Ounce
-3.0	1	piece	Cupcake, Chocolate, Hostess
-3.0	1	piece	Brownie, Chocolate, Frozen, Weight Watchers
-3.0	1/2	piece	Cake, Chocolate w/o Frosting (12 Pieces/Cake)
-3.0	1/2	piece	Cake, Devil's Food, Deluxe, Duncan Hines
-3.0	1/2	cookie	Wendy's Chocolate Chip Cookie
-3.0	1/2	piece	Cake, Boston Cream, Supreme, Pepperidge Farm
-3.0	1/4	piece	Burger King Great Danish
-3.0	1	piece	Sopaipilla
-3.0	1/2	piece	Cake, Chocolate w/Frosting (12 Pieces/Cake)
-3.0	1/2	piece	Cake, Dutch Apple, Streusel Swirl, Pillsbury
-3.5	1/2	piece	Snack Cake, Suzy Q's
-3.5	2	pieces	Cookie Dough, Chocolate Chip, Pillsbury
-3.5	1/2	piece	Cake, Angel Food, w/Glaze
-3.5	1	piece	Brownie, w/o Frosting
-3.5	1	piece	Cake, Golden Layer, Pepperidge Farm
-3.5	1	piece	Cake, Chocolate Fudge Snack, Sara Lee
-3.5	1	piece	Chocolate Eclair, Good Humor
-3.5	2	cookies	Cookies, Chocolate Chip, Duncan Hines
-3.5	1/2	piece	Cake, Sponge, w/Icing
-3.5	1	cookies	Cookies, Chocolate Chip Oatmeal, Pillsbury
-3.5	1/2	piece	Cake, German Chocolate, Moist, Betty Crocker
-3.5	1	piece	Brownie, w/Frosting
-3.5	2	cookies	Cookies, Peanut Butter'n Fudge, Duncan Hines
-3.5	3	cookies	Cookies, Milano Distinctive, Pepperidge Farm
-3.5	1	piece	Cupcake, w/o Frosting
-3.5	1/2	piece	Carl's Jr. Chocolate Cake
-4.0	1/2	piece	Cake, Chocolate Mint Plus, Pillsbury
-4.0	3	cookies	Cookies, Chocolate Chip, Pepperidge Farm
-4.0	1	piece	Cake, Pound, Original, Sara Lee
-4.0	3	cookies	Cookies, Chessmen, Pepperidge Farm
-4.0	2	cookies	Cookies
-4.0	2	cookies	Cookies, Chocolate Chip
-4.0	2	cookies	Cookies, Sandwich, Mystic Mint
-4.0	1	piece	Cupcake, w/Frosting
-4.0	3	cookies	Cookies, Bordeaux, Pepperidge Farm
-4.0	1/2	serving	Mousse, Chocolate, Light, Sara Lee
-4.5	3	cookies	Cookies, Pirouettes, Chocolate-Laced, Pepperidge Farm
-4.5	1	piece	Cake, Sponge
-5.0	1	piece	Cake, Pound
-5.5	2	pieces	Snack Cake, Apple Delight, Little Debbie

Nutripoints	Serving Size		Food Name—Grains
-5.5	1/2	piece	Cheesecake, Classic Snack, Sara Lee
-6.5	2	pieces	Snack Cake, Oatmeal Creme Pie, Little Debbie
-7.0	2	pieces	Snack Cake, Peanut Butter Bar, Little Debbie
-8.5	2	pieces	Snack Cake, Star Crunch, Little Debbie

LEGUME/NUT/SEED GROUP

Nutripoints	Serving Size		Food Name—Legumes/Nuts/Seeds
34.5	1	bar	Snack Bar, DrSoy Protein Bar (*)
31.0	8	fl oz	Milk Drink, Juice Plus+ Complete® (w/water) (*)
28.5	1	bar	Snack Bar, Clif Luna Bar (*)
21.0	1	bar	Snack Bar, Pria, Power Bar (*)
18.0	2	cups	Bean Sprouts, Mung, Fresh
17.0	1 1/2	cups	Soup, French Market, Nutripoint Recipe
16.5	1	bar	Snack Bar, Pria Carb Select, Power Bar (*)
15.5	1	burger	Hamburger, Vegan, Natural Touch
15.0	1	serving	Hamburger, Vegetarian, Better 'N Burgers, Worthington
14.5	2	servings	Pepperoni, Veggie Pizza, Yves
14.5	1	serving	Hamburger, Vegetarian, Spicy Black Bean, Worthington
14.0	1	piece	Frankfurter, Linketts, Loma Linda Foods
14.0	1	bar	Snack Bar, PR Nutrition Bar (*)
14.0	1	cup	Peas, Green, No Salt Added, Canned, Del Monte
14.0	1	cup	Peas, Frozen, Cooked
14.0	1 1/2	cups	Soup, Minestrone, Health Valley
13.5	1	cup	Beans, Navy, Cooked
13.5	1	cup	Soup, Lentil, Nutripoint Recipe
13.0	3/4	cup	Chili, South/Border Vegetarian, Nutripoint Recipe
13.0	1	bar	Snack Bar, Breakthrough, Honey Graham (*)
12.5	8	fl oz	Milk Drink, Soy Protein, Health Source (*)
12.5	2	pieces	Hot Dog, Veggie Dogs, Yves
12.0	1	cup	Peas, Green, Frozen, Birds Eye
11.5	1/2	cup	Chili, Vegetarian, Health Valley Fat Free
11.0	1	cup	Pigeon Peas, Green, Cooked
10.5	2	cups	Bean Sprouts, Mung, Arrowhead Mills
10.5	2	patties	Sausage Patty, Breakfast, Frozen, Morningstar Farms
10.0	4	links	Sausage Links, Veggie, Morningstar Farms
10.0	1/2	cup	Soup, Pea, Split Green, Health Valley
9.5	1	bar	Snack Bar, Atkins Advantage Bar (*)
9.5	3/4	cup	Beans, Lima, Cooked
9.5	8	fl oz	Milk, Soy, Silk Light Organic
9.0	2	cups	Milk, Soy, Light Original, 8th Continent
9.0	1	cup	Peas, Black-Eyed, Canned
8.5	1/2	cup	Beans, Kidney, Cooked
8.5	3	slices	Bacon, Veggie Canadian, Yyves
8.5	1	bar	Snack Bar, Balance Bar 40-30-30 (*)
8.5	4	wt oz	Vegeburger, Loma Linda Foods
8.5	3/4	cup	Beans, Cooked
8.5	1	cup	Peas, Black-Eyed, Cooked

Nutripoints	Serving Size		Food Name—Legumes/Nuts/Seeds
8.5	4	pieces	Chicken Nuggets, Vegetarian, Morningstar Farms
8.0	3	slices	Ham, Meatless, Wham, Worthington
8.0	1	cup	Lentils, Cooked
8.0	1/4	cup	Dip, Bean, Black, Nutripoint Recipe
8.0	1/2	cup	Soup, Lentil, Health Valley
8.0	1	cup	Cowpeas, Cooked
8.0	1/2	cup	Peas, Split
8.0	4	slices	Bologna Slices, Veggie, Yves
8.0	1/2	cup	Beans, Garbanzo, Cooked
8.0	1	serving	Hamburger, Vegetarian, Grillers, Fzn, Morningstar Farms
7.5	1/2	cup	Beans, Baked, w/Tomato Sauce
7.5	1	wt oz	Soybeans, Dry, Arrowhead Mills
7.5	1	cup	Peas, Canned
7.5	1	pat	Hamburger, (Vege) Harvest Burger, Green Giant
7.5	1	cup	Soup, Bean, Black, Health Valley
7.5	8	fl oz	Milk, Soy, Power Dream, Imagine Foods
7.5	8	fl oz	Milk, Soy, Soyamel, Worthington
7.0	3	slices	Bologna, Vegetarian, Bolono, Worthington
7.0	4	slices	Turkey Slices, Veggie, Yves
7.0	2	cups	Milk, Soy, Light Vanilla, 8th Continent
7.0	2	wt oz	Bologna, Slices, Frozen, Loma Linda
7.0	3/4	cup	Soybeans, Cooked
7.0	1	bar	Snack Bar, Genisoy Xtreme (*)
6.5	8	fl oz	Milk, Soy, Silk Organic
6.5	1	bar	Snack Bar, DrSoy Healthy Snacker Bar (*)
6.5	1/2	cup	Beans, Pinto, Cooked
6.5	2	wt oz	Beef, Roast, Slices, Frozen, Loma Linda
6.5	1	bar	Snack Bar, Genisoy (*)
6.5	1	cup	Lentils and Rice, Herbed, Nutripoint Recipe
6.5	1/2	cup	Peas, Sweet, 50% Less Salt, Canned, Green Giant
6.5	1/2	cup	Peas, Sweet, Canned, Green Giant
6.5	2	wt oz	Turkey, Slices, Frozen, Loma Linda Foods
6.5	1	cup	Soup, Lentil Curry, Couscous, Nile Spice Foods
6.0	1/2	cup	Hamburger Crumbles, Vegetarian, Morningstar Farms
6.0	1	bar	Breakfast Bar, Atkins (*)
6.0	1/2	cup	Peas, Sweet, Early Garden, Canned, Del Monte
6.0	1	cup	Soup, Hearty Lentil & Vegetable, Wolfgang Puck's
6.0	2	pieces	Sausage, Meatless, Prosage Patties, Worthington
5.5	2	wt oz	Chicken, Slices, Frozen, Loma Linda Foods
5.5	1	burger	Hamburger, Vegetarian, Boca Burger
5.5	1	wt oz	Beans, Adzuki, Dry, Arrowhead Mills
5.5	8	fl oz	Milk, Soy Dream, Vanilla, Imagine Foods
5.5	2	wt oz	Salami, Slices, Frozen, Loma Linda Foods

Nutripoints	Serving Size		Food Name—Legumes/Nuts/Seeds
5.5	1	bar	Snack Bar, Clif Bar (*)
5.5	1/2	bar	Snack Bar, Clif Builder's Bar (*)
5.5	1	serving	Meal Bar, All Flavors, South Beach Diet
5.5	1	cup	Soup, Lentil
5.5	1	burger	Hamburger, Vegetarian, Dr. Praeger's
5.5	1/2	portion	Enchiladas, Mexican, Legume
5.0	2	Tbls	Seeds, Flax
5.0	1	bar	Snack Bar, Slim-Fast Optima (*)
5.0	1/2	cup	Tofu
5.0	1	cup	Soup, Minestrone, Healthy Choice
5.0	1	cup	Soup, Bean, Black
5.0	1/2	cup	Chili, Bean
5.0	1	wt oz	Soybean Nuts, Roasted, Salted
5.0	1	patty	Chicken Patty, Vegetarian, Morningstar Farms
4.5	1	piece	Frankfurter, Vegetarian, Lowfat, Big Franks, Loma Linda
4.5	1/2	portion	Mexican Style Dinner, Frozen, Morton
4.5	1	serving	Burrito, Beans/Rice/Cheese, Lowfat, Cedarlane
4.5	1	cup	Soup, Lentil, w/Ham
4.5	4	pieces	Bacon Strips, Veggie, Morningstar Farms
4.5	8	fl oz	Milk, Soy, Silk Chocolate Organic
4.5	1/4	cup	Seeds, Sunflower, Unsalted
4.5	8	fl oz	Milk, Soy, Original Flavor, 8th Continent
4.5	1	cup	Peas, Early June, Canned, Le Sueur
4.5	1	cup	Chili, Vegetarian Burrito Flavor, Health Valley
4.0	1/2	cup	Beans, Kidney, Best Light, Canned, Bush's
4.0	1/2	cup	Tuno, Meatless Tuna, Worthington
4.0	1	cup	Soup, Pea, Split Naturals, Hain
4.0	1/2	portion	Enchiladas, Beef/Cheese
4.0	1/2	portion	Taco Bell Bean Burrito w/Green Sauce
4.0	8	fl oz	Milk, Soy, Light Chocolate, 8th Continent
4.0	1/2	serving	Taco Bell Bean Burrito w/Red Sauce
4.0	1	cup	Chili, Meatless, Lowfat, Worthington
4.0	1	cup	Soup, Pea
4.0	1	cup	Soup, Hot and Sour, Nutripoint Recipe
4.0	3	wt oz	Soyburger Patty
4.0	1/2	cup	Chili, Vegetarian, Canned, Worthington
4.0	1/2	cup	Butter Beans, Frozen, Pictsweet
4.0	1	cup	Soup, Minestrone, Progresso
3.5	2	Tbls	Dip, Bean
3.5	5	pieces	Chicken, Buffalo Wings, Vegetarian, Morningstar Farms
3.5	1	serving	Taco Bell Tostada, Fresco Style
3.5	1	wt oz	Soybeans, Roasted, Unsalted
3.5	5	pieces	Chik Nuggets, Meatless, Loma Linda

Nutripoints	Serving Size		Food Name—Legumes/Nuts/Seeds
3.5	1	patty	Chicken, (Vege) Chick Patties, Morningstar Farms
3.5	1	cup	Soup, Bean
3.5	8	fl oz	Milk, Soy, Vanilla, 8th Continent
3.5	1	cup	Beans, Refried, Old El Paso
3.5	1/2	cup	Beans, Boston Baked
3.5	1/2	serving	Del Taco Half Pound Red or Green Burrito
3.5	1	piece	Frankfurter, Vegetarian, Big Franks, Loma Linda
3.5	1	serving	Taco Bell Bean Burrito, Fresco Style
3.0	1/3	cup	Chili, Vegetarian Low Fat Texas Style, Health Valley
3.0	1/2	cup	Chili w/Lentils, Vegetarian, Health Valley
3.0	1/2	cup	Beans, w/Pork
3.0	1/2	burger	Soyburger, w/Bun
3.0	1	cup	Chili w/Beans, Spicy Vegetarian, Health Valley
3.0	1/2	serving	Chili, Vegetarian, ZonePerfect
3.0	1/2	serving	Subway Veggie-Max Sandwich (6")
3.0	2	wt oz	Chic-ketts, Meatless, Worthington
3.0	1/2	serving	Del Taco Veggie Works Burrito
3.0	1/2	cup	Beans, Chili, Loma Linda
3.0	1	cup	Soup, Lentil, Lenticchie, Alessi (dry mix)
3.0	1	serving	Del Taco Red or Green Bean/Cheese Burrito
2.5	1/2	cup	Beans, Vegetarian Style, Van Camp's
2.5	8	wt oz	Soup, Green Pea, Campbell's
2.5	1	serving	Veggie Burger, 365 Organic, Whole Foods
2.5	1/2	serving	Burrito, Bean/Cheese
2.5	3	slices	Salami, Meatless, Worthington
2.5	1/2	cup	Soup, Pea, Split Green, Progresso
2.5	1	wt oz	Seeds, Pumpkin & Squash, Roasted, Unsalted
2.5	1	wt oz	Seeds, Pumpkin & Squash, Roasted, Salted
2.5	1	serving	Del Taco Soft Taco
2.5	1	serving	Taco Bell Pintos & Cheese, Green Sauce
2.5	1	serving	Taco Bell Pintos & Cheese, Red Sauce
2.0	1/2	cup	Soup, Chunky Old Fashioned Bean 'n Ham, Campbell's
2.0	1/4	cup	Trail Mix
2.0	1/2	serving	Del Taco Big Fat Taco
2.0	1/4	serving	Del Taco Deluxe Taco Salad
2.0	1	cup	Milk, Soy, Natural, Edensoy
2.0	2	Tbls	Seeds, Sunflower, Hulled, Arrowhead Mills
2.0	1	piece	Chicken, Veggie, Italian Marinara
2.0	1/2	cup	Beans, Refried
2.0	1/2	portion	Beans, w/Frankfurters Dinner, Frozen, Morton
2.0	1/2	cup	Beans, Lima, Baby, w/Butter, Frozen, Green Giant
2.0	1/2	serving	Sandwich, Peanut Butter, Whole Wheat
2.0	1/4	cup	Seeds, Pumpkin & Squash

Nutripoints	Serving Size		Food Name—Legumes/Nuts/Seeds
2.0	1/2	serving	Taco Bell Burrito Supreme w/Red Sauce
2.0	1/2	serving	Taco Bell Burrito Supreme w/Green Sauce
2.0	2	wt oz	Nut Meat, Nuteena, Loma Linda Foods
2.0	1/2	cup	Beans, w/Pork, Van Camp's
2.0	1/2	cup	Chili, Vegetarian, Worthington
2.0	1	serving	Del Taco Regular Taco
2.0	1	serving	Del Taco Carnitas Taco
1.5	1	cup	Chili, Vegetarian, Natural Touch
1.5	1/2	cup	Beans, w/Pork In Tomato Sauce, Campbell's
1.5	1/2	cup	Beans, w/Pork, Showboat, Bush's
1.5	8	fl oz	Milk, Soy, Chocolate, 8th Continent
1.5	25	nuts	Peanuts, Oil Roasted, Unsalted
1.5	1	cup	Salad, Three Bean
1.5	2	Tbls	Peanut Butter, Chunky, No Salt, Health Valley
1.5	2	Tbls	Peanut Butter, Chunky, Health Valley
1.5	1/2	serving	Beans, Red w/Southwest Cornbread, Fzn, Moosewood
1.5	2	Tbls	Peanut Butter, 25% less fat, Laura Scudder's Natural
1.5	1/2	serving	Sandwich, Peanut Butter, White
1.5	1	wt oz	Sesame Butter (tahini)
1.5	12	nuts	Cashews, Dry Roasted, Unsalted
1.5	1	patty	Vegi-Patties, Frozen, Lifestream
1.5	18	nuts	Almonds, Raw
1.5	1	wt oz	Cashews, Dry Roasted, Unsalted, Planter's
1.5	1/2	serving	Burger King Veggie Burger
1.5	1/2	serving	Taco Bell Beef Burrito w/Green Sauce
1.5	1	wt oz	Peanuts, Dry Roasted, Unsalted, Planter's
1.5	1	serving	Taco Bell Bean/Cheese Taco, Fresco Style
1.0	1/2	cup	Beans, Home Style, Campbell's
1.0	25	nuts	Peanuts, Oil Roasted, Salted
1.0	1	serving	Frankfurter, Vegetarian, Worthington
1.0	1	wt oz	Peanuts, Dry Roasted, Salted, Planter's
1.0	1	Tbls	Peanut Butter, Unsalted
1.0	1	wt oz	Mixed Nuts, Dry Roast, Unsalted
1.0	1	Tbls	Peanut Butter, No Salt Added, Natural, Smucker's
1.0	1	burger	Cheeseburger, Vegetarian, Boca Burger
1.0	1	wt oz	Pine Nuts, Pignolia
1.0	1	Tbls	Peanut Butter, Low Sodium
1.0	1	wt oz	Butternuts
1.0	2	Tbls	Peanut Butter, 25% less fat, Skippy
1.0	2	Tbls	Peanut Butter, 30% less fat, Peter Pan Smart Choice
1.0	2	Tbls	Peanut Butter, Reduced Fat, Jiff
1.0	1	Tbls	Peanut Butter, Natural, Smucker's

Nutripoints	Serving Size		Food Name—Legumes/Nuts/Seeds
1.0	1	wt oz	Peanuts, Spanish, Salted, Planter's
1.0	1/2	cup	Chili, Bean/Beef
1.0	1/2	serving	Taco Bell Beef Burrito w/Red Sauce
1.0	1	cup	Milk, Soy, Natural Creamy Original, Vitasoy
1.0	1	wt oz	Mixed Nuts, Oil Roasted, Salted
1.0	1	wt oz	Pistachios, Raw
1.0	1	wt oz	Peanuts, Cocktail, Planter's
1.0	25	nuts	Peanuts, Dry Roasted, Salted, Frito-Lay
1.0	1/4	portion	Burrito Dinner, Frozen, Patio
0.5	1	Tbls	Peanut Butter
0.5	1	serving	Del Taco Ultimate Taco
0.5	1	wt oz	Cashews, Dry Roasted, Salted
0.5	1	cup	Milk, Non-Dairy, Soy, West Soy
0.5	1	wt oz	Cashews, Oil Roasted, Unsalted
0.5	1	Tbls	Almond Butter, Salted
0.5	1/2	serving	Sandwich, Peanut Butter/Jelly, Whole Wheat
0.5	1/2	cup	Beans, Baked, Barbecue, B&M
0.5	1	wt oz	Peanuts, Honey Roasted
0.5	1/2	serving	Taco, Bean/Cheese
0.5	1/2	serving	Del Taco Regular Taco Salad
0.5	1/2	serving	Burrito, Bean/Beef, Green, Frozen, Patio
0.5	8	fl oz	Milk, Soy, Solait, Miller Farms
0.5	1/2	serving	Burrito, Bean/Beef, Red Chili, Frozen, Patio
0.5	1/2	serving	Enchiladas, Chicken w/Sour Cream Sauce
0.5	8	nuts	Macadamia Nuts, Oil Roasted, Salted
0.5	1/2	serving	Sandwich, Peanut Butter/Jelly, White
0.5	1	wt oz	Filberts, Oil Roasted, Salted
0.5	2	Tbls	Peanut Butter, Skippy Reduced Fat
0.5	12	nuts	Walnuts, Black
0.5	1	wt oz	Almonds, Blanched, Blue Diamond
0.5	1	wt oz	Cashews, Oil Roasted, Salted
0.5	1	wt oz	Cashew Butter, Salted
0.5	12	nuts	Almonds, Oil Roasted, Salted
0.0	6	nuts	Brazil Nuts, Unsalted
0.0	1/2	serving	Burrito, Red Hot, Frozen, Patio
0.0	1/2	serving	Burrito, Beef/Cheese
0.0	12	nuts	Walnuts, English or Persian
0.0	2	crackers	Cracker, Peanut Butter Sandwich
0.0	1	burger	Hamburger, Veggie, Grillers Prime, Fzn, Morningstar Farms
0.0	1	Tbls	Peanut Butter, Creamy, Skippy
0.0	1/4	portion	Mexican Dinner, Frozen, Patio
0.0	1	cup	Milk, Soy, Soymoo, Health Valley
0.0	1/3	serving	Wendy's Taco Supreme Salad

Nutripoints	Serving Size		Food Name—Legumes/Nuts/Seeds
0.0	15	nuts	Pecans, Unsalted, Raw
0.0	1	Tbls	Peanut Butter, Creamy, Jif
0.0	1	Tbls	Peanut Butter, Super Chunk, Skippy
0.0	1	burger	Tofu Burger, Frozen, Island Spring Oriental
0.0	1/2	portion	Burrito, Chicken, Frozen, Weight Watchers
0.0	1/4	cup	Seeds, Sesame
0.0	1/4	cup	Pistachios, Dry Roasted, Salted
0.0	1/2	portion	Burrito, Bean/Beef, Frozen, Patio
0.0	1/2	portion	Burrito, Beefsteak, Frozen, Weight Watchers
0.0	1/3	portion	Mexican Style Combo Dinner, Frozen, Patio
0.0	1	Tbls	Peanut Butter, Crunchy, Peter Pan
0.0	1/2	serving	Enchiladas, Bean/Cheese
0.0	1	bar	Candy Bar, Peanut, Planters
0.0	1/2	portion	Fiesta Dinner, Frozen, Patio
-0.5	1/2	portion	Combination Dinner, Frozen, Patio
-0.5	1	wt oz	Candy, Peanut Butter Morsels
-0.5	1	wt oz	Pecans, Oil Roasted, Salted
-0.5	1	wt oz	Walnuts, Baking, Diamond
-1.0	5	wt oz	Burrito, Beef/Bean, Patio
-1.0	4	fl oz	Cream, Soy, Solait, Miller Farms
-1.0	1	wt oz	Peanuts, Yogurt-Covered
-1.0	1/2	cup	Beans, Refried, w/Sausage, Old El Paso
-1.0	1	wt oz	Peanuts, Chocolate Covered
-1.0	1/3	portion	Mexican Combination Dinner, Frozen, Swanson
-1.0	6	pieces	Almonds, Chocolate-Covered
-1.0	2	cookies	Cookies, Peanut Butter
-1.0	1/3	portion	Enchiladas, Cheese Ranchero, Van de Kamp's
-1.0	1	wt oz	Filberts, Dry Roasted, Salted
-1.5	1	wt oz	Nuts, Mixed, w/Peanuts, Planter's
-1.5	1	serving	Jack In the Box Taco
-1.5	2	pieces	Candy Bar, Twix Peanut Butter
-1.5	6	pieces	Almonds, Sugar-Coated
-2.0	1/2	cup	Frozen Dessert, Lowfat, Tofutti
-2.0	1/2	serving	Jack In the Box Super Taco
-2.0	1	wt oz	Candy, Reese's Pieces
-2.5	1	wt oz	Candy, Caramel w/Nuts, Chocolate-Covered
-3.0	1	wt oz	Candy, Peanut Brittle
-3.0	1	wt oz	Candy Bar, Milk Chocolate w/Peanuts
-3.5	1	piece	Candy, Peanut Butter Cup
-3.5	1/2	piece	Pie, Pecan

MILK/DAIRY GROUP

Nutripoints	Serving	Size	Food Name
34.0	8	fl oz	Milk Drink, Spiru-Tein (w/skim milk) (*)
25.5	1	bar	Snack Bar, Pure Protein (*)
23.5	1	bar	Snack Bar, Marathon, Snickers (*)
23.5	3/4	cup	Egg, Scrambled, Garden, Egg Beaters, Nutripoint Recipe (*)
23.5	1/4	cup	Egg Substitute, Better 'n Eggs (*)
23.0	16	fl oz	Milk Drink, MET-Rx White Box Protein Powder (w/water) (*)
22.5	8	fl oz	Milk Drink, Shake Mix, ZonePerfect (*)
22.5	12	fl oz	Milk Drink, MET-Rx Total Nutrition Drink Powder (w/water) (*)
20.5	8	fl oz	Milk Drink, Shake Mix, Slim-Fast Optima (*)
19.5	1	bar	Snack Bar, Protein Plus, Power Bar, All Flavors (*)
18.5	12	fl oz	Milk Drink, MET-Rx RTD-51 (*)
18.5	1	bar	Snack Bar, Barbell Energy Bar (*)
17.5	1	serving	Milk Drink, Smart Fuel Protein Anytime Mix (*)
17.5	1/2	cup	Egg Substitute, Egg Beaters, Fleischmann's (*)
16.0	12	fl oz	Milk Drink, Slim-Fast Optima (*)
15.0	1	bar	Snack Bar, Bio-X Bar (*)
15.0	8	fl oz	Milk Drink, Ready to Drink, ZonePerfect (*)
13.5	10	fl oz	Milk Drink, Diet, Lite, Sego (*)
13.5	1/2	cup	Egg Substitute, Egg Beaters, Veg. Omelette Mix, Fleischmann's (*)
13.5	11	fl oz	Milk Drink, Atkins Ready to Drink Shakes (*)
13.0	10	fl oz	Milk Drink, Nestle Sweet Success (*)
13.0	8	fl oz	Milk Drink, Slim Fast (*)
12.5	1	cup	Milk Drink, Glucerna (*)
12.0	15	fl oz	Milk Drink, MET-Rx RTD-40 (*)
12.0	1	cup	Instant Breakfast, w/Low-Fat Milk, No Sugar, Carnation (*)
11.5	2	cups	Milk, Instant Nonfat Dry, Carnation
11.5	8	fl oz	Milk Drink, Ultra Slim Fast (*)
11.0	1	serving	Milk Drink, Balance 40-30-30 (mixed w/water) (*)
10.5	1	piece	Cheese Substitute, Pasteurized Process, Formagg
10.5	1/4	cup	Milk, Nonfat Dry
10.5	11	fl oz	Yogurt Drink, Nouriche Light, All Flavors, Yoplait
10.0	8	fl oz	Milk Drink, Boost High Protein (*)
10.0	1/2	cup	Egg Substitute, Egg Watchers, Tofutti (*)
10.0	1/2	cup	Egg Substitute, Scramblers (*)
10.0	1	bar	Snack Bar, MetaForm (*)
9.5	1	cup	Milk, Skim
9.5	8	fl oz	Milk Drink, Ensure Light (*)
9.5	1/2	cup	Milk, Canned, Skim, Evaporated
9.5	1	cup	Buttermilk, Skim

Nutripoints	Serving Size		Food Name—Milk/Dairy
9.0	5	wt oz	Yogurt, Frozen, TCBY
9.0	1	cup	Yogurt, Nonfat, Plain, Dannon
9.0	3/4	cup	Milk, Evaporated Skimmed, Carnation
9.0	1	bar	Snack Bar, Tiger's Milk (*)
9.0	1	bar	Snack Bar, VO2 MAX (*)
8.5	8	fl oz	Milk Drink, Ensure High Protein (*)
8.0	11	fl oz	Milk Drink, MET-Rx Carb Count RTD
8.0	10	fl oz	Milk Drink, Carnation Instant Breakfast (*)
8.0	8	fl oz	Milk Drink, Ensure (*)
8.0	8	fl oz	Milk Drink, Ensure w/Fiber (*)
8.0	1	cup	Milk, Lowfat (1%)
8.0	4	fl oz	Sustacal (*)
8.0	1	serving	McDonald's Lowfat Milk Jug
7.5	8	fl oz	Milk Drink, Boost Breeze (*)
7.5	6	fl oz	Milk Drink, Diet, Sego (*)
7.5	1	cup	Milk, Lowfat (2%), Hi-Calcium, Borden
7.5	1	bar	Snack Bar, MET-Rx Big-100 Meal Replacement (*)
7.0	8	wt oz	Yogurt, Lowfat, Plain
7.0	8	fl oz	Milk Drink, Resource (*)
6.5	1/4	cup	Cream, Sour, New Way, Nutripoint Recipe
6.5	1/4	cup	Sauce, Banana Mint, Nutripoint Recipe
6.5	8	fl oz	Milk Drink, Resource Plus (*)
6.5	1	bar	Snack Bar, SmartZone, Hershey's
6.5	11	fl oz	Milk Drink, MET-Rx RTD Lite
6.0	12	fl oz	Smoothie, All Flavors, Horizon Organic
6.0	1/2	cup	Instant Breakfast, Chocolate, Carnation (*)
6.0	4	wt oz	Egg Substitute, Egg Beaters, Cheez, Fleischmann's (*)
6.0	12	fl oz	Milk Drink, MET-Rx Protein Plus Powder (w/water)
6.0	6	whole	Egg Whites
6.0	4	fl oz	Milk Drink, Muscle Milk, Cytomax (*)
6.0	1/2	bar	Snack Bar, Promax Carb Conscious (*)
6.0	6	fl oz	Yogurt Drink, Nouriche, All Flavors, Yoplait
6.0	1	bar	Snack Bar, MET-Rx Protein Plus (*)
6.0	1	cup	Milk, Lowfat (2%), Protein Fortified
6.0	1/2	cup	Instant Breakfast, Vanilla, Carnation (*)
5.5	1/2	bar	Snack Bar, Promax (*)
5.5	1/2	cup	Mousse, Key Lime, Nutripoint Recipe
5.5	1/4	cup	Cheese, Ricotta, Precious Fat Free
5.5	8	fl oz	Milk Drink, NutraStart (*)
5.5	8	fl oz	Milk Drink, Sustical High Protein (*)
5.5	3/4	cup	Egg, Scrambled, Garden, Nutripoint Recipe
5.5	1/2	portion	Cannelloni, Florentine, Frozen, Celentano
5.5	1/2	cup	Casserole, Five Cheese, Nutripoint Recipe

Nutripoints	Serving Size		Food Name—Milk/Dairy
5.5	1/2	cup	Cheese, Cottage, Dry
5.5	8	wt oz	Yogurt, Lowfat, Plain, Dannon
5.5	6	wt oz	Yogurt, Light, All Flavors, Yoplait
5.5	8	wt oz	Yogurt, Light 'N Fit Smoothie, Dannon
5.5	1/4	cup	Cheese, Cream, Honey, Nutripoint Recipe
5.0	6	wt oz	Yogurt, Light 'N Fit Creamy, Dannon
5.0	1	cup	Buttermilk, Regular
5.0	8	fl oz	Milk Drink, Ensure Plus (*)
4.5	1/2	cup	Egg Substitute, Second Nature
4.5	1/2	cup	Cheese, Cottage, Lowfat (1%)
4.5	1	wt oz	Wendy's Imitation Parmesan Cheese
4.5	12	fl oz	Milk Drink, Nutrament (*)
4.5	8	fl oz	Milk Drink, Sustical Plus (*)
4.5	8	wt oz	Yogurt, Light 'N Fit, Dannon
4.0	1	wt oz	Cocoa Mix, Hot, Sugar-Free, Swiss Miss
4.0	1/2	cup	Cocoa Mix, Ovaltine, Chocolate Flavor
4.0	1/2	serving	Milk Drink, Gatorade Nutrition Shake (*)
4.0	2	slices	Cheese, Non-Fat, Processed American or Swiss
4.0	1	cup	Milk Substitute, Non-Dairy, Vitamite
4.0	16	fl oz	Milk Drink, Alba
4.0	1	cup	Yogurt, Fat-Free Light, Columbo
3.5	1/2	cup	Mousse, Cheesecake, Sans Sucre de Paris
3.5	2	wt oz	Cheese, Low Cal
3.5	6	wt oz	Yogurt, Ultra Low-Carb, All Flavors, Yoplait
3.0	8	wt oz	Yogurt, Light 'N Fit Smoothie Carb Control, Dannon
3.0	4	wt oz	Cheese, Cottage, Lowfat (2%)
3.0	2	cups	Cocoa Mix, Hot, Sugar Free, Carnation
3.0	1	cup	Pudding, Low Cal
3.0	8	wt oz	Yogurt, Light 'N Fit Carb Control, Dannon
2.5	2	pieces	Cheese, Reduced Calorie, Laughing Cow
2.5	6	wt oz	Yogurt, Natural Flavors Vanilla, Dannon
2.5	1	cup	Cocoa Mix, Sugar Free, Quik, Nestle
2.5	1/3	cup	Banana Flambé, Nutripoint Recipe
2.5	8	wt oz	Yogurt, Whole Milk, Plain
2.5	1	cup	Milk, Whole (3.3%)
2.5	1	cup	Milk, Chocolate, Lowfat (1%)
2.5	6	fl oz	Milk, Chocolate, Lowfat (2%)
2.0	1/2	portion	Manicotti, Frozen, Celentano
2.0	6	wt oz	Yogurt, Fruit
2.0	1	cup	Milk, Whole (3.7%)
2.0	1/2	portion	Shells, Stuffed, Frozen, Celentano
2.0	1/2	cup	Pudding, Sustacal
2.0	3/4	cup	Yogurt, Fat Free, All Flavors, Horizon Organic

Nutripoints	Serving Size		Food Name—Milk/Dairy
2.0	6	fl oz	Yogurt, YoBaby Drinkable, Stonyfield Farm Organic
2.0	1/4	cup	Dressing, Honey Yogurt, Nutripoint Recipe
2.0	1	cup	Pudding Mix, Vanilla, Sugar-Free, Instant, Jell-O
1.5	1	cup	Yogurt, Lowfat, Swiss Style Plain, Lite-Line, Borden
1.5	1/4	portion	Shells, Frozen, Broccoli Stuffed, Celentano
1.5	1	cup	Soup, Cream
1.5	4	wt oz	Yogurt, Frozen
1.5	1	cup	Milk, Goat
1.5	1/2	cup	Cheese, Cottage
1.5	1	cup	Ice Cream, Extra Light, Blue Bell
1.5	1	wt oz	Wendy's Imitation Cheese, Salad Bar
1.5	1/2	cup	Cheese, Cottage, Lowfat, Weight Watchers
1.5	1	cup	Yogurt, Blended Multipack, Columbo
1.0	3/4	cup	Yogurt, Blended Lowfat, All Flavors, Horizon Organic
1.0	1/2	cup	Milk, Canned, Evaporated, Unsweetened
1.0	1/2	cup	Milk, Evaporated, Carnation
1.0	1	Tbls	Malted Milk Powder
1.0	1/4	cup	Cream, Sour, Blend, Weight Watchers
1.0	1/4	cup	Pudding, Banana
1.0	1/2	portion	Shells, Stuffed, 3 Cheese, Frozen, Le Menu
1.0	1	cup	Cocoa Mix, Hot, 70 Calorie, Carnation
1.0	1/2	portion	Ravioli, Baked Cheese, Frozen, Weight Watchers
1.0	4	wt oz	Yogurt, Lowfat, Fruit On Bottom, All Flavors, Dannon
1.0	1/2	cup	Yogurt, Frozen, Lowfat, Peach, Blue Bell
1.0	1/2	portion	Enchiladas, Cheese Dinner, Frozen, Patio
0.5	1	cup	Yogurt Drink, Lowfat, Dan'Up, All Flavors, Dannon
0.5	4	wt oz	Yogurt, Lowfat, Nuts/Raisins/Fruit, Dannon
0.5	3	wt oz	Cheese, Ricotta, Low-Fat
0.5	2	Tbls	Dressing, Yogurt
0.5	1	wt oz	Cheese, Mozzarella, Low-Fat
0.5	1/2	portion	Manicotti, 3 Cheese, Tomato Sauce, Le Menu
0.5	1/3	portion	Manicotti, Cheese, w/Meat Sauce, Fzn, Budget Gourmet
0.5	6	wt oz	Yogurt, Fruit on the Bottom, Dannon
0.5	1	wt oz	Cheese, Grated, Parmesan
0.5	1/2	portion	Ravioli, Cheese, Slim, Frozen, Budget Gourmet
0.5	1/2	portion	Cannelloni, Cheese, Lean Cuisine, Frozen, Stouffer's
0.5	1	piece	Pie, Fruit Yogurt, Nutripoint Recipe
0.5	6	wt oz	Yogurt, Original, All Flavors, Yoplait
0.5	1	wt oz	Cheese, Swiss, Reduced Fat, Kraft
0.5	1	wt oz	Cheese, Mozzarella, Skim, Land O'lakes

0.5	1/2	serving	Del Taco Cheddar Quesadilla
0.0	1/2	portion	Manicotti, Cheese, Frozen, Weight Watchers

Nutripoints	Serving Size		Food Name—Milk/Dairy
0.0	4	wt oz	Yogurt, Whips, All Flavors, Yoplait
0.0	2	wt oz	Cheese, American, Pasteurized Process, Lite-Line
0.0	1/2	serving	Ice Cream Sundae, Strawberry
0.0	1	cup	Chocolate, Hot
0.0	1/2	cup	Yogurt, Frozen, Lowfat, Raspberry, Blue Bell
0.0	1	cup	Yogurt, Colombo Classic w/Fruit on Bottom
0.0	4	wt oz	Yogurt, Lowfat, Nuts/Raisins/Vanilla, Dannon
0.0	1	wt oz	Cheese, Parmesan, Imitation, Grated, Formagg
0.0	1/2	serving	Sandwich, Grilled Cheese, White
0.0	2	pieces	Cheese, Laughing Cow
0.0	1/2	portion	Tortellini, Cheese, w/Tomato Sauce, Frozen Stouffer's
0.0	4	fl oz	Yogurt, Fzn, 97% Fat Free, Strawberry Passion, Colombo
0.0	4	wt oz	Yogurt, Yumsters, Yoplait
0.0	4	wt oz	Dairy Queen Frozen Dessert
0.0	4	fl oz	Yogurt, Frozen, 96% Fat Free, Vanilla Dream, Colombo
0.0	4	wt oz	Yogurt, Trix, Yoplait
0.0	6	wt oz	Yogurt, Creamy Fruit Blends, Dannon
0.0	4	wt oz	Yogurt, Grande!, All Flavors, Yoplait
-0.5	4	fl oz	Ice Cream, Simple Pleasures, (w/Simplesse)
-0.5	6	wt oz	Yogurt, Custard Style, All Flavors, Yoplait
-0.5	2	wt oz	Cheese, Mozzarella, Pasteurized Process, Lite-Line
-0.5	1/2	cup	Milk, Instant Natural Malted, Carnation
-0.5	6	fl oz	Yogurt Drink, Frusion Smoothie, Dannon
-0.5	1/2	cup	Yogurt, Frozen, Almond Amaretto, Brice's
-0.5	4	wt oz	Yogurt, Lowfat, Strawberry, Borden
-0.5	4	wt oz	Yogurt, Lowfat, Cherry Vanilla, Borden
-0.5	4	wt oz	Yogurt, Lowfat, Peach, Borden
-0.5	2	pieces	Cheese, Swiss, Pasteurized Process, Lite-Line
-0.5	1/2	cup	Milk, Chocolate
-0.5	2.25	wt oz	Yogurt, Go-GURT!, All Flavors, Yoplait
-0.5	1/2	portion	Enchiladas, Cheese Ranchero, Frozen, Weight Watchers
-0.5	1	wt oz	Cheese, Sharp Cheddar, Pasteurized Process, Lite-Line
-0.5	3	fl oz	Yogurt, Fzn, 94% Fat Free, Caramel Pecan Chunk, Colombo
-0.5	4	wt oz	Ice Cream, Simple Pleasures, Coffee
-0.5	4	wt oz	Yogurt, Lowfat, Boysenberry, Yoplait
-0.5	4	wt oz	Yogurt, Lowfat, Strawberry, Yoplait
-0.5	1	wt oz	Cheese, Pasteurized Process, Reduced Sodium, Lite-Line
-0.5	1/2	portion	Pasta Shells, Cheese Stuffed, w/Meat Sauce, Stouffer's
-0.5	1	wt oz	Cheese, Swiss
-0.5	1/2	cup	Pudding, Tapioca
-0.5	1	wt oz	Cheese, Gjetost
-1.0	1/2	cup	Milkshake, Vanilla
-1.0	1	wt oz	Cheese, American, Light N'Lively, Kraft

Nutripoints	Serving Size		Food Name—Milk/Dairy
-1.0	1	wt oz	Cheese, Provolone
-1.0	1	wt oz	Cheese, Swiss, Light N'Lively, Kraft
-1.0	1/2	cup	Ice Milk, Vanilla
-1.0	1/4	cup	Cream, Sour, Slender Choice
-1.0	1/2	portion	Enchiladas Ranchero, Cheese, Frozen, Weight Watchers
-1.0	4	wt oz	Yogurt, Banana Custard Style, Yoplait
-1.0	1	wt oz	Cheese, Edam
-1.0	2	wt oz	Cheese, Mozzarella, Low Fat, Alpine Lace
-1.0	1	serving	McDonald's Soft Serve Cone
-1.0	3	fl oz	Yogurt, Fzn, 94% Fat Free, Bavarian Choc. Crunch, Colombo
-1.0	1	bar	Snack Bar, Melaleuca Access Activity bar
-1.0	1/2	serving	Dairy Queen Cone - Medium
-1.0	1	wt oz	Cheese, Monterey Jack, Reduced Fat, Kraft
-1.0	1	wt oz	Cheese, Camembert
-1.0	1/2	cup	Soup, Cheese
-1.0	1	wt oz	Cheese, Cheddar, Mild, Reduced Fat, Kraft
-1.0	1/2	serving	Ice Cream Sundae, Hot Fudge
-1.0	1/2	piece	Pie, Boston Cream
-1.0	1/2	serving	Burger King Chocolate Shake
-1.0	1/2	cup	Milkshake, Chocolate
-1.0	1	wt oz	Cheese, Gruyere
-1.0	1	wt oz	Wendy's Potato Chili Cheese
-1.5	1/4	serving	Dairy Queen Parfait
-1.5	1/4	serving	Dairy Queen Malt - Medium
-1.5	2	wt oz	Cheese, Monterey Jack, Low Fat, Alpine Lace
-1.5	1	wt oz	Cheese Spread
-1.5	1	wt oz	Cheese, Mozzarella
-1.5	1/2	cup	Pudding, Vanilla
-1.5	1	cup	Cocoa Mix, Hot, Regular, Swiss Miss
-1.5	3	fl oz	Yogurt, Fzn, 90% Fat Free, Peanut Butter Cup, Colombo
-1.5	1	wt oz	Cheese Food Substitute, Low Cholesterol, Lite-Line
-1.5	3	fl oz	Yogurt, Fzn, 92% Fat Free, Mocha Swiss Almond, Colombo
-1.5	1/4	cup	Cream, Sour, Light, Dairy Blend, Land O'Lakes
-1.5	1	wt oz	Cheese, Mozzarella, Skim, Kraft
-1.5	1	piece	Frozen Dessert, Chocolate, Pudding Pops, Jello
-1.5	1/2	serving	McDonald's Strawberry Sundae
-1.5	1/4	serving	Dairy Queen Freeze (1 Cup)
-1.5	1	wt oz	Cheese, Gouda
-1.5	1/2	serving	McDonald's Hot Caramel Sundae
-1.5	1/2	serving	McDonald's Hot Fudge Sundae
-1.5	1	wt oz	Cheese, Brick
-1.5	1	serving	McDonald's Vanilla Reduced Fat Ice Cream Cone
-1.5	1/2	cup	Carl's Jr. Shakes - Reg. Size

Nutripoints	Serving Size		Food Name—Milk/Dairy
-1.5	2	Tbls	Cream, Non-Dairy, Imitation, Liquid, Vegetable Oil
-1.5	1/4	serving	Dairy Queen Chipper Sandwich
-1.5	1/4	serving	Dairy Queen Heath Blizzard
-1.5	1	wt oz	Cheese, American, Pasteurized Process, Kraft
-1.5	1	wt oz	Cheese, Parmesan, Grated, Kraft
-1.5	1	wt oz	Cheese, Muenster
-1.5	1/2	serving	Ice Cream Cone, Vanilla
-1.5	1	wt oz	Cheese, Monterey Jack
-1.5	1	serving	Mousse, Chocolate, Frozen, Weight Watchers
-1.5	1/2	piece	Pie, Pumpkin Custard, Mrs. Smith's
-2.0	1/2	cup	Ice Cream, Dutch Chocolate, Borden
-2.0	1	bar	Frozen Dessert, Vanilla, Lite Bar, Dove
-2.0	4	wt oz	Yogurt, Strawberry All Natural, Breyer's
-2.0	1	wt oz	Cheese, Romano
-2.0	1	wt oz	Cheese, Blue
-2.0	1/4	cup	Cream, Non-Dairy, Mocha Mix
-2.0	1/2	cup	Yogurt, Soft Frozen Peach, Yoplait
-2.0	2	wt oz	Cheese, Ricotta
-2.0	1	wt oz	Cheese, Swiss, Natural, Kraft
-2.0	1	wt oz	Cheese, Colby
-2.0	1	wt oz	Cheese, Swiss, Low Fat, Alpine Lace
-2.0	1/2	serving	Ice Cream Sundae, Caramel
-2.0	1/2	portion	Cheesecake, Strawberry, Frozen, Weight Watchers
-2.0	1/2	cup	Ice Milk, Chocolate, Borden
-2.0	1	wt oz	Cheese, Cheddar
-2.0	1/2	cup	Cocoa Mix, Chocolate, Quik, Nestle
-2.0	1/2	piece	Cake, Cheese, w/Fruit Topping
-2.0	1/2	cup	Ice Cream, Regular Fat, Vanilla
-2.0	1	cup	Pudding Mix, Americana Tapioca, Jell-O
-2.0	1	cup	Milk Drink Mix, Non-Fat, Hot Cocoa, Swiss Miss
-2.0	1/2	cup	Eggnog
-2.0	1/2	serving	Carl's Jr. Sunrise Sandwich w/Bacon
-2.0	2	fl oz	Milk, Sweetened Condensed, Canned
-2.0	4	wt oz	Yogurt, Pineapple All Natural, Breyer's
-2.0	1/2	cup	Ice Milk, Vanilla, Borden
-2.0	1	wt oz	Cheese, Brie
-2.0	1	wt oz	Cheese, Pimento
-2.0	1/4	cup	Ice Cream, Vanilla, Rich
-2.0	1/2	cup	Ice Milk, Strawberry, Borden
-2.0	1/2	cup	Milk Drink Mix, Strawberry, Quik, Nestle
-2.0	1/4	cup	Milk, Sweetened Condensed, Carnation
-2.0	1	piece	Yogurt, Frozen, Lowfat, Chocolate, Tuscan Pop
-2.0	1/4	cup	Wendy's Chocolate Pudding

Nutripoints	Serving Size		Food Name—Milk/Dairy
-2.0	1/2	serving	Cheesecake, Frozen, Weight Watchers
-2.5	1	wt oz	Cheese, Feta
-2.5	1/4	serving	Dairy Queen Shake - Medium
-2.5	1/2	cup	Ice Cream, Non-Dairy, Vanilla, Mocha Mix
-2.5	1	wt oz	Cheese, Muenster, Land O'lakes
-2.5	1	wt oz	Cheese, Swiss, Low Sodium, Kraft
-2.5	1/2	piece	Pie, Boston Cream Classic, Betty Crocker
-2.5	1/2	serving	Dairy Queen Sundae - Medium
-2.5	1/2	serving	Burger King Vanilla Shake
-2.5	1	wt oz	Cheese, Swiss, Process, Borden
-2.5	1/2	bar	Ice Cream Bar, Non-Dairy, Chocolate Covered, Mocha Mix
-2.5	1/2	piece	Pie, Yogurt
-2.5	1/2	cup	Pudding, Fat-Free, Swiss Miss (all flavors)
-2.5	1/2	cup	Pudding, Tapioca, Healthy Choice Lowfat
-2.5	1	wt oz	Cheese, Swiss, Sargento
-2.5	1	cup	Pudding Mix, Vanilla, Jell-O
-2.5	1/2	serving	Wendy's Breakfast Sandwich
-2.5	1	wt oz	Cheese, American, Process, Borden
-2.5	1	serving	Ice Cream Sandwich
-2.5	1/4	serving	Carl's Jr. Sunrise Sandwich w/Sausage
-2.5	1/2	serving	Ice Cream Sandwich, Good Humor
-2.5	1	wt oz	Cheese, Swiss, Processed
-2.5	1	piece	Pie, Boston Cream, Frozen, Weight Watchers
-2.5	1/4	cup	Wendy's Butterscotch Pudding
-2.5	1	serving	Dairy Queen DQ Sandwich
-2.5	1	wt oz	Cheese Spread, Pasteurized Process Slices, Velveeta
-3.0	1/2	cup	Topping, Lite, Cool Whip
-3.0	1	wt oz	Cheese, Cheddar, Low Sodium, Tillamook
-3.0	1	wt oz	Cheese, American, Processed
-3.0	1/4	cup	Cream, Half and Half
-3.0	1/2	cup	Soufflé, Cheese
-3.0	1/2	piece	Pie, Vanilla Cream
-3.0	1	wt oz	Cheese, Neufchatel, Philadelphia Brand
-3.0	1/2	piece	Ice Cream Bar, Chocolate Peanut Butter, Haagen-Dazs
-3.0	1	wt oz	Cheese Spread, Pasteurized Process, Velveeta
-3.0	1/2	serving	McDonald's Chocolate Milk Shake
-3.0	1	wt oz	Cheese, Cheddar, Tillamook
-3.0	1/2	serving	McDonald's Vanilla Milk Shake
-3.0	2	Tbls	Cream, Non-Dairy, Imitation, Powder
-3.0	1/4	cup	Milk, Condensed, Sweetened, Eagle Brand
-3.0	1	wt oz	Cheese, Limburger
-3.0	1/2	serving	McDonald's Strawberry Milk Shake
-3.0	1/2	piece	Cake, Cheese, Plain

Nutripoints	Serving Size		Food Name—Milk/Dairy
-3.0	1/2	piece	Jack In the Box Cheesecake
-3.0	1	wt oz	Cheese, Roquefort
-3.0	1	wt oz	Cheese, Cheddar, Natural Mild, Kraft
-3.0	1	wt oz	Cheese, Natural Colby, Kraft
-3.0	1/2	serving	Sandwich, Egg Salad, Whole Wheat Bread
-3.5	1/2	cup	Ice Cream, Sorbet & Cream, Key Lime, Haagen-Dazs
-3.5	1/2	cup	Ice Cream, Vanilla, Louis Sherry
-3.5	6	fl oz	Ice Cream Soda
-3.5	1/2	cup	Ice Cream, Vanilla, Soft Serve
-3.5	1	wt oz	Cheese, Mozzarella, Casino, Kraft
-3.5	1/2	cup	Pudding, Chocolate
-3.5	1/2	serving	Sandwich, Egg Salad, White Bread
-3.5	1	wt oz	Cheese, Cheddar, Sharp, Cracker Barrel
-3.5	1	wt oz	Cheese, Gouda, Kraft
-3.5	1/4	cup	Ice Cream, Coffee, Haagen-Dazs
-3.5	1	wt oz	Cheese, Monterey Jack, Kraft
-3.5	1/2	serving	Dairy Queen Dipped Cone - Medium
-3.5	1/2	serving	Wendy's Frosty Dairy Dessert
-3.5	1	wt oz	Cheese Spread, Cheez Whiz, Kraft
-3.5	1/2	cup	Pudding, Tapioca, Jello Fat Free
-3.5	2	Tbls	Cream, Non-Dairy, Coffee Mate, Carnation
-3.5	1	bar	Ice Cream Bar, Eskimo Pie
-3.5	1/4	serving	Dairy Queen Mr. Misty Freeze
-3.5	1/4	serving	Jack In the Box Scrambled Egg Platter
-3.5	1/4	cup	Ice Cream, Choc/Choc Chip, Haagen-Dazs
-3.5	1/2	piece	Pie, Custard
-3.5	1/4	bar	Dairy Queen Buster Bar
-3.5	1/4	serving	Dairy Queen Peanut Buster Parfait
-3.5	1/4	cup	Cream, Sour
-3.5	1/2	cup	Ice Cream, Strawberry, Borden
-3.5	1	wt oz	Candy Bar, Milk Chocolate
-3.5	1/2	serving	Dairy Queen Mr. Misty Float
-3.5	4	wt oz	Pudding, Choc. Pudding Snacks, Jell-O
-3.5	1/2	bar	Dairy Queen Dilly Bar
-3.5	1/2	serving	Burger King Breakfast Croissan'wich w/Ham
-3.5	1	wt oz	Cheese, Monterey Jack, Casino Brand
-4.0	1/2	cup	Custard
-4.0	2	Tbls	Cream, Non-Dairy, Imitation, Liquid
-4.0	1/4	cup	Ice Cream, Vanilla, Haagen-Dazs
-4.0	1/2	cup	Ice Cream, French Vanilla, Meadow Gold
-4.0	1/4	cup	Sauce, Custard
-4.0	1/2	cup	Sherbet, Orange, Borden
-4.0	1/2	cup	Dairy Queen Float

Nutripoints	Serving Size		Food Name—Milk/Dairy
-4.0	1	wt oz	Cheese, Swiss, Pasteurized Process, Kraft
-4.0	1/2	bar	Ice Cream Bar, Vanilla/Almonds, Haagen-Dazs
-4.0	1/2	cup	Ice Cream, Vanilla, Party Time, Knudsen
-4.0	1/2	muffin	McDonald's Egg McMuffin
-4.0	1/4	cup	Ice Cream, Vanilla Swiss Almond, Haagen-Dazs
-4.0	1/2	cup	Ice Cream, Buttered Pecan, Borden's
-4.0	1/4	cup	Ice Cream, Chocolate, Schrafft's
-4.0	4	wt oz	Pudding, Chocolate, Snack Pack, Hunts
-4.0	4	wt oz	Pudding, Vanilla, Snack Pack, Hunts
-4.0	1/2	serving	Burger King Scrambled Egg Platter w/Bacon
-4.0	1/4	serving	Burger King Scrambled Egg Platter w/Sausage
-4.0	1/2	bar	Ice Cream Bar, Vanilla/Milk Chocolate, Haagen-Dazs
-4.0	1/2	serving	Burger King Breakfast Croissan'wich w/Bacon
-4.0	1	wt oz	Cheese, Neufchatel
-4.5	1/4	cup	Cheese Fondue
-4.5	1/2	serving	Burger King Scrambled Egg Platter
-4.5	1/4	piece	Quiche, Cheese/Bacon
-4.5	4	pieces	Fried Cheese Sticks
-4.5	1/4	cup	Topping, Non-Dairy, Cool Whip, Birds Eye
-4.5	1/2	serving	McDonald's Biscuit w/Bacon, Egg & Cheese
-4.5	2	Tbls	Cream, Non-Dairy, Cremora
-5.0	1/2	cup	Ice Cream Butter Pecan, Meadow Gold
-5.0	2	Tbls	Cheese, Cream
-5.5	1/2	serving	Burger King Breakfast Croissan'wich w/Sausage
-5.5	1/4	cup	Sauce, Cheese
-5.5	1/4	cup	Topping, Whipped, La Creme
-5.5	2	Tbls	Cream, Sour, Imitation
-6.0	2	Tbls	Cream, Coffee, Light
-6.0	1/4	cup	Topping, Extra Creamy, Cool Whip, Birds Eye
-6.0	1/2	piece	Quiche, Cheese
-6.5	1/4	cup	Cream, Whipped
-6.5	2	Tbls	Cream, Whipping, Light
-7.0	1/2	serving	Wendy's Omelet #1 (eggs, Ham, Cheese)
-7.0	2	Tbls	Cream, Heavy
-7.0	1/2	cup	Egg Foo Young
-8.0	1/2	serving	Egg, Omelet, w/Ham/Cheese (3 Eggs)
-9.0	1/4	cup	Egg Salad
-10.0	1/2	serving	Wendy's Omelet #3 (eggs, Ham, Cheese, Onion)
-10.0	1/2	serving	Wendy's Omelet #2 (eggs, Ham, Cheese, Mushroom)
-10.5	1/4	cup	Sauce, Zabaglione
-10.5	1	egg	Egg, Devilled
-11.0	1	serving	Carl's Jr. Scrambled Eggs
-11.5	2	whole	Egg, Boiled

Nutripoints	Serving Size		Food Name—Milk/Dairy
-11.5	2	whole	Egg, Hard
-11.5	2	whole	Egg, Poached
-11.5	1	serving	Wendy's Omelet #4 (eggs, Mushroom, Green Pepper, Onion)
-12.5	1	whole	Egg, Fried
-13.5	1	whole	Egg, Scrambled
-15.0	2	whole	Egg Yolk

MEAT/FISH/POULTRY

Nutripoints	Serving Size		Food Name—Meat/Fish/Poultry
16.0	2	sticks	Scallop Kabob, Nutripoint Recipe
13.5	6	wt oz	Clams, Mixed Species, Raw (‡)
13.0	3	wt oz	Red Snapper, Vera Cruz Style, Nutripoint Recipe
13.0	12	whole	Oysters, Eastern, Raw (‡)
12.0	6	wt oz	Clams, Raw (‡)
10.5	4	wt oz	Salmon, Lettuce Wrapped, w/Herb Sauce, Nutripoint Recipe
9.5	1	portion	Chicken La Russe w/Veg, Cm
8.5	4	wt oz	Venison, Baked
8.5	1	cup	Chicken Stir Fry, Nutripoint Recipe
8.0	1	cup	Clams, Canned
8.0	4	whole	Oysters, Pacific, Raw (‡)
8.0	1/2	cup	Tuna, Chunk Light, Water, Low Sodium, Chicken of the Sea
7.5	3/4	cup	Tuna, Canned In Water
7.5	6	wt oz	Pike, Baked
7.5	3	wt oz	Salmon, Steamed/Poached
7.5	4	wt oz	Halibut, Baked
7.0	1	serving	McDonald's Caesar Salad w/Grilled Chicken
7.0	6	wt oz	Red Snapper, Baked
7.0	1	serving	Beef, Carne Asada, Nutripoint Recipe
7.0	1/2	cup	Tuna, Light Chunk, In Water, Bumble Bee
7.0	6	wt oz	Bass, Freshwater, Baked
7.0	3	wt oz	Beef Liver, Fried (†)
7.0	4	wt oz	Halibut, w/Yellow Bell Pepper Sauce, Nutripoint Recipe
6.5	3	wt oz	Oysters, Broiled w/Butter
6.5	3/4	cup	Tuna, Chunk Light, Water, Chicken of the Sea
6.5	6	wt oz	Venison, w/Juniper Berry Sauce, Nutripoint Recipe
6.5	1/2	cup	Tuna, White Solid, In Water, Bumble Bee
6.5	4	wt oz	Turkey, Breast Slices, Turkey Store
6.5	4	wt oz	Turkey, Breast Tenderloins, Turkey Store
6.5	4	wt oz	Turkey, Ground Breast Meat, Turkey Store
6.5	3.5	wt oz	Abalone
6.5	1/2	cup	Salmon, Canned In Water
6.5	3	wt oz	Swordfish, Baked
6.5	3	wt oz	Tuna, Fresh, Broiled
6.5	3/4	cup	Chicken Salad, Nutripoint Recipe
6.5	3	wt oz	Fish, Crunchy, Nutripoint Recipe
6.0	1/2	portion	Chicken Primavera, Frozen, Celentano
6.0	6	wt oz	Clams, Steamed/Boiled

‡ ***Caution:** high risk for contamination*

† ***Cholesterol:** excessively high*

Nutripoints	Serving Size		Food Name—Meat/Fish/Poultry
6.0	1	cup	Soup, Healthy Classics, Chicken Noodle, Progresso
6.0	1	portion	Ginger Chicken Dinner, Cm
6.0	4	wt oz	Quail, w/o Skin
6.0	6	wt oz	Sole, Baked
6.0	1/2	cup	Tuna, Lite Chunk Light, Water & Oil, Chicken of the Sea
5.5	4	slices	Ham, Slices, Jubilee, Oscar Mayer
5.5	1/2	cup	Tuna, Solid White, In Water, Star-Kist
5.5	4	wt oz	Pheasant, w/o Skin
5.5	4	wt oz	Sturgeon, Steamed
5.5	3/4	cup	Soup, Chicken Gumbo
5.5	1/2	cup	Tuna, Solid White, Water, Chicken of the Sea
5.5	3	wt oz	Moose
5.5	1 1/2	cups	Soup, Chicken, Home Style, Progresso
5.5	1	cup	Soup, Healthy Request, Vegetable Beef, Campbell's
5.5	3	wt oz	Salmon, Baked/Broiled
5.5	3	wt oz	Chicken, Cajun, Nutripoint Recipe
5.0	1	whole	Hamburger, Aerobics, Nutripoint Recipe
5.0	1/2	cup	Tuna, Diet Albacore, Chunk White, Water, Low Sodium, Chicken/Sea
5.0	1	serving	Subway Barbeque Chicken Sandwich (6")
5.0	3	wt oz	Clams, Smoked, Canned In Oil
5.0	4	wt oz	Ham, Lean, Baked, Canned, 4% Fat
5.0	1/2	cup	Tuna Salad, Nutripoint Recipe
5.0	1	portion	Ham Dinner, Frozen, Morton
5.0	1	serving	McDonald's Chicken Salad Oriental
5.0	1	serving	Pizza, Chicken & Vegetable, Fzn, South Beach Diet
5.0	1	slice	Pizza Hut Chicken Supreme Thin 'N Crispy Pizza
5.0	3	wt oz	Trout, Baked
5.0	1	serving	Subway Savory Turkey Breast Sandwich (6")
5.0	2	pieces	Enchiladas, Chicken, Nutripoint Recipe
5.0	1/2	portion	Beef Teriyaki, Frozen, Chun King
4.5	1	serving	Subway Turkey Pastrami Sandwich (6")
4.5	3	wt oz	Clams, Breaded, Fried
4.5	2	wt oz	Liverwurst (†)
4.5	6	wt oz	Crab, Hard-shell, Steamed (†)
4.5	3/4	cup	Salmon, Pink, Chunk, Skinless/Boneless, Water, Chicken of the Sea
4.5	3	pieces	Sardines, Canned In Oil
4.5	1	cup	Soup, Clam Chowder, New England Milk Base
4.5	1	serving	Subway Roast Beef Sandwich (6")
4.5	4	wt oz	Chicken, Grilled w/Mango Sauce, Nutripoint Recipe
4.5	3	wt oz	Abalone, Floured, Fried
4.5	1	cup	Soup, Healthy Classics, Beef Vegetable, Progresso
4.5	4	wt oz	Smelt, Rainbow, Baked

† *Cholesterol: excessively high*

Nutripoints	Serving Size		Food Name—Meat/Fish/Poultry
4.5	1	cup	Soup, Chicken, w/Ribbon Pasta, Pritikin
4.5	4	wt oz	Ocean Perch, Baked
4.5	3	slices	Bacon, Canadian Style, Oscar Mayer
4.0	3	wt oz	Turkey, Light Meat Baked w/o Skin
4.0	3	wt oz	Chicken Breast, Baked w/o Skin
4.0	3	wt oz	Beef Round Steak, Lean, Broiled
4.0	1/2	serving	Sandwich, Chicken Salad, Whole Wheat Bread
4.0	1	cup	Soup, Beef
4.0	3	wt oz	Anchovy, Canned
4.0	1/2	cup	Salmon, Pink, Bumble Bee
4.0	4	wt oz	Shark, Mixed Species, Raw
4.0	3	wt oz	Beef Hart, Braised
4.0	1	serving	Beef, Sliced, Frozen, Morton
4.0	4	wt oz	Snails
4.0	1	whole	Sandwich, Turkey, Nutripoint Recipe
4.0	1	cup	Soup, Chunky Beef, Campbell's
4.0	2	wt oz	Braunschweiger (†)
4.0	3	wt oz	Beef Flank Steak, Lean, Broiled
4.0	1	serving	Taco Bell Beef Enchirito, Fresco Style
4.0	1/2	cup	Tuna, Tonno, Solid Light, Oil, Chicken of the Sea
4.0	6	wt oz	Scallops, Baked/Broiled
4.0	5	wt oz	Orange Roughy, Raw
4.0	4	wt oz	Perch Fillet, Broiled/Baked
4.0	1	portion	Turkey, w/Dressing, Frozen, Morton
4.0	3	wt oz	Mackerel, Baked
4.0	1	portion	Turkey Dinner, Frozen, Morton
4.0	3	wt oz	Beef Top Loin, Lean, Broiled
4.0	1/2	serving	Subway Seafood Sensation Sandwich (6")
4.0	1/2	cup	Tuna, Albacore Solid White, Oil, Chicken of the Sea
3.5	6	pieces	Sardines, Canned, Tomato Sauce
3.5	1	serving	Subway Honey Mustard Ham Sandwich (6")
3.5	1	serving	Subway Club Sandwich (6")
3.5	3	wt oz	Veal Cutlet/Steak, Lean, Braised
3.5	3	wt oz	Fish, Smoked
3.5	1	cup	Soup, Seafood Gumbo
3.5	3	wt oz	Lamb Roast, Leg, Baked
3.5	4	wt oz	Pork, Light, Rich Meat Service
3.5	1	serving	Subway Oven Roasted Chicken Breast Sandwich (6")
3.5	1	serving	Taco Bell Steak Gordita Baja, Fresco Style
3.5	3	wt oz	Flounder, Baked
3.5	3	wt oz	Halibut Fillet, Batter-Fried
3.5	1	serving	Subway Cheese Steak Sandwich (6")

† *Cholesterol: excessively high*

Nutripoints	Serving Size		Food Name—Meat/Fish/Poultry
3.5	1	cup	Beef Stew
3.5	1	serving	Taco Bell Chicken Gordita Baja, Fresco Style
3.5	1/2	portion	Beef, Frozen Dinner
3.5	1/2	cup	Salmon, Red, Chunk, Skinless/Boneless, Chicken of the Sea
3.5	1	serving	Beef w/Broccoli & Asian Style Noodles, Fzn, South Beach Diet
3.5	1/2	pieces	Sandwich, Chicken Salad, White Bread
3.5	1	serving	Carl's Jr. Chicken Salad (take-Out)
3.5	1/2	serving	Sandwich, Tuna Salad, Whole Wheat
3.5	1	serving	Pizza, Pepperoni, Fzn, South Beach Diet
3.5	4	wt oz	Cod, Baked
3.5	3	wt oz	Beef Tenderloin Fillet, Lean, Broiled
3.5	4	wt oz	Turkey, White, Canned, Premium Chunk, Swanson
3.5	3	wt oz	Beef Chuck Roast, Lean, Braised
3.5	3	wt oz	Turkey, Light/Dark Meat, w/o Skin, Baked
3.5	1	portion	Chicken Oriental, Frozen, Healthy Choice
3.5	1	serving	Del Taco Chicken Soft Taco
3.5	1/2	portion	Turkey, Frozen Dinner
3.5	3	slices	Turkey Breast Slices, Louis Rich
3.5	1	portion	Chicken Parmigiana, Frozen, Healthy Choice
3.5	1/2	cup	Tuna, Chunk Light, Oil, Chicken of the Sea
3.5	4	wt oz	Chicken, Marinated Hawaiian, Nutripoint Recipe
3.5	1/2	serving	Burrito, Chicken
3.5	3	slices	Luncheon Meat, Honeyloaf
3.5	1	cup	Tuna Noodle Casserole
3.5	4	wt oz	Chicken, Lemon, Nutripoint Recipe
3.5	1	serving	Beef w/Cheesy Broccoli, Fzn, South Beach Diet
3.0	1	cup	Oyster Stew
3.0	1	serving	Taco Bell Beef Gordita Baja, Fresco Style
3.0	4	wt oz	Chicken, Fried, Lowfat, Nutripoint Recipe
3.0	3	wt oz	Turkey, Dark Meat, Baked w/o Skin
3.0	3	wt oz	Rabbit, Wild
3.0	3	wt oz	Squirrel
3.0	3	wt oz	Hamburger Patty, Lean, Broiled
3.0	1/2	cup	Salmon, Red Sockeye, Bumble Bee
3.0	1	cup	Chicken Ala King w/Rice, Dining Lite
3.0	1	cup	Beef, Macaroni and Tomato Sauce
3.0	1	portion	Chicken, Sweet & Sour, Frozen, Healthy Choice
3.0	1/2	serving	Sandwich, Tuna Salad, White
3.0	5	wt oz	Catfish, Baked
3.0	3	wt oz	Lamb Shoulder, Lean, Baked
3.0	1	serving	Del Taco Big Fat Chicken Taco
3.0	1	serving	Salmon w/Basil, Fzn, Lean Cuisine
3.0	1/2	cup	Tuna Salad

Nutripoints	Serving Size		Food Name—Meat/Fish/Poultry
3.0	1	serving	Taco Bell Chicken Burrito Supreme, Fresco Style
3.0	1/2	burger	Hamburger w/Bun/Lettuce/Tomato, Fast Food
3.0	1	portion	Beef Sirloin Tips, Frozen, Healthy Choice
3.0	1	serving	McDonald's California Cobb Salad w/Grilled Chicken
3.0	1	serving	Taco Bell Steak Burrito Supreme, Fresco Style
3.0	1/2	serving	Subway Classic Tuna Sandwich (6")
3.0	3	wt oz	Pork Chop, Loin, Lean, Baked
3.0	3	wt oz	Turkey Roll, Light Meat
3.0	3	wt oz	Rabbit, Domestic, Breaded, Fried
3.0	1	serving	Subway Onion Chicken Teriyaki Sandwich (6")
3.0	5	wt oz	Grouper, Baked
3.0	1/2	portion	Beef Pepper Oriental, Frozen, Chun King
3.0	1/4	serving	Del Taco Deluxe Chicken Salad
3.0	1	patty	Sausage Patty
3.0	3	wt oz	Salmon, Smoked
3.0	1/2	portion	Chicken, Imperial, Frozen, Chun King
3.0	1/2	serving	Soup, Beef Lentil, ZonePerfect
2.5	3	pieces	Beef Jerky
2.5	1	serving	Chicken w/Broccoli & Cauliflower, Fzn, South Beach Diet
2.5	3	wt oz	Chicken Breast, Fried w/o Bread, w/Skin
2.5	1/2	serving	Subway Turkey Breast, Ham & Bacon Melt Sandwich (6")
2.5	1	serving	Taco Bell Grilled Steak Soft Taco, Fresco Style
2.5	1	serving	Chicken & Penne w/Broccoli, Fzn, South Beach Diet
2.5	4	wt oz	Ocean Perch Fillet, Frozen, Gorton's
2.5	1/2	cup	Tuna Helper, Prepared
2.5	3	wt oz	Beef Rib Eye, Lean, Broiled
2.5	1/2	cup	Chicken Fricassee
2.5	1/2	portion	Ham, Frozen Dinner
2.5	1	serving	Taco Bell Fiesta Chicken Burrito Supreme, Fresco Style
2.5	1	serving	Taco Bell Chicken Enchirito, Fresco Style
2.5	1/2	serving	Subway Meatball Marinara Sandwich (6")
2.5	1	whole	Green Pepper, Stuffed w/Meat
2.5	1/3	serving	Del Taco Macho Chicken Burrito
2.5	1	cup	Soup, Healthy Request, Chicken Noodle, Campbell's
2.5	3.5	wt oz	Turkey, Burger Patties, Turkey Store
2.5	1	serving	Taco Bell Soft Chicken Taco, Fresco Style
2.5	3	wt oz	Beef Porterhouse Steak, Lean, Broiled
2.5	6	wt oz	Lobster, Steamed/Boiled
2.5	1/2	portion	Chicken, Low Cal, Frozen Dinner
2.5	6	wt oz	Sushi/Raw Fish
2.5	1	portion	Chicken & Pasta Divan, Frozen, Healthy Choice
2.5	1	serving	Chicken w/Cashews & Snap Peas, Fzn, South Beach Diet
2.5	1	cup	Soup, Turkey Vegetable, Campbell's

Nutripoints	Serving Size		Food Name—Meat/Fish/Poultry
2.5	3	wt oz	Carp, Smoked
2.5	1/2	serving	Sandwich, Turkey, Whole Wheat Bread
2.5	1/2	serving	Jack In the Box Club Pita
2.5	1/2	serving	Wendy's Ultimate Chicken Grill Sandwich
2.5	4	wt oz	Haddock, Baked
2.5	1	taco	Taco, Beef/Cheese
2.5	3	wt oz	Chicken Leg, Baked w/o Skin
2.5	3	wt oz	Beef T-Bone Steak, Lean, Choice, Broiled
2.5	1	serving	Chicken w/Green Beans Almondine, Fzn, South Beach Diet
2.5	3.5	wt oz	Turkey, Light Meat and Skin, Baked
2.0	3	wt oz	Rabbit, Stewed
2.0	1/2	cup	Chicken Salad
2.0	6	wt oz	Mussels, Cooked
2.0	1	cup	Soup, Chicken Vegetable, Couscous, Nile Spice Foods
2.0	1/2	serving	Del Taco Spicy Chicken Burrito
2.0	1/2	serving	Sandwich, Chicken, Whole Wheat Bread
2.0	1/2	portion	Fish Dinner, Frozen, Morton
2.0	3	wt oz	Salmon, Baked w/Butter
2.0	1	serving	Chicken w/Couscous & Vegetables, Fzn, South Beach Diet
2.0	3	wt oz	Beef Round Steak, Medium Fat, Broiled
2.0	1/2	serving	Jack In the Box Chicken Fajita Pita
2.0	1/4	serving	Del Taco Macho Combo Burrito
2.0	1	portion	Lasagna, Tuna, Spinach Noodles & Vegetables, Fzn, Stouffer's
2.0	1	cup	Soup, Chicken Vegetable, Campbell's
2.0	3	wt oz	Chicken Thigh, Fried w/o Breading
2.0	1	cup	Wendy's Taco Beef Salad
2.0	3	wt oz	Chicken Liver, Stewed
2.0	1	serving	Del Taco Big Fat Steak Taco
2.0	1/2	serving	Del Taco Del Combo Burrito
2.0	4	wt oz	Whiting, Broiled, Baked
2.0	1	portion	Chicken, Vegetables w/Vermicelli, Frozen, Stouffer's
2.0	1	serving	Chicken, Lemongrass, Fzn, Lean Cuisine
2.0	3/4	cup	Chicken w/Dumplings
2.0	1	piece	Shrimp Etouffé (1 Pc=1.5 C)
2.0	1/2	portion	Beef Salisbury Steak, Frozen Dinner
2.0	4	wt oz	Luncheon Meat, Turkey Ham
2.0	1/2	portion	Fish, w/Chips, Frozen, Morton
2.0	1/2	serving	Sandwich, Chicken, White Bread
2.0	1/2	portion	Pork, Sweet and Sour, Frozen, Chun King
2.0	6	wt oz	Cod, Smoked
2.0	1	portion	Turkey Breast, Frozen, Healthy Choice
2.0	6	wt oz	Squid, Raw

Nutripoints	Serving Size		Food Name—Meat/Fish/Poultry
2.0	1	portion	Egg Rolls, Restaurant, Frozen, Chun King
2.0	1/2	portion	Peppers, Sweet, Stuffed, Frozen, Celentano
2.0	3	wt oz	Beef Ribs, Baked
2.0	1/2	taco	Taco, Chicken
2.0	6	wt oz	Haddock, Smoked
2.0	1	portion	Veal Parmigiana, Frozen, Morton
2.0	1/2	serving	Wendy's Chicken Sandwich
2.0	1/2	cup	Tuna, Canned In Oil
2.0	1/2	portion	Chicken Parmigiana, Frozen, Celentano
2.0	1/2	serving	McDonald's Chicken McGrill Sandwich
2.0	3	wt oz	Beef Brisket, Lean, Braised
2.0	3	wt oz	Ham, Baked, Canned, 13% Fat
2.0	1/2	portion	Beef Szechuan, Frozen, Chun King
2.0	3	wt oz	Veal Roast, Lean, Braised
2.0	1/2	serving	Sandwich, BLT, Whole Wheat Bread
2.0	3	pieces	Chicken Wing, Baked w/Out Skin
2.0	3/4	cup	Beefaroni
2.0	1/2	portion	Pork, Frozen Dinner
2.0	3	wt oz	Octopus, Fried
2.0	1	serving	Pork w/Pecans & Green Beans, Fzn, South Beach Diet
2.0	1	portion	Chicken Au Gratin, Slim, Frozen, Budget Gourmet
1.5	1	portion	Beef Oriental Pepper Steak, Frozen, Healthy Choice
1.5	1/2	serving	Sandwich, Corned Beef, Rye Bread
1.5	1/2	portion	Meatloaf, Frozen Dinner
1.5	3	wt oz	Chicken Leg, Fried w/o Bread, w/Skin
1.5	1	portion	Chicken Breast, Marsala w/Vegetables, Frozen, Stouffer's
1.5	1/2	serving	Chicken Dijon, ZonePerfect
1.5	1/2	portion	Beef Steak, Chopped, Frozen, Weight Watchers
1.5	1/2	portion	Chicken Chow Mein, Frozen, Chun King
1.5	3	wt oz	Duck, Baked, w/o Skin
1.5	1/2	cup	Herring, Canned
1.5	1/2	serving	Sandwich, Turkey, White Bread
1.5	3	wt oz	Beef Flank Steak, Medium Fat, Choice, Broiled
1.5	3	wt oz	Barracuda, Baked/Broiled
1.5	1	portion	Chicken Breast, Glazed, Frozen, Le Menu
1.5	3	slices	Bacon, Canadian
1.5	1/2	serving	Subway Cold Cut Combo Sandwich (6")
1.5	1/2	portion	Sole, Stuffed, Newburg Sauce, Frozen, Weight Watchers
1.5	1	cup	Soup, Chicken w/Noodles, Low Sodium, Campbell's
1.5	3	wt oz	Capon, Baked, w/Skin
1.5	3	wt oz	Chicken Breast, Fried w/o Skin
1.5	1	portion	Chicken A L'orange, w/Almonds and Rice, Frozen, Stouffer's
1.5	1/2	serving	Jack In the Box Beef Fajita Pita

Nutripoints	Serving Size		Food Name—Meat/Fish/Poultry
1.5	1/2	serving	Carl's Jr. Charbroiler Barbeque Chicken Sandwich
1.5	1	cup	Soup, Chicken
1.5	1	portion	Sole Au Gratin, Frozen, Healthy Choice
1.5	1	serving	Del Taco Steak Del Carbon Taco
1.5	1	serving	Taco Bell Soft Beef Taco, Fresco Style
1.5	1/2	portion	Chicken, Frozen Dinner
1.5	1	serving	Fajita, Beef
1.5	1/2	cup	Tuna, Chunk Light, In Oil, Star-Kist
1.5	1	portion	Chicken Tenders, Sweet 'n Sour, Frozen, Weight Watchers
1.5	1	slice	Pizza Hut Meat Lover's Thin 'N Crispy Pizza
1.5	1/2	piece	Hamburger w/Bun, Fast Food Small Plain
1.5	1/2	serving	Del Taco Chicken Works Burrito
1.5	3	wt oz	Hamburger Patty, Lean, Fried
1.5	1	serving	Chicken Marsala w/Broccoli, Weight Watchers Smart Ones
1.5	1/4	cup	Bacon Bits, Imitation
1.5	1	serving	Chicken, Roasted w/Vegetables, Uncle Ben's
1.5	6	pieces	Sardines, Canned, Mustard Sauce
1.5	1	cup	Chicken Chow Mein w/Rice, Dining Lite
1.5	1	portion	Salisbury Steak, Frozen, Healthy Choice
1.5	3	wt oz	Eel, Smoked
1.5	1	portion	Fish Fillet, Divan, Frozen, Stouffer's
1.5	1/2	cup	Chicken, Creamed
1.5	1/2	portion	Tortellini, Veal w/Tomato Sauce, Frozen, Stouffer's
1.5	3	whole	Oysters, Fried
1.5	3	wt oz	Eel
1.5	1/2	serving	Del Taco Carnitas Burrito
1.5	1	portion	Beef, Sliced, w/Gravy, Frozen, Morton
1.5	1	portion	Chicken Imperial, Frozen, Weight Watchers
1.5	1/2	serving	Wendy's New Beef Chili
1.5	1	burger	McDonald's McLean Deluxe Hamburger
1.0	1	serving	Chicken Pecan, Fzn, Lean Cuisine
1.0	1	portion	Chicken, Mandarin, Slim, Frozen, Budget Gourmet
1.0	3	wt oz	Bonito, Canned
1.0	1/2	serving	Dairy Queen Fish Fillet
1.0	1/2	serving	Sandwich, BLT, White Bread
1.0	1/4	cup	Hamburger Helper, Prepared
1.0	1	cup	Soup, Beef Noodle
1.0	4	wt oz	Ham, Canned, Armour Golden Star
1.0	4	wt oz	Turkey Breast, Roasted, No Sodium Added, Mr. Turkey
1.0	3.5	wt oz	Turkey, Dark Meat and Skin, Baked
1.0	3	wt oz	Turkey Breast, Sliced, Mr. Turkey
1.0	3	wt oz	Scallops, Fried
1.0	4	slices	Turkey Ham, Louis Rich

Nutripoints	Serving Size		Food Name—Meat/Fish/Poultry
1.0	4	slices	Salami, Pork
1.0	6	wt oz	Crab, Canned
1.0	1	serving	Del Taco Crispy Fish Taco
1.0	3	wt oz	Chicken Breast, Fried w/Batter, w/Skin
1.0	3	wt oz	Barracuda, Breaded/Floured, Fried
1.0	1/2	serving	Del Taco Steak Works Burrito
1.0	1/2	serving	Dairy Queen Fish Fillet w/Cheese
1.0	3	wt oz	Beef Swiss Steak
1.0	3	wt oz	Perch, Fried w/ Breading
1.0	1/2	cup	Ham Salad
1.0	1	serving	Fajita, Chicken
1.0	1/2	serving	Fish, Sandwich, Fast Food
1.0	1/2	burger	Wendy's Small Hamburger
1.0	3	wt oz	Chicken Thigh, Baked w/o Skin
1.0	1/2	serving	Sandwich, Roast Beef, Hot
1.0	1	serving	Taco Bell Steak Fajita
1.0	3	links	Sausage Links, Healthy Choice
1.0	1/2	burger	Wendy's Jr. Hamburger
1.0	1/2	serving	Taco Bell Double Beef Burrito Supreme w/Red Sauce
1.0	1/2	serving	Sandwich, Sloppy Joe w/Bun
1.0	1/2	serving	Taco Bell Double Beef Burrito Supreme w/Green Sauce
1.0	1	cup	Soup, Chunky Beef & Potato, Healthy Choice
1.0	1	serving	Turkey Breast, Grilled, Fzn, Healthy Choice
1.0	1	cup	Soup, Old Fashioned Chicken Noodle, Healthy Choice
1.0	1/2	serving	Arby's Super Roast Beef Sandwich
1.0	2	wt oz	Veal Patty, Fried
1.0	3	wt oz	Beef Short Ribs, Lean, Braised
1.0	1	piece	Chicken Thigh, Baked w/Out Skin
1.0	1/2	serving	Chicken Teriyaki, Uncle Ben's Rice Bowl
1.0	1/2	serving	Del Taco Del Classic Chicken Burrito
1.0	1/2	burger	Wendy's Small Cheeseburger
1.0	1	portion	Veal Parmigiana Patty, Frozen, Weight Watchers
1.0	4	wt oz	Turkey Sausage, Lean Italian, Jennie-O, Turkey Store
1.0	1/2	portion	Lobster Newburg, Frozen Dinner
1.0	1	cup	Soup, Chowder, Fish
1.0	1/2	serving	Subway Italian BMT Sandwich (6")
1.0	3	wt oz	Swordfish Fillet, Breaded, Fried
1.0	1	portion	Beef Sirloin, w/Herb Sauce, Slim, Frozen, Budget Gourmet
1.0	3	wt oz	Veal Cutlet, Medium Fat, Braised
1.0	1/2	serving	Carl's Jr. California Roast Beef 'n Swiss
1.0	1	portion	Chicken Tenderloins In Peanut Sauce, Frozen, Stouffer's
1.0	1/2	burger	Wendy's Jr. Cheeseburger
1.0	1	portion	Beef Sirloin Salisbury Steak, Slim, Frozen, Budget Gourmet

Nutripoints	Serving Size		Food Name—Meat/Fish/Poultry
1.0	3	slices	Pastrami, Turkey
1.0	1	portion	Enchiladas, Sirloin, Ranchero, Slim, Budget Gourmet
1.0	1	portion	Turkey Breast, Sliced, Mushroom Sauce, Frozen, Stouffer's
1.0	1/2	serving	Jack In the Box Grilled Chicken Fillet
1.0	3	wt oz	Beef Tenderloin, Medium Fat, Broiled
1.0	3	wt oz	Salmon Patty, Fried
1.0	4	wt oz	Turkey Roll, Light/Dark Meat
1.0	1/4	serving	Del Taco Macho Beef Burrito
1.0	1/2	portion	Chicken Cacciatore, Frozen, Budget Gourmet
1.0	1/2	cup	Chicken, Sweet and Sour
1.0	1/2	serving	Wendy's Mediterranean Chicken Salad
1.0	1/2	cup	Chicken, Canned
1.0	1/2	serving	Del Taco Deluxe Del Beef Burrito
0.5	2	pieces	Herring, Pickled
0.5	1	portion	Enchiladas, Chicken, Suiza, Slim, Budget Gourmet
0.5	1/2	portion	Chicken Teriyaki, Frozen, Budget Gourmet
0.5	1/2	portion	Chicken, Sweet & Sour, w/Rice, Frozen, Budget Gourmet
0.5	1/2	serving	Dairy Queen Double Hamburger
0.5	1/3	serving	Wendy's Mandarin Chicken Salad
0.5	3	wt oz	Carp, Baked/Broiled
0.5	2	wt oz	Pate, Chicken Liver, Canned
0.5	1/2	serving	Arby's King Roast Beef Sandwich
0.5	1/2	serving	Carl's Jr. Charbroiler Chicken Club Sandwich
0.5	1/2	serving	Soup, Chicken Gumbo, ZonePerfect
0.5	1/2	serving	Wendy's Chicken Club Sandwich
0.5	1	portion	Fajita, Chicken, Frozen, Weight Watchers
0.5	1	cup	Carl's Jr. Old Fashioned Chicken Noodle Soup
0.5	1	piece	Arby's Junior Roast Beef Sandwich
0.5	1/2	serving	McDonald's McChicken Sandwich
0.5	1/2	serving	Wendy's Homestyle Chicken Fillet
0.5	3	wt oz	Veal Roast, Medium Fat, Braised
0.5	4	wt oz	Beef, Light, Rich Meat Service
0.5	1/2	serving	Del Taco Del Beef Burrito
0.5	1/2	serving	Arby's Regular Roast Beef Sandwich
0.5	1	portion	Chicken Oriental, Frozen, Stouffer's
0.5	1	cup	Soup, Beef, Campbell's
0.5	1/2	pie	Turkey Pot Pie
0.5	1/2	cup	Chop Suey, Beef/Pork
0.5	1/2	portion	Beef Meatloaf Dinner, Frozen, Morton
0.5	1/2	portion	Fajita, Beef, Weight Watchers
0.5	1	cup	Soup, Chunky Steak 'n Potato, Campbell's
0.5	1	portion	Turkey, Divan, Frozen, Le Menu
0.5	1	cup	Soup, Chunky Chicken Noodle, Campbell's

Nutripoints	Serving Size		Food Name—Meat/Fish/Poultry
0.5	3	wt oz	Fish, Fried
0.5	1	portion	Fish Fillet, Au Gratin, Frozen, Weight Watchers
0.5	1/2	serving	Sandwich, Ham/Cheese, Whole Wheat
0.5	1/3	serving	Wendy's Homestyle Chicken Strips Salad
0.5	3	wt oz	Lamb Roast, Leg, Med. Fat, Baked
0.5	1/2	serving	Dairy Queen Single Hamburger
0.5	1/2	pie	Beef Pot Pie
0.5	1	portion	Chicken Cacciatore w/Vermicelli, Frozen, Stouffer's
0.5	1	piece	Taco Bell Chicken Fajita
0.5	2	wt oz	Beef Chuck Roast, Medium Fat, Baked
0.5	1	portion	Shrimp Creole, Frozen, Healthy Choice
0.5	1/2	serving	Dairy Queen Double Hamburger w/Cheese
0.5	1/2	portion	Beef Sirloin Tips, w/Burgundy Sauce, Frozen, Budget Gourmet
0.5	1	burger	McDonald's Hamburger
0.5	3	wt oz	Ham, Chopped
0.5	1/2	portion	Chicken, Fried, w/Corn, Frozen, Morton
0.5	1/2	serving	Burger King Ham and Cheese Specialty Sandwich
0.5	1/2	portion	Beef Salisbury Steak Dinner, Frozen, Morton
0.5	6	pieces	Burger King Chicken Tenders
0.5	1/2	pie	Chicken Pot Pie
0.5	4	pieces	Fish Sticks
0.5	1	serving	Chicken & Pasta w/Mushroom Sauce, Michelina's Lean Gourmet
0.5	1/2	portion	Turkey Breast, Sliced, Frozen, Budget Gourmet
0.5	3	wt oz	Beef Top Loin, Medium Fat, Broiled
0.5	1/2	serving	Beef Jardine, ZonePerfect
0.5	1/2	serving	Sandwich, Ham/Cheese, Rye
0.5	1/2	serving	Dairy Queen Single Hamburger w/Cheese
0.5	1	portion	Catfish, Fillets, Light, Mrs. Paul's
0.5	3	wt oz	Pike Fillet, Breaded, Fried
0.5	1/2	burger	Wendy's Single Hamburger w/Everything
0.5	1/2	portion	Scallops & Shrimp Mariner, Frozen, Budget Gourmet
0.5	2	wt oz	Beef Rump Roast, Baked
0.5	1/2	burger	Burger King Hamburger
0.5	2	slices	Bologna, Pork
0.5	3	wt oz	Goat
0.5	1/2	burger	Wendy's Single Cheese Hamburger w/Everything
0.5	1	portion	Turkey, Glazed, Slim, Frozen, Budget Gourmet
0.5	1	cup	Soup, Chicken Noodle
0.5	1/2	burger	Wendy's Plain Single Hamburger
0.0	3	wt oz	Pompano, Baked/Broiled
0.0	15	pieces	Shrimp, Steamed
0.0	1	portion	Beef Salisbury Steak, w/Potatoes, Frozen, Morton
0.0	1/2	portion	Beef Pot Roast, Yankee, Frozen, Budget Gourmet

Nutripoints	Serving Size		Food Name—Meat/Fish/Poultry
0.0	2	wt oz	Chicken Fried Steak
0.0	1	portion	Chicken Ala King, Frozen, Weight Watchers
0.0	1/4	serving	Sandwich, Submarine (12")
0.0	3	wt oz	Hamburger Patty, Broiled
0.0	1/2	burger	Cheeseburger w/Bun, Fast Food, Small Plain
0.0	1/4	serving	Dairy Queen Triple Hamburger w/Cheese
0.0	1/2	serving	Sandwich, Ham/Cheese, White
0.0	1/2	burger	Wendy's Plain Single Hamburger w/Cheese
0.0	1	portion	Beef Stroganoff, Slim, Frozen, Budget Gourmet
0.0	1	piece	Chicken Thigh, Meat & Skin, Baked
0.0	3	wt oz	Shark, Mixed Species, Batter-Dipped & Fried
0.0	3	wt oz	Catfish, Fried w/Breading
0.0	1/2	portion	Veal Parmigiana, Frozen, Budget Gourmet
0.0	1/2	portion	Chicken, Fried, Dinner, Frozen, Morton
0.0	1/2	burger	Carl's Jr. Old Time Star Hamburger
0.0	1	serving	Chicken, Parmesan w/Garden Veg, Weight Watchers Smart Ones
0.0	2	wt oz	Pork Roast, Baked
0.0	1/4	serving	Dairy Queen Triple Hamburger
0.0	1	wt oz	Wendy's Sliced Pepperoni
0.0	1	burger	Carl's Jr. Happy Star Hamburger
0.0	1/2	cup	Beef Stroganoff
0.0	1/2	piece	Chicken Kiev
0.0	1/2	portion	Tuna Noodle Casserole, Frozen, Stouffer's
0.0	1/2	burger	Jack In the Box Jumbo Jack
0.0	3/4	cup	Pork, Sweet and Sour
0.0	2	pieces	Chicken Wing, Fried w/o Breading
0.0	1/2	serving	Del Taco Chicken Cheddar Quesadilla
0.0	1/2	serving	Dairy Queen Chicken Breast Fillet
0.0	1	portion	Egg Rolls, Chicken, Frozen, Chun King
0.0	1	portion	Beef Oriental, w/Vegetables and Rice, Frozen, Stouffer's
0.0	3	wt oz	Beef Porterhouse Steak, Medium Fat, Choice, Broiled
0.0	1/2	serving	Sandwich, Ham Salad, Whole Wheat
0.0	1/2	serving	Dairy Queen Chicken Breast Fillet w/Cheese
0.0	1	wt oz	Pork Skins
0.0	2	cups	Soup, Clam Chowder, Manhattan Tomato Base
0.0	1/2	portion	Pepper Steak, w/Rice, Frozen, Budget Gourmet
0.0	1/2	portion	Beef Salisbury Steak, Romana, Frozen, Weight Watchers
0.0	4	wt oz	Chicken, White and Dark, Premium Chunk, Canned, Swanson
0.0	4	wt oz	Turkey, White & Dark, Canned, Premium Chunk, Swanson
0.0	3	wt oz	Squid, Fried
0.0	1/2	cup	Chicken Ala King
0.0	1	portion	Ham, Asparagus Au Gratin, Slim, Frozen, Budget Gourmet
0.0	1/3	serving	Wendy's Spicy Chicken Fillet

Nutripoints	Serving Size		Food Name—Meat/Fish/Poultry
0.0	1	portion	Egg Rolls, Shrimp, Frozen, Chun King
0.0	1/2	serving	Taco Bell Beef Enchirito w/Red Sauce
0.0	1/2	portion	Meatballs, Italian, w/Noodles/Peppers, Frozen, Budget Gourmet
0.0	1/2	burger	Burger King Cheeseburger
0.0	2	wt oz	Ham and Cheese Loaf/Roll
0.0	1	portion	Chicken Ala King, w/Rice, Frozen, Stouffer's
0.0	1/2	burger	Burger King Whopper Jr. Sandwich
0.0	1	burger	Jack In the Box Hamburger
0.0	1	piece	Chicken Thigh, Meat & Skin, Fried, Batter
0.0	1	taco	Taco Bell Soft Taco
0.0	1/2	serving	Arby's Beef 'n Cheddar Sandwich
0.0	1	cup	Soup, Cream of Chicken
0.0	1/2	burger	Wendy's Philly Swiss Hamburger
0.0	1	serving	Chicken Breast, Roasted, Fzn, Healthy Choice
0.0	1	portion	Haddock Fillet, Light, Mrs. Paul's
0.0	1	portion	Beef Szechwan, w/Noodles and Vegetables, Frozen, Stouffer's
0.0	3	wt oz	Goose, Meat and Skin, Baked
0.0	1/2	serving	Wendy's Fish Sandwich
0.0	2	wt oz	Sausage, Polish
0.0	1/2	portion	Enchiladas, Beef Ranchero, Frozen, Weight Watchers
0.0	1	portion	Western Dinner, Frozen, Morton
0.0	2	wt oz	Salami, Beef
0.0	1/2	burger	McDonald's Cheeseburger
0.0	1	portion	Beef Salisbury Steak, Frozen, Le Menu
0.0	2	wt oz	Ham, Minced
0.0	1/3	burger	Wendy's Classic Hamburger
0.0	2	pieces	Chicken Wing, Meat & Skin, Baked
0.0	1/2	serving	Taco Bell Beef Enchirito w/Green Sauce
0.0	1/2	serving	Jack In the Box Cheeseburger
-0.5	3	wt oz	Beef Tongue, Simmered
-0.5	3	wt oz	Veal Chop, Medium Fat, Fried
-0.5	1	portion	Egg Rolls, Shrimp/Meat, Frozen, Chun King
-0.5	1/2	cup	Hash
-0.5	1/2	serving	Carl's Jr. Country Fried Steak Sandwich
-0.5	2	wt oz	Pork Chop, Broiled
-0.5	2	pieces	Meatballs
-0.5	4	wt oz	Chicken, Chunk White, Premium, Canned, Swanson
-0.5	1	portion	Beef Stew, Frozen, Stouffer's
-0.5	1/3	burger	Wendy's Classic Hamburger w/Cheese
-0.5	1	taco	Taco Bell Super Combo Taco
-0.5	4	wt oz	Yellowtail, Raw
-0.5	1/2	burger	Burger King Whopper Jr. Sandwich w/Cheese
-0.5	1	portion	Veal Primavera, Frozen, Stouffer's

Nutripoints	Serving Size		Food Name—Meat/Fish/Poultry
-0.5	1/2	serving	Jack In the Box Hot Club Supreme
-0.5	1/2	portion	Turkey A La King, w/Rice, Frozen, Budget Gourmet
-0.5	1	serving	Fish, Herb Baked, Fzn, Healthy Choice
-0.5	1/2	portion	Enchiladas, Beef Dinner, Frozen, Patio
-0.5	1	piece	Chicken Wing, Meat & Skin, Fried, Batter
-0.5	3	wt oz	Lobster, Floured/Breaded, Fried
-0.5	1/2	portion	Chicken Pie, Frozen, Stouffer's
-0.5	3	wt oz	Meatloaf
-0.5	1	serving	Dairy Queen All White Chicken Nuggets
-0.5	1/4	burger	Wendy's Bacon Swiss Hamburger
-0.5	3	wt oz	Beef T-Bone Steak, Medium Fat, Broiled
-0.5	1	portion	Veal Marsala, Frozen, Le Menu
-0.5	2	wt oz	Sausage, Italian
-0.5	1	cup	Soup, New England Clam Chowder w/Milk, Campbell's
-0.5	3	wt oz	Cod, Floured/Breaded, Fried
-0.5	1/2	portion	Beef Pie, Frozen, Stouffer's
-0.5	1/2	serving	Sandwich, Ham Salad, White
-0.5	1/2	portion	Enchiladas, Chicken, Suiza, Frozen, Weight Watchers
-0.5	2	pieces	Jack In the Box Egg Rolls-5 Piece
-0.5	1/2	portion	Seafood Newberg, Frozen, Budget Gourmet
-0.5	1	serving	Chicken Alfredo Florentine, Michelina's Lean Gourmet
-0.5	4	wt oz	Turkey Roll, White, Cooked, Mr. Turkey
-0.5	1/2	portion	Chicken Parmigiana Patty, Frozen, Weight Watchers
-0.5	1/2	portion	Beef Pie, Frozen, Morton
-0.5	1	portion	Cod Fillets, Light, Mrs. Paul's
-0.5	1	taco	Taco Bell Supreme Soft Taco
-0.5	1/2	serving	Jack In the Box Taquitos (7 Pieces)
-0.5	3	wt oz	Flounder, Fillet, Breaded, Fried
-0.5	1/2	burger	Carl's Jr. Famous Star Hamburger
-0.5	1/2	serving	Burger King Chicken Specialty Sandwich
-0.5	1/2	burger	McDonald's Quarter Pounder
-0.5	1/2	portion	Beef Sirloin Salisbury Steak, Frozen, Budget Gourmet
-0.5	1/2	pie	Turkey, Pie, Frozen, Morton
-0.5	1	portion	Green Pepper, Stuffed, w/Beef & Tomato Sauce, Fzn, Stouffer's
-0.5	1	serving	Beef, Roasted Sirloin, Michelina's Lean Gourmet
-0.5	3	wt oz	Carp, Floured/Breaded, Fried
-0.5	1/2	pie	Chicken, Pie, Frozen, Morton
-0.5	3	wt oz	Pompano, Floured/Breaded, Fried
-0.5	1/2	piece	Frankfurter, Pork & Beef, w/Bun
-0.5	1/2	muffin	McDonald's Sausage McMuffin
-0.5	1	piece	Kentucky Fried Chicken, Chicken Keel, Extra Crispy
-0.5	2	wt oz	Lamb Chop, Loin, Med. Fat, Baked
-0.5	1	serving	Fish Fillet, Florentine, Frozen, Stouffer's

Nutripoints	Serving Size		Food Name—Meat/Fish/Poultry
-0.5	1	portion	Turkey, w/Dressing & Potatoes, Frozen, Swanson
-0.5	1	piece	Pork Chop, Pan-Fried
-1.0	1	piece	Kentucky Fried Chicken, Chicken Keel
-1.0	3	wt oz	Haddock, Floured/Breaded, Fried
-1.0	3	wt oz	Pork Feet, Pickled
-1.0	1/2	portion	Turkey Breast, Stuffed, Frozen, Weight Watchers
-1.0	1/2	cup	Beef, Creamed Chipped
-1.0	1/2	serving	Burger King Fish Filet Sandwich
-1.0	1	serving	Beef Stroganoff, Fzn, Healthy Choice
-1.0	1	portion	Beef Salisbury Steak, In Gravy, Frozen, Stouffer's
-1.0	4	wt oz	Fish Sticks, Crunchy, Frozen, Mrs. Paul's
-1.0	1/2	portion	Beef Stroganoff, Frozen, Weight Watchers
-1.0	2	pieces	Luncheon Meat, Picnic Loaf, Oscar Mayer
-1.0	1	piece	Flounder Fillet, Light, Mrs. Paul's
-1.0	1/2	portion	Tortellini, Veal, Alfredo, Frozen, Stouffer's
-1.0	1	portion	Fish Fillet, Batter Dipped, Frozen, Mrs. Paul's
-1.0	1	portion	Beef Salisbury Steak, w/Italian Sauce, Frozen, Stouffer's
-1.0	2	wt oz	Luncheon Meat, Pimento Loaf
-1.0	1/2	portion	Chicken Divan, Frozen, Stouffer's
-1.0	1/2	burger	Burger King Whopper Sandwich w/Cheese
-1.0	1/2	burger	McDonald's Big Mac
-1.0	2	pieces	Jack In the Box Egg Rolls- 3 Piece
-1.0	1/2	serving	Carl's Jr. Filet of Fish Sandwich
-1.0	3	slices	Bacon, Low-Salt, Oscar Mayer
-1.0	2	slices	Luncheon Meat, Pickle and Pimiento Loaf
-1.0	1/2	portion	Chicken, w/Fettucini, Frozen, Budget Gourmet
-1.0	1	serving	Chicken, Country Herb, Fzn, Healthy Choice
-1.0	3	wt oz	Lamb Shoulder, Med. Fat, Baked
-1.0	4	wt oz	Lobster, Baked/Broiled w/Butter
-1.0	3	wt oz	Duck, Meat and Skin, Baked
-1.0	3	pieces	Jack In the Box Chicken Strips-6 Piece
-1.0	4	slices	Turkey, Luncheon Loaf, Louis Rich
-1.0	1/2	pie	Turkey Pie, Frozen, Stouffer's
-1.0	1	wt oz	Pate, de Foie Gras, Canned (goose liver)
-1.0	1/2	serving	Corn Dog
-1.0	1	serving	Dairy Queen Hot Dog
-1.0	1/2	portion	Beef Sirloin Tips w/Country Style Vegetables, Fzn, Budget Gourmet
-1.0	3	pieces	Shrimp, Fried
-1.0	1/2	serving	McDonald's Filet-O-Fish Sandwich
-1.0	3	wt oz	Clams, Fried, Light Batter, Mrs. Paul's
-1.0	1	piece	Ocean Perch Fillet, Light, Mrs. Paul's
-1.0	1/2	serving	Dairy Queen Hot Dog w/Chili
-1.0	1/2	pie	Turkey Pot Pie, Swanson

Nutripoints	Serving Size		Food Name—Meat/Fish/Poultry
-1.0	2	wt oz	Beef Short Ribs, Medium Fat, Braised
-1.0	2	pieces	Sausage, Summer
-1.0	2	pieces	Jack In the Box Chicken Strips-4 Piece
-1.0	1/2	serving	Jack In the Box Fish Supreme
-1.0	1/2	burger	Carl's Jr. Western Bacon Cheeseburger
-1.0	1/2	pie	Chicken Pot Pie, Frozen, Swanson
-1.0	1/2	cup	Crab Salad
-1.0	1	serving	Frankfurter, Chicken, w/Bun
-1.0	2	wt oz	Bratwurst
-1.0	1	portion	Enchiladas Suiza, Chicken, Van de Kamp's
-1.0	1/2	burger	McDonald's Quarter Pounder w/Cheese
-1.0	1/2	burger	Jack In the Box Bacon Cheeseburger
-1.0	3	wt oz	Crab, Soft Shell, Fried
-1.0	4	wt oz	Fish Fillet, Light Recipe, Frozen, Gorton's
-1.0	1/2	burger	Burger King Bacon Double Cheeseburger
-1.0	1	taco	Taco Bell Taco
-1.0	1	piece	Kentucky Fried Chicken
-1.0	1/2	burger	Jack In the Box Double Cheeseburger
-1.0	1	piece	Kentucky Fried Chicken, Side Breast, Extra Crispy
-1.0	1	piece	Sole Fillet, Light, Mrs. Paul's
-1.0	1/2	piece	Chicken, Fried, Homestyle, Frozen, Swanson
-1.0	3	slices	Bacon, Fried
-1.5	1/2	serving	Dairy Queen Hot Dog w/Cheese
-1.5	3	wt oz	Sausage, Italian, 1 Link
-1.5	1/4	burger	Carl's Jr. Double Western Bacon Cheeseburger
-1.5	2	wt oz	Spam
-1.5	1	cup	Soup, Chicken Noodle, Campbell's
-1.5	3	pieces	Pork Spareribs
-1.5	1	piece	Kentucky Fried Chicken, Side Breast
-1.5	3	wt oz	Kielbasa
-1.5	1	serving	McDonald's Chicken McNuggets
-1.5	8	wt oz	Soup, Oyster Stew, w/Milk, Campbell's
-1.5	1/3	serving	Wendy's Chicken BLT Salad
-1.5	1	cup	Soup, Chicken Rice
-1.5	1/2	burger	Carl's Jr. Super Star Hamburger
-1.5	1	piece	Kentucky Fried Chicken, Drumstick, Extra Crispy
-1.5	1/2	serving	Taco Bell Taco Bellgrande
-1.5	3	slices	Bacon, Low-Sodium, No Sugar, Bryan
-1.5	1/2	pie	Beef Pot Pie, Frozen, Swanson
-1.5	2	wt oz	Luncheon Meat, Beef
-1.5	4	pieces	Wendy's Crispy Chicken Nuggets (vegetable Oil)
-1.5	3	wt oz	Chicken, Smoked Sliced, Buddig
-1.5	1	Tbls	McDonald's Bacon Bits

Nutripoints	Serving Size		Food Name—Meat/Fish/Poultry
-1.5	1/2	piece	Veal Parmigiana
-1.5	2	slices	Luncheon Meat, Head Cheese
-1.5	1/2	portion	Beef Stroganoff, w/Parsley Noodles, Frozen, Stouffer's
-1.5	1/2	cup	Chicken Pot Pie, Claim Jumper
-1.5	1/2	burger	Jack In the Box Jumbo Jack w/Cheese
-1.5	1/2	serving	Wendy's Chicken Strips Sandwich
-1.5	1/2	serving	Jack In the Box Chicken Supreme
-1.5	1/2	serving	Dairy Queen Hounder w/Chili
-1.5	1/2	taco	Taco Bell Taco Light
-1.5	3.75	wt oz	Fish Sticks, Crispy Crunchy, Mrs. Paul's
-1.5	1	piece	Fish Almondine, Frozen Dinner
-1.5	1	cup	Carl's Jr. Boston Clam Chowder Soups
-1.5	2	wt oz	Bologna, Turkey
-1.5	1/2	serving	McDonald's Biscuit w/Sausage
-1.5	1	cup	Soup, Cream of Chicken, 1/3 Less Salt, Campbell's
-1.5	1	piece	Kentucky Fried Chicken, Drumstick
-1.5	3	wt oz	Halibut, Smoked
-1.5	6	wt oz	Squid, Boiled
-1.5	1	piece	Fish Fillet, Crispy Crunchy, Frozen, Mrs. Paul's
-2.0	3	slices	Salami, Turkey Cotto, Louis Rich
-2.0	1/4	burger	Jack In the Box Ultimate Cheeseburger
-2.0	2	slices	Salami, Cotto, Oscar Mayer
-2.0	4	pieces	Wendy's Crispy Chicken Nuggets (animal Oil)
-2.0	2	wt oz	Knockwurst
-2.0	3	slices	Bacon, Bryan
-2.0	2	pieces	Frog Legs, Fried
-2.0	1/2	portion	Chicken Breast Portions, Fried, Frozen, Swanson
-2.0	1/2	portion	Chicken & Egg Noodles, w/Broccoli, Frozen, Budget Gourmet
-2.0	2	wt oz	Beef Sirloin Steak, Broiled
-2.0	3	wt oz	Corned Beef, Smoked Sliced, Buddig
-2.0	4	wt oz	Pastrami, Land O' Frost
-2.0	1/2	portion	Chicken, Southern Fried Patty, Frozen, Weight Watchers
-2.0	3	slices	Bacon, Oscar Mayer
-2.0	1/3	serving	Wendy's Chicken Fried Steak
-2.0	1/2	serving	Dairy Queen Hounder w/Cheese
-2.0	3	wt oz	Corned Beef, Libby's
-2.0	12	wt oz	Chicken Fettucini Alfredo, Uncle Ben's Pasta Bowl
-2.0	1	piece	Kentucky Fried Chicken, Thigh, Extra Crispy
-2.0	3	wt oz	Beef, Smoked, Sliced, Buddig
-2.0	1/2	serving	Dairy Queen Hounder
-2.0	1	piece	Kentucky Fried Chicken, Wing, Extra Crispy
-2.0	1	cup	Soup, Cream of Chicken, Campbell's
-2.0	4	wt oz	Beef, Land O' Frost

Nutripoints	Serving Size		Food Name—Meat/Fish/Poultry
-2.0	4	wt oz	Ham, Turkey, Mr. Turkey
-2.0	2	slices	Luncheon Meat, Olive Loaf, Oscar Mayer
-2.0	4	wt oz	Sole Fillet, Fishmarket Fresh, Frozen, Gorton's
-2.5	1	cup	Soup Mix, Chicken Noodle, w/Chicken Meat, Lipton
-2.5	1	cup	Soup Mix, Chicken Rice, Lipton
-2.5	4	slices	Salami, Hard (Genoa), Oscar Mayer
-2.5	4	wt oz	Scrod, Baked, Stuffed, Frozen, Gorton's
-2.5	3	slices	Bacon, West Virginia Brand, Hygrade's
-2.5	1/2	burger	Jack In the Box Swiss & Bacon Burger
-2.5	2	slices	Bologna, Turkey, Louis Rich
-2.5	1	patty	Carl's Jr. Sausage Patty
-2.5	1/3	portion	Meatballs, Swedish, w/Noodles, Frozen, Budget Gourmet
-2.5	1	piece	Kentucky Fried Chicken, Chicken Wing
-2.5	1	serving	Frankfurter, Beef
-2.5	1	piece	Kentucky Fried Chicken, Thigh
-2.5	2	slices	Bologna, Bryan
-2.5	2	links	Sausage Link, Pork
-2.5	1/2	portion	Beef Salisbury Steak, Homestyle, Frozen, Swanson
-2.5	2	slices	Bologna, Beef, Bryan
-2.5	3	pieces	Beef, Breakfast Strip, Lean 'n Tasty, Oscar Mayer
-2.5	2	wt oz	Beef Prime Rib, Baked
-2.5	2	wt oz	Pastrami, Beef
-2.5	3	slices	Bacon, Sliced, Farmland
-2.5	1	portion	Enchiladas, Beef, Shredded, Van de Kamp's
-2.5	1/2	serving	Jack In the Box Breakfast Jack
-2.5	2	wt oz	Luncheon Meat, Olive Loaf, Eckrich
-2.5	1/2	serving	Jack In the Box Supreme Crescent Breakfast
-2.5	1/2	serving	Beef, Barbecue, Sandwich, w/Bun
-2.5	1	serving	Frankfurter, Bryan
-2.5	3	wt oz	Corned Beef
-2.5	7	pieces	Jack In the Box Shrimp - 15 Piece
-2.5	7	pieces	Jack In the Box Shrimp - 10 Piece
-2.5	1	serving	Frankfurter, Original Brown & Serve, Beef, Swift
-3.0	1	patty	Wendy's Sausage Patty
-3.0	2	wt oz	Sausage, Little, Jones
-3.0	1	serving	Frankfurter, Oscar Mayer
-3.0	1/2	serving	Jack In the Box Sausage Crescent Breakfast
-3.0	2	wt oz	Sandwich, Steak, Frozen, Steak-Um
-3.0	1	serving	Frankfurter, With Cheese, Oscar Mayer
-3.0	2	wt oz	Liverwurst, Original, Jones
-3.0	1/2	serving	Jack In the Box Canadian Crescent Breakfast
-3.5	1	serving	Frankfurter, Original Brown & Serve, Pork, Swift
-3.5	1	serving	Frankfurter, Beef, Eckrich

Nutripoints	Serving Size		Food Name—Meat/Fish/Poultry
-3.5	1	cup	Soup, Mushroom, Beefy, Campbell's
-3.5	1	serving	Frankfurter, Beef, Oscar Mayer
-3.5	1	serving	Frankfurter, Turkey
-3.5	2	slices	Luncheon Meat, Oscar Mayer
-3.5	2	wt oz	Bologna, Beef
-3.5	1	piece	McDonald's Pork Sausage
-3.5	2	slices	Bologna, Oscar Mayer
-3.5	2	wt oz	Ham, Deviled, Underwood
-3.5	2	wt oz	Sausage, Pork, Jimmy Dean
-3.5	1	serving	Frankfurter, Eckrich
-3.5	2	slices	Bologna, Garlic, Eckrich
-3.5	2	slices	Bologna, Beef, Oscar Mayer
-3.5	3	wt oz	Crab Cake
-3.5	3	wt oz	Ham, Land O' Frost
-3.5	1	serving	Frankfurter, Chicken, Tyson
-3.5	1	serving	Frankfurter, Pork & Beef
-3.5	3	slices	Bacon, Premium Sizzlean, Swift
-3.5	3	pieces	Sausage, Vienna
-3.5	2	wt oz	Paté
-3.5	3	wt oz	Shrimp, Fried, Frozen, Mrs. Paul's
-4.0	1	serving	Frankfurter, Ball Park
-4.0	2	slices	Bologna, Eckrich
-4.0	1/2	muffin	McDonald's Sausage McMuffin w/ Egg
-4.0	2	wt oz	Salami, Cooked, Armour
-4.0	2	wt oz	Frankfurter, Beef, Ball Park
-4.0	1	serving	Frankfurter, Beef, Armour
-4.0	1	wt oz	Salami, Cotto Beef, Eckrich
-4.0	1	wt oz	Salt Pork, Raw
-4.0	2	slices	Bologna, Beef, Armour
-4.5	1/2	serving	McDonald's Biscuit w/Sausage & Egg
-4.5	2	wt oz	Treet
-5.0	3	wt oz	Chicken, Land O' Frost
-5.0	1	wt oz	Pepperoni
-6.0	1	wt oz	Pepperoni, Gallo
-52.0	3	wt oz	Sweetbreads (organ meats)

OTHER GROUPS

FAT/OIL GROUP

Nutripoints	Serving Size		Food Name—Fats/Oils
8.0	1/4	cup	Dressing, Blue Cheese, Nutripoint Recipe
7.5	1/4	cup	Dip, Slim Guacamole, Nutripoint Recipe
3.5	1/4	cup	Dressing, Lite, Ranch, Nutripoint Recipe
2.5	1/4	cup	Dressing, Lite, 16 Island, Nutripoint Recipe
2.5	2	Tbls	Dressing, Vinaigrette, Orange, Nutripoint Recipe
2.0	2	Tbls	Dressing, Caper, Nutripoint Recipe
1.5	1/4	cup	Sauce Mix, Stroganoff, Prepared w/Milk/Water
1.5	1/4	cup	Mayo Mix, Lite, Nutripoint Recipe
1.0	1/4	cup	Sauce Mix, Mushroom, Prepared w/Milk
1.0	2	Tbls	Margarine-like Spread, Smart Beat Squeeze
1.0	1	fl oz	Margarine, 20% Corn Oil, Smart Beat
1.0	1/4	cup	Gravy, Beef, Canned
0.0	1/4	cup	Gravy Mix, Chicken, Prepared
0.0	1/4	cup	Sauce Mix, Curry, w/Milk
0.0	1/4	cup	Sauce Mix, Sweet and Sour, Prepared
0.0	2	Tbls	Mayonnaise, Light, Kraft
0.0	1/4	cup	Gravy, Mushroom, Canned
0.0	1	Tbls	Margarine, Take Control Light
0.0	1	Tbls	Dressing, Lite Red French, Wish-Bone
0.0	1	Tbls	Dressing, Non-Fat, Healthy Sensation (all flavors)
0.0	1	Tbls	Mayonnaise, Non-Fat, Kraft Free
0.0	1	Tbls	Margarine, Benecol Light
0.0	1/4	cup	Gravy, Turkey, Canned
-0.5	1	Tbls	Sauce, Tartar, Sauce Works, Kraft
-0.5	2	Tbls	Dip, Clam
-0.5	1/4	cup	Gravy Mix, Turkey, Prepared
-0.5	1/4	cup	Gravy Mix, Mushroom, Prepared
-0.5	2	Tbls	Dressing, Russian, Low Cal
-0.5	1	Tbls	Dressing, Lite Italian, Wish-Bone
-0.5	1	Tbls	Dressing, Non-Fat, Kraft Free (all flavors)
-0.5	1	Tbls	Dressing, Non-Fat, Take Heart, Hidden Valley (all flavors)
-1.0	1/4	cup	Sauce, White
-1.0	2	Tbls	Dressing, Salad, Low Cal
-1.0	1	Tbls	Margarine, Take Control

Nutripoints	Serving Size		Food Name—Fats/Oils
-1.0	1	Tbls	Margarine, Low Cal
-1.5	1	Tbls	Margarine, Benecol
-1.5	2	Tbls	Dressing, Low Cal, French
-1.5	1/4	cup	Gravy, Chicken, Canned
-1.5	2	Tbls	Dressing, Vinaigrette, Lite, Nutripoint Recipe
-1.5	1/4	cup	Kentucky Fried Chicken, Gravy
-2.0	1/4	cup	Gravy, Mix, Pork, Prepared
-2.0	4	Tbls	Margarine, Sweet Unsalted, Heart Beat
-2.0	2	Tbls	Margarine, Reduced Cal, Unsalted, Weight Watchers
-2.0	1	Tbls	Margarine, Promise
-2.0	1	Tbls	Margarine, Family Spread, Mrs. Filbert's
-2.0	1	Tbls	Dressing, French, Catalina, Kraft
-2.5	1	Tbls	Margarine, Safflower, Hain
-2.5	2	Tbls	Margarine, Extra Light, Promise
-2.5	2	Tbls	Margarine, Brummel & Brown Spread
-2.5	2	Tbls	Dressing, Thousand Island, Low Cal
-2.5	1	Tbls	Dressing, French, Kraft
-2.5	2	Tbls	Margarine, Reduced Cal Spread, Blue Bonnet
-2.5	1	Tbls	Margarine, 37% Light, Smart Balance
-2.5	2	Tbls	Dressing, Russian
-2.5	1	Tbls	Margarine, Omega Plus w/Flax, Smart Balance
-2.5	1	Tbls	Margarine, Unsalted, Mazola
-2.5	2	Tbls	Margarine, Corn Oil Spread, Light, Mazola
-2.5	2	Tbls	Margarine, Diet Imitation, Mazola
-2.5	1	Tbls	Mayonnaise, Canola Oil, Smart Beat
-2.5	2	Tbls	Margarine, Diet, Soft, Parkay
-2.5	2	Tbls	Margarine, Soft, Spread, Touch of Butter, Kraft
-2.5	1	Tbls	Oil, Hazelnut
-2.5	2	Tbls	Margarine, Reduced Cal, Weight Watchers
-2.5	1	Tbls	Margarine, Hard, Coconut, Safflower and Palm
-2.5	1	Tbls	Mayonnaise, Cholesterol Free, Kraft
-2.5	1	Tbls	Oil, Almond
-2.5	2	Tbls	Margarine, Diet, Fleischmann's
-2.5	1	Tbls	Dressing, Mayonnaise Type
-2.5	1	Tbls	Oil, Canola, Puritan
-2.5	1	Tbls	Oil, Vegetable, Puritan
-2.5	1	Tbls	Margarine, Stick, Unsalted, Fleischmann
-2.5	2	Tbls	Margarine, Reduced Cal, Diet, Mazola
-2.5	1	Tbls	Oil, Walnut
-2.5	1	Tbls	Oil, Safflower
-2.5	2	Tbls	McDonald's French Dressing
-2.5	1	Tbls	Margarine, Parkay
-2.5	1/4	cup	Sauce Mix, Teriyaki, Prepared

Nutripoints	Serving Size		Food Name—Fats/Oils
-2.5	1	Tbls	Oil, Linseed
-2.5	1	Tbls	Margarine, Whipped Spread, Parkay
-2.5	1	Tbls	Margarine, Cookery, Parkay
-2.5	1	Tbls	Margarine, Squeeze, Parkay
-2.5	1	Tbls	Margarine, Corn Oil
-2.5	2	Tbls	Mayonnaise, Low Cal
-2.5	1	Tbls	Mayonnaise, Cholesterol Free, Miracle Whip
-2.5	1	Tbls	Margarine, Mazola
-2.5	1	Tbls	Oil, Sunflower
-2.5	1	Tbls	Margarine, Soft, Corn Oil, Mrs. Filbert's
-2.5	1	Tbls	Margarine, Stick, Land O'lakes
-2.5	1/4	cup	Gravy
-2.5	1/4	cup	Gravy Mix, Chicken, Prepared w/Milk/Butter
-2.5	1/4	cup	Gravy Mix, Turkey, Prep w/Milk & Butter
-2.5	2	Tbls	Margarine, Whipped, Imperial
-2.5	2	Tbls	Dressing, Italian
-2.5	2	Tbls	Mayonnaise, Light Reduced Cal, Kraft
-2.5	1	Tbls	Margarine, I Can't Believe It's Not Butter
-2.5	1	Tbls	Mayonnaise
-2.5	1	Tbls	Oil, Puritan
-2.5	1	Tbls	Oil, Safflower, Hollywood
-2.5	1	Tbls	Oil, Sunlite
-3.0	1	Tbls	Margarine, Soft, Blue Bonnet
-3.0	1	Tbls	Margarine, Stick, Blue Bonnet
-3.0	1	Tbls	Margarine, Stick, Fleischmann's
-3.0	2	Tbls	Dressing, Thousand Island
-3.0	1	Tbls	Margarine, Stick, Imperial
-3.0	1	Tbls	Oil, Soybean
-3.0	4	Tbls	Margarine, Heart Beat
-3.0	1	Tbls	Margarine
-3.0	2	Tbls	Mayonnaise, Light Reduced Cal, Hellman's
-3.0	1	Tbls	Margarine, Country Crock Spread, Shedd's
-3.0	1	Tbls	Oil, Olive
-3.0	2	Tbls	Dressing, Green Goddess
-3.0	1	Tbls	Oil, Corn, Mazola
-3.0	1	Tbls	Oil, Sesame
-3.0	1	Tbls	Margarine, Liquid, Soybean & Cottonseed
-3.0	1	Tbls	Oil, Olive, Bertolli
-3.0	1	Tbls	Margarine, Soft, Chiffon
-3.0	1	Tbls	Oil, Corn, Crisco
-3.0	1	Tbls	Oil, Crisco
-3.0	1	Tbls	Mayonnaise, Imitation, Soybean
-3.0	1	Tbls	Margarine, Soft Imperial

Nutripoints	Serving Size		Food Name—Fats/Oils
-3.0	1	Tbls	Oil, Wesson
-3.0	2	Tbls	McDonald's 1000 Island Dressing
-3.0	1	Tbls	Margarine, Soybean, Willow Run (Shedd's)
-3.0	1	Tbls	Oil, Peanut
-3.0	2	Tbls	Mayonnaise, Light, Miracle Whip
-3.0	2	Tbls	McDonald's Ranch Dressing
-3.0	1	Tbls	Dressing, Salad, Miracle Whip, Kraft
-3.0	1	Tbls	Dressing, Oil & Vinegar
-3.0	2	Tbls	Dressing, French
-3.0	1	Tbls	Dressing, French, Home Recipe
-3.0	1	Tbls	Jack In the Box Bleu Cheese Dressing
-3.0	1	Tbls	Margarine, 67% Light, Smart Balance
-3.0	1	Tbls	Mayonnaise, Real, Best Foods
-3.0	1	Tbls	Mayonnaise, Blue Plate
-3.0	1	Tbls	Crisco, Butter Flavored
-3.0	1	Tbls	Oil, Wheat Germ

- - -

-3.0	2	Tbls	Dressing, Blue Cheese
-3.0	1	Tbls	Jack In the Box Buttermilk House Dressing
-3.0	1	Tbls	Oil
-3.0	3	wt oz	Wendy's Sausage Gravy
-3.0	2	Tbls	Dressing, Ranch/Buttermilk
-3.5	1	Tbls	Jack In the Box Thousand Island Dressing
-3.5	1	Tbls	McDonald's Bleu Cheese Dressing
-3.5	4	Tbls	McDonald's Newman's Own Lowfat Balsamic Vinaigrette Dressing
-3.5	1	Tbls	Dressing, Oil & Vinegar, Kraft
-3.5	1	Tbls	Shortening, Crisco
-3.5	1	Tbls	Shortening, Soybean and Cottonseed
-3.5	2	Tbls	Sauce, Tartar
-3.5	2	Tbls	Taco Bell Sour Cream
-3.5	1	Tbls	Mayonnaise, Real, Kraft
-3.5	1	Tbls	Mayonnaise, Real, Hellmann's
-3.5	2	wt oz	Wendy's Imitation Sour Topping
-3.5	1	Tbls	Mayonnaise, Imitation, Milk Cream
-3.5	1	Tbls	Oil, Cottonseed
-3.5	1	Tbls	Dressing, Salad, Reduced Cal, Miracle Whip
-3.5	1/4	cup	Gravy, Mushroom, Franco-American
-3.5	2	Tbls	Dressing, Salad
-4.0	1	Tbls	Taco Bell Ranch Dressing
-4.0	1	Tbls	Shortening, Soybean and Palm
-4.0	1/4	cup	Gravy Mix, Brown, French's
-4.0	1	Tbls	Margarine, Soft, Low Salt, Country Morning Blend, Land O'Lakes
-4.0	1/4	cup	Gravy, Chicken, Franco-American

Nutripoints	Serving Size		Food Name—Fats/Oils
-4.0	1/4	cup	Gravy Mix, Mushroom, French's
-4.0	1	Tbls	Fat, Goose
-4.0	1	Tbls	Fat, Chicken
-4.5	2	Tbls	Jack In the Box Reduced Calorie French Dressing
-4.5	1	Tbls	Fat, Turkey
-4.5	1	Tbls	Fat, Duck
-4.5	2	Tbls	Dressing, Low Cal, Blue Cheese
-4.5	1/4	cup	Gravy Mix, Chicken, McCormick's
-4.5	1	Tbls	Shortening, Lard and Vegetable Oil
-5.0	1	Tbls	Lard
-5.0	1	Tbls	Oil, Palm
-5.0	1	Tbls	Dip, Onion
-5.0	1/4	cup	Sauce, Hollandaise
-5.5	1/4	cup	Sauce Mix, Béarnaise, w/Milk-Butter
-5.5	1	Tbls	Fat, Mutton Tallow
-5.5	1	Tbls	Oil, Cocoa Butter
-6.0	1	Tbls	Wendy's Creamy Peppercorn Dressing
-6.5	1	Tbls	Fat, Beef Tallow
-6.5	1	Tbls	Butter, Unsalted
-6.5	1	Tbls	Butter, Sweet, Cream, Unsalted, Land O'Lakes
-6.5	1	Tbls	Oil, Palm Kernel
-7.0	1	Tbls	Butter, Sweet, Light Salt, Land O'Lakes
-7.0	1	Tbls	Oil, Coconut
-7.5	1	Tbls	Butter, Salted

SUGAR GROUP

Nutripoints	Serving Size		Food Name—Sugars
13.5	8	fl oz	Sports Drink, Zing (*)
10.0	8	fl oz	Energy Drink, Red Bull (*)
8.5	1	serving	Sports Powder, AminoVital Fast Charge
8.5	8	fl oz	Energy Drink, SoBe No Fear (*)
5.5	1	serving	Energy Gel, GU (*)
5.0	8	fl oz	Sports Drink, AminoVital Shake Mix (*)
4.5	1	serving	Sports Gel, Accelerade Accel Gel (*)
3.5	2	Tbls	Molasses, Blackstrap
3.5	1	serving	Sports Drink, Cytomax Energy and Recovery Drink (*)
3.0	6	fl oz	Fruit Drink, Tang
2.5	12	fl oz	Sports Drink, Gatorade Energy Drink (*)
2.0	12	fl oz	Sports Drink, Accelerade Powder Mix (*)
1.5	20	fl oz	Sports Drink, AminoVital Ready to Drink (*)
0.5	12	fl oz	Sports Drink, Endurox R4 (*)
-1.0	4	Tbls	Jelly, Low Cal, All Flavors
-1.0	6	pieces	Ginger Snaps
-1.5	1	serving	Power Gel, Power Bar
-2.0	1	wt oz	Halvah, Plain
-2.0	1	wt oz	Candy Bar, Diet
-2.0	1	wt oz	Candy, M&M's Peanut
-2.0	8	fl oz	Sports Drink, Power Bar Recovery Drink
-2.0	1	bar	Candy Bar, Kit Kat
-2.0	1/2	bar	Candy Bar, Baby Ruth
-2.0	500	ml	Sports Drink, Lucozade (*)
-2.5	1/2	piece	Pie, Chocolate Cream
-2.5	1	piece	Fudge, Peanut Butter
-2.5	1	bar	Candy Bar, Butterfinger
-3.0	8	fl oz	Sports Drink, Powerade
-3.0	2	Tbls	Molasses
-3.0	1	piece	Candy, Peanut Butter Cups, Reese's
-3.0	1	wt oz	Chocolate, Unsweetened, Baker's
-3.0	1	piece	Brownie/Blondie, Fat-Free, Pepperidge Farm
-3.0	17	pieces	Gummy Bears
-3.0	1	piece	Candy, Pralines
-3.0	1	piece	Cake, Choco-Bake, Nestle'
-3.0	1/2	bar	Candy Bar, Snickers
-3.0	1/2	bar	Candy Bar, Mr. Goodbar
-3.0	10	pieces	Gum
-3.5	1	bar	Candy, Milk Chocolate w/Almonds, Hershey's

Nutripoints	Serving Size		Food Name—Sugars
-3.5	1/2	bar	Candy Bar, Mars Bar
-3.5	1	piece	Fudge, Divinity
-3.5	6	pieces	Candy, Kisses, Hershey's
-3.5	1	piece	Fudge, Chocolate w/Nuts
-3.5	1	pieces	Fudge, Vanilla, w/Nuts
-3.5	2	Tbls	Jelly, All Flavors
-3.5	2	tsp	Syrup, Sorghum
-3.5	3	pieces	Candy, Caramels
-3.5	2	Tbls	Sauce, Chocolate Fudge
-4.0	2	pieces	Candy Bar, Twix Caramel
-4.0	1	wt oz	Candy, Brach Toffees
-4.0	1	bar	Candy Bar, Chocolit
-4.0	2	Tbls	Syrup, Maple Low Cal
-4.0	1	bar	Candy Bar, 3 Musketeers
-4.0	1	bar	Candy Bar, $100,000
-4.0	1	piece	Fudge, Vanilla
-4.0	1/2	bar	Candy Bar, Milky Way
-4.0	8	fl oz	Sports Drink, Accelerade Ready to Drink
-4.0	1	wt oz	Candy, Brach Royals
-4.0	1/2	bar	Candy Bar, Three Musketeers
-4.0	1	piece	Frozen Dessert, Creamsicle
-4.0	1	wt oz	Chocolate, Baking
-4.0	8	fl oz	Drink Mix, Rainbow Punch, Sweetened, Kool-Aid
-4.5	1.4	wt oz	Candy Bar, Nestle' Crunch
-4.5	3	Tbls	Sugar, Powdered
-4.5	1	wt oz	Chocolate, Semi-Sweet, Baker's
-4.5	1	wt oz	Candy, Semi-Sweet Morsels, Nestle'
-4.5	10	pieces	Gum, Doublemint, Wrigley's
-4.5	2	Tbls	Sauce, Butterscotch
-4.5	5	pieces	Candy, Rolo
-4.5	1	fl oz	Syrup, Lite, Aunt Jemima
-4.5	2	Tbls	Frosting
-4.5	1/2	piece	Pie, Chiffon
-4.5	1	wt oz	Chocolate, Sweet or Dark
-4.5	1	wt oz	Candy, M&M's Chocolate
-4.5	1	wt oz	Chocolate, Semi-Sweet
-4.5	2	Tbls	Frosting, Chocolate
-5.0	2	tsp	Syrup, Cane
-5.0	2	Tbls	Syrup, Maple
-5.0	2	Tbls	Marmalade
-5.0	2	Tbls	Sugar, Brown
-5.0	8	fl oz	Drink Mix, Strawberry, Sweetened, Kool-Aid
-5.0	2	Tbls	Syrup, Corn

Nutripoints	Serving Size		Food Name—Sugars
-5.0	2	Tbls	Sauce, Chocolate
-5.0	2	pieces	Frozen Dessert, Popsicle
-5.0	2	Tbls	Sauce, Butterscotch, Smucker's
-5.0	12	fl oz	Soft Drink, Ginger Ale
-5.0	2	Tbls	Sugar, Raw
-5.0	12	fl oz	Soft Drink, w/o Caffeine
-5.5	2	Tbls	Sugar, Cinnamon
-5.5	1	wt oz	Fudge, Chocolate
-5.5	1/2	cup	Mousse, Chocolate
-5.5	12	fl oz	Soft Drink, Lemon Lime, w/o Caffeine
-5.5	4	pieces	Marshmallows, Jet-Puffed (large), Kraft
-5.5	1	cup	Dairy Queen Mr. Misty Kiss (1/2 Cup)
-5.5	8	fl oz	Sports Drink, Gatorade Endurance Hydration Formula (*)
-5.5	1	fl oz	Syrup, Original, Aunt Jemima
-5.5	2	Tbls	Honey
-5.5	28	pieces	Candy, Gum Drop, Small
-5.5	2	Tbls	Topping, Marshmallow Cream
-5.5	12	fl oz	Tonic Water, Sweetened
-5.5	12	fl oz	Soft Drink, 7-Up
-5.5	12	fl oz	Soft Drink, Cream Soda
-5.5	12	fl oz	Soft Drink, Dr. Pepper
-5.5	1/2	cup	Dairy Queen Mr. Misty - Medium (1 Cup)
-5.5	8	fl oz	Quinine Water
-5.5	15	pieces	Jelly Beans
-5.5	3	Tbls	Sugar, Maple
-5.5	4	pieces	Candy, Marshmallow (large)
-5.5	1	wt oz	Candy, Taffy, Plain
-5.5	4	Tbls	Sugar, White Confectioner's
-6.0	5	pieces	Gum, Bubble, Original, Hubba Bubba
-6.0	1	wt oz	Candy, Chocolate Chips
-6.0	10	pieces	Candy, Spear O Mint, Life Savers
-6.0	10	pieces	Candy, Wild Cherry, Life Savers
-6.0	2	tsp	Syrup, Butter Blends
-6.0	1	wt oz	Candy, Hard
-6.0	2	Tbls	Sugar, White
-6.0	12	fl oz	Soft Drink, Coke w/Caffeine
-6.0	1	fl oz	Syrup, Butterlite, Aunt Jemima
-6.0	12	fl oz	Root Beer
-6.5	8	fl oz	Iced Tea Mix, Sugar & Lemonade Flavor, Nestea
-6.5	12	fl oz	Soft Drink, Mountain Dew
-6.5	2	cups	Gatorade
-7.0	12	fl oz	Soft Drink, w/Caffeine
-7.5	8	fl oz	Tea Mix, Iced, Lipton

ALCOHOL GROUP

Nutripoints	Serving Size		Food Name—Alcohol
5.0	12	fl oz	Beer, Alcohol-Free, Clark's
4.0	12	fl oz	Beer, Near
1.0	12	fl oz	Beer, Nonalcoholic
-5.5	12	fl oz	Beer, Light
-7.5	3	fl oz	Pina Colada
-8.0	12	fl oz	Beer
-8.5	1.5	fl oz	Cordials/liqueurs
-8.5	2	fl oz	Grasshopper
-9.0	8	fl oz	Wine Cooler
-9.5	2	fl oz	Gold Cadillac
-9.5	8	fl oz	Screwdriver
-10.0	6	fl oz	Tequila Sunrise
-10.5	6	fl oz	Rum and Carbonated Beverage
-11.0	6	fl oz	Bloody Mary
-11.0	8	fl oz	Gin and Tonic
-11.5	2	fl oz	Mai Tai
-12.0	3	fl oz	Alexander
-12.5	2	fl oz	Stinger
-12.5	3	fl oz	Rum, Hot Buttered
-13.0	2	fl oz	Black Russian
-13.0	4	fl oz	Wine, Sweet
-13.0	2	fl oz	White Russian
-13.0	2	fl oz	Bacardi
-13.5	6	fl oz	Singapore Sling
-13.5	6	fl oz	Champagne
-13.5	3	fl oz	Manhattan
-13.5	3	fl oz	Margarita
-14.0	6	fl oz	Wine, Table
-14.0	8	fl oz	Tom Collins
-14.0	6	fl oz	Wine, Light
-14.5	6	fl oz	Wine Spritzer
-14.5	3	fl oz	Daiquiri
-14.5	6	fl oz	Wine, Chinese
-14.5	8	fl oz	Slow Gin Fizz

Nutripoints	Serving Size		Food Name—Alcohol
-15.0	2	fl oz	Mint Julep
-15.5	2	fl oz	Old Fashioned
-15.5	6	fl oz	Gin Rickey
-15.5	3	fl oz	Martini
-16.5	2	fl oz	Vodka
-16.5	2	fl oz	Whiskey
-16.5	2	fl oz	Rum
-17.0	6	fl oz	Bourbon or Scotch w/Soda
-17.0	2	fl oz	Alcohol, 68 Proof
-17.0	3	fl oz	Brandy
-17.5	2	fl oz	Gin
-19.0	3	fl oz	Whiskey Sour

CONDIMENT GROUP

Nutripoints	Serving Size		Food Name—Condiments
4.0	1/4	cup	Sauce, Picante
3.5	1	cup	Soup, Chicken Broth, Low Sodium, Campbell's
3.0	2	wt oz	Wendy's Picante Sauce
2.5	1	Tbls	Peppers, Green, Hot Chili
2.5	1/4	lemon	Lemon
2.5	1	tsp	Paprika
2.0	1	Tbls	Taco Bell Salsa
2.0	1	tsp	Chili Powder
1.5	1	Tbls	Sauce, Steak
1.5	1	tsp	Parsley, Dried
1.5	1	tsp	Pepper, Cayenne/Red
1.0	2	pieces	Onion, Green
1.0	2	Tbls	Taco Bell Pico de Gallo
1.0	1	tsp	Chives, Raw
1.0	2	Tbls	Dressing, Lite, Zero, Nutripoint Recipe
1.0	1	tsp	Sauce, Worcestershire
1.0	1	tsp	Cinnamon
1.0	1	tsp	Oregano
1.0	1	Tbls	Juice, Lemon, ReaLemon
1.0	1	Tbls	Sauce, Chili
1.0	1	Tbls	Juice, Lemon
1.0	1/4	cup	Endive, Raw
1.0	1/4	lime	Lime
0.5	1	tsp	Marjoram
0.5	1	tsp	Celery Seed
0.5	1	tsp	Basil
0.5	1	tsp	Seasoning, Poultry
0.5	1	tsp	Turmeric
0.5	1	tsp	Garlic Powder
0.5	1	tsp	Curry Powder
0.5	1	tsp	Thyme
0.5	2	Tbls	Ketchup, Low Sodium, Heinz
0.5	1	tsp	Ginger
0.5	1	tsp	Chili Seasoning Mix, McCormick's
0.5	1	tsp	Dill Weed

Nutripoints	Serving Size		Food Name—Condiments
0.5	1	Tbls	Mayonnaise, Reduced Cal, Light N' Lively
0.5	1	tsp	Bouillon, Chicken, Low-Sodium, Lite-Line, Borden
0.5	1	tsp	Pepper, Black
0.5	1	tsp	Caraway Seed
0.5	1	tsp	Sage
0.5	1	tsp	Bay Leaves
0.5	1	Tbls	Juice, Lime
0.5	1	tsp	Cloves
0.5	1	tsp	Tarragon
0.5	1	tsp	Rosemary
0.5	1	Tbls	Dressing, Mustard, Spicy, Nutripoint Recipe
0.5	1	tsp	Mustard, Dry
0.5	1	piece	Pepper, Jalapeno
0.5	1	tsp	Allspice, Ground
0.5	1	tsp	Onion Powder
0.5	1	piece	Garlic, Raw
0.5	1/2	cup	Coriander, Raw
0.0	1	Tbls	Sauce, BBQ
0.0	1	Tbls	McDonald's Barbeque Sauce
0.0	1	tsp	Taco Bell Taco Hot Sauce
0.0	2	Tbls	Sandwich, Manwich, Original, Hunts
0.0	1	Tbls	Vinegar
0.0	1	tsp	Taco Bell Taco Sauce
0.0	1	cup	Broth, Beef
0.0	1	tsp	Vanilla Extract
0.0	1	Tbls	McDonald's Oriental Dressing
0.0	1	Tbls	McDonald's Lite Vinaigrette Dressing
0.0	1	tsp	Salt
0.0	1	tsp	Salt, Iodized, Morton
0.0	1	tsp	Salt, Lite
0.0	1	tsp	Mustard
0.0	1	cup	Broth, Chicken
0.0	1	Tbls	Horseradish
0.0	1	cup	Broth, No-Chicken Organic, Imagine Foods
0.0	1	Tbls	Seasoning, Shake 'n Bake Original Chick
0.0	1	cup	Broth, Chicken, Organic Free Range, Imagine Foods
0.0	1	Tbls	McDonald's Sweet & Sour Sauce
0.0	1	tsp	Nutmeg

Nutripoints	Serving Size		Food Name—Condiments
0.0	2	Tbls	Sauce, Juniper Berry, Nutripoint Recipe
0.0	1	tsp	Sauce, Soy
-0.5	1/3	gram	Oil, Pam Spray
-0.5	1	Tbls	McDonald's Hot Mustard Sauce
-0.5	2	Tbls	Ketchup, Heinz
-0.5	1	Tbls	Mustard, Bold 'n Spice, French's
-0.5	1	Tbls	Sauce, Teriyaki
-0.5	2	Tbls	Dressing, Ranch, Free, Kraft
-0.5	1	Tbls	Mustard, Yellow, Prepared, French's
-0.5	1	tsp	Sauce, Soy, Kikkoman
-0.5	1	Tbls	Mustard, w/Horseradish, French's
-0.5	1	Tbls	Dressing, Italian, Light, Bernstein's
-0.5	1	Tbls	Sauce, BBQ, All-Natural Original Flavor, Hunts
-0.5	2	Tbls	Dressing, Italian, Free, Kraft
-0.5	2	Tbls	Butter Mix, Imitation, Butter Buds

-1.0	2	Tbls	Dressing, French, Free, Kraft
-1.0	1	wt oz	Pickles, Sweet Butter Chips, Vlasic
-1.0	1	Tbls	Seasoning, Shake 'n Bake for Pork
-1.0	2	Tbls	Dressing, Ranch, Take Heart, Hidden Valley
-1.0	1	Tbls	Sauce, BBQ, Hickory Smoke Flavor, Open Pit
-1.0	1	Tbls	Sauce, Heinz 57
-1.5	1	Tbls	Sauce, BBQ, All-Natural Hot & Zesty, Hunts
-1.5	1	Tbls	Sauce, BBQ, Onion Bits, Kraft
-1.5	2	Tbls	Taco Bell Jalapeno Peppers
-1.5	1	Tbls	Sauce, BBQ, Original Flavor, Open Pit
-1.5	1	Tbls	Sauce, Sweet and Sour
-2.0	1	tsp	Bouillon, Beef, Wyler's, Borden
-2.0	1	cup	Bouillon, Chicken, Wyler's, Borden
-2.5	1	Tbls	Sauce, BBQ, Kraft

MISCELLANEOUS GROUP

Nutripoints	Serving Size		Food Name--Miscellaneous
14.5	3	wt oz	Chlorella (powder or w/water -- standard quantity is for powder)
5.5	6	fl oz	Postum
4.5	1	packet	Yeast, Dry Active
3.5	1	Tbls	Yeast, Brewers
2.0	1	Tbls	Protein Powder
2.0	8	fl oz	Drink Mix, Grape, Sugar-Free, Kool-Aid
2.0	2	bar	Frozen Dessert, Fudgesicle, Sugar-Free, Good Humor
2.0	8	fl oz	Fruit Drink Mix, Crystal Light (all flavors)
1.5	8	fl oz	Drink Mix, Tropical Punch, Sugar Free, Kool-Aid
1.0	8	fl oz	Drink Mix, Orange, Sugar Free, Crystal Light
1.0	8	fl oz	Lemonade Mix, Sugar Free, Country Time
1.0	8	fl oz	Fruit Drink Mix, Wild Grape, Sugar Free, Wyler's
1.0	1	Tbls	Carob Powder
0.5	2	Tbls	Creamer, Non-Dairy, Fat-Free, Mocha Mix
0.5	2	bars	Frozen Dessert, Popsicle, Sugar-Free, Good Humor
0.5	1	cup	Coffee, Decaffeinated
0.5	1	tsp	Baking Powder
0.5	6	fl oz	Tea, Herb
0.5	1	cup	Consommé
0.5	1	Tbls	Cocoa Powder
0.5	0.25	wt oz	Yeast, Active Dry, Fleischmann's
0.0	1	cup	Tea, Decaffeinated
0.0	1	Tbls	Cornstarch
0.0	12	fl oz	Soft Drink, Diet, w/o Caffeine
0.0	1	tsp	Baking Soda
0.0	6	fl oz	Club Soda
0.0	8	fl oz	Perrier Mineral Water
-1.0	1	piece	Bouillon Cube
-1.0	1	cup	Soup, Wonton
-1.5	1	serving	Soup Mix, Chicken Noodle, Dehydrated
-1.5	2	Tbls	Soup Mix, Onion, Dehydrated
-2.0	8	fl oz	Sports Drink, All Sport
-2.0	8	fl oz	Tea, Arizona Herbal w/Honey
-2.5	8	fl oz	Tea Mix, Iced, Lemon, Sugar-Free, Lipton
-3.0	1	cup	Tea, American Black
-3.0	1	Tbls	Gravy, Dehydrated
-3.0	12	fl oz	Soft Drink, Diet, w/Caffeine
-4.0	1	cup	Coffee
-4.0	12	fl oz	Coffee, Caffe' Vanilla, Frappuccino Light, Starbuck's

Nutripoints	Serving Size		Food Name--Miscellaneous
-4.5	9.5	fl oz	Coffee, Frappuccino, Starbuck's
-5.0	12	fl oz	Coffee, Caffe' Latte, Starbuck's
-5.0	12	fl oz	Coffee, Caffe' Mocha, Starbuck's
-5.0	12	fl oz	Coffee, Cappuccino, Starbuck's
-5.5	12	fl oz	Coffee, Mocha Frappuccino, Starbuck's
-10.0	1	tsp	Coffee, International
-11.5	1	Tbls	Caviar

ALPHABETICAL RATINGS

Food Name	Nutripoints	Serving Size		Nutrigroup
Abalone	**6.5**	3.5	wt oz	Meat/Fish/Poultry
Abalone, Floured, Fried	**4.5**	3	wt oz	Meat/Fish/Poultry
Alcohol, 68 Proof	**-17.0**	2	fl oz	Alcohol
Alexander	**-12.0**	3	fl oz	Alcohol
Alfalfa Sprouts, Arrowhead Mills	**13.0**	1	cup	Vegetable
Alfalfa Sprouts, Raw	**17.5**	2	cups	Vegetable
Allspice, Ground	**0.5**	1	tsp	Condiment
Almond Butter, Salted	**0.5**	1	Tbls	Legume/Nut/Seed
Almonds, Blanched, Blue Diamond	**0.5**	1	wt oz	Legume/Nut/Seed
Almonds, Chocolate-Covered	**-1.0**	6	pieces	Legume/Nut/Seed
Almonds, Oil Roasted, Salted	**0.5**	12	nuts	Legume/Nut/Seed
Almonds, Raw	**1.5**	18	nuts	Legume/Nut/Seed
Almonds, Sugar-Coated	**-1.5**	6	pieces	Legume/Nut/Seed
Amaranth, Dry, Arrowhead Mills	**5.0**	1	wt oz	Grain
Anchovy, Canned	**4.0**	3	wt oz	Meat/Fish/Poultry
Apple Butter	**2.0**	2	Tbls	Fruit
Apple Crisp	**-1.0**	1/4	cup	Fruit
Apple, Fresh	**4.5**	1	whole	Fruit
Apples, Dried, Chunks, Sun-Maid	**2.5**	2	wt oz	Fruit
Apples, Escalloped, Frozen, Stouffer's	**-0.5**	1/2	portion	Fruit
Apples, Glazed, Raspberry Sauce, Frozen, Budget Gourmet	**10.5**	1/2	portion	Fruit
Applesauce, Natural Style, Mott's	**3.0**	1/2	cup	Fruit
Applesauce, No Sugar	**3.5**	1/2	cup	Fruit
Applesauce, Nutripoint Recipe	**3.0**	1/2	cup	Fruit
Applesauce, Unsweetened, Musselman	**2.0**	1/2	cup	Fruit
Applesauce, w/Sugar	**-0.5**	1/2	cup	Fruit
Apricot Nectar, Canned	**4.5**	4	fl oz	Fruit
Apricot, Fresh	**13.5**	3	whole	Fruit
Apricots, Canned In Heavy Syrup	**2.5**	1/2	cup	Fruit
Apricots, Canned, Unsweetened	**11.0**	1/2	cup	Fruit
Apricots, Dried	**11.0**	6	pieces	Fruit
Apricots, Dried, Del Monte	**7.5**	6	pieces	Fruit
Apricots, Dried, Sun-Maid	**8.0**	6	pieces	Fruit
Arby's Beef 'n Cheddar Sandwich	**0.0**	1/2	serving	Meat/Fish/Poultry

Food Name—Alphabetical	Nutripoints	Serving Size		Nutrigroup
Arby's Junior Roast Beef Sandwich	**0.5**	1	serving	Meat/Fish/Poultry
Arby's King Roast Beef Sandwich	**0.5**	1/2	serving	Meat/Fish/Poultry
Arby's Regular Roast Beef Sandwich	**0.5**	1/2	serving	Meat/Fish/Poultry
Arby's Super Roast Beef Sandwich	**1.0**	1/2	serving	Meat/Fish/Poultry
Artichoke Hearts, Marinated	**3.0**	1/4	cup	Vegetable
Artichoke, Cooked	**12.5**	1	whole	Vegetable
Asparagus, 50-Percent Less Salt, Canned, Green Giant	**14.5**	1	cup	Vegetable
Asparagus, Canned	**32.5**	8	stalks	Vegetable
Asparagus, Cuts, Canned, Green Giant	**14.0**	1/2	cup	Vegetable
Asparagus, Fresh	**44.0**	8	stalks	Vegetable
Asparagus, Frozen, Cooked	**27.0**	8	stalks	Vegetable
Asparagus, Marinated, Nutripoint Recipe	**38.5**	8	stalks	Vegetable
Avocado, California	**2.0**	1/4	fruit	Fruit
Avocado, Florida	**4.0**	1/4	fruit	Fruit
Bacardi	**-13.0**	2	fl oz	Alcohol
Bacon Bits, Imitation	**1.5**	1/4	cup	Meat/Fish/Poultry
Bacon Strips, Veggie, Morningstar Farms	**4.5**	4	slices	Legume/Nut/Seed
Bacon, Bryan	**-2.0**	3	slices	Meat/Fish/Poultry
Bacon, Canadian	**1.5**	3	slices	Meat/Fish/Poultry
Bacon, Canadian Style, Oscar Mayer	**4.5**	3	slices	Meat/Fish/Poultry
Bacon, Fried	**-1.0**	3	slices	Meat/Fish/Poultry
Bacon, Low-Salt, Oscar Mayer	**-1.0**	3	slices	Meat/Fish/Poultry
Bacon, Low-Sodium, No Sugar, Bryan	**-1.5**	3	slices	Meat/Fish/Poultry
Bacon, Oscar Mayer	**-2.0**	3	slices	Meat/Fish/Poultry
Bacon, Premium Sizzlean, Swift	**-3.5**	3	slices	Meat/Fish/Poultry
Bacon, Sliced, Farmland	**-2.5**	3	slices	Meat/Fish/Poultry
Bacon, Veggie Canadian, Yyves	**8.5**	3	slices	Legume/Nut/Seed
Bacon, West Virginia Brand, Hygrade's	**-2.5**	3	slices	Meat/Fish/Poultry
Bagel	**2.0**	1	whole	Grain
Bagel, Plain, Lender's	**2.0**	2	whole	Grain
Bagel, Pumpernickel	**3.5**	1	whole	Grain
Bagel, Raisin 'n Honey, Lender's	**2.0**	1	whole	Grain
Bagel, Whole Grain, Natural Ovens Bakery	**5.5**	1	bagel	Grain
Bagel, Whole Wheat	**4.0**	1	whole	Grain
Baking Powder	**0.5**	1	tsp	Miscellaneous
Baking Soda	**0.0**	1	tsp	Miscellaneous
Bamboo Shoots, Canned	**16.5**	1	cup	Vegetable
Bamboo Shoots, Raw	**17.0**	1/2	cup	Vegetable
Banana	**7.5**	1/2	fruit	Fruit
Banana Flambé, Nutripoint Recipe	**2.5**	1/3	cup	Milk/Dairy
Banana Gladje, Nutripoint Recipe	**6.0**	1/3	cup	Fruit
Banana Split	**-1.5**	1/4	serving	Fruit

Food Name—Alphabetical	Nutripoints	Serving Size		Nutrigroup
Barley, Uncooked	**4.0**	1/4	cup	Grain
Barracuda, Baked/Broiled	**1.5**	3	wt oz	Meat/Fish/Poultry
Barracuda, Breaded/Floured, Fried	**1.0**	3	wt oz	Meat/Fish/Poultry
Basil	**0.5**	1	tsp	Condiment
Bass, Freshwater, Baked	**7.0**	6	wt oz	Meat/Fish/Poultry
Bay Leaves	**0.5**	1	tsp	Condiment
Bean Sprouts, Mung, Arrowhead Mills	**10.5**	2	cups	Legume/Nut/Seed
Bean Sprouts, Mung, Fresh	**18.0**	2	cups	Legume/Nut/Seed
Beans, Adzuki, Dry, Arrowhead Mills	**5.5**	1	wt oz	Legume/Nut/Seed
Beans, Baked, Barbecue, B&M	**0.5**	1/2	cup	Legume/Nut/Seed
Beans, Baked, w/Tomato Sauce	**7.5**	1/2	cup	Legume/Nut/Seed
Beans, Boston Baked	**3.5**	1/2	cup	Legume/Nut/Seed
Beans, Chili, Loma Linda	**3.0**	1/2	cup	Legume/Nut/Seed
Beans, Cooked	**8.5**	3/4	cup	Legume/Nut/Seed
Beans, Garbanzo, Cooked	**8.0**	1/2	cup	Legume/Nut/Seed
Beans, Green 50-Percent Less Salt, Canned, Green Giant	**8.0**	1	cup	Vegetable
Beans, Green Cooked	**24.5**	1	cup	Vegetable
Beans, Green, Cut, Frozen, Birds Eye (Large Portion)	**15.5**	1	cup	Vegetable
Beans, Green, Cut, Frozen, Birds Eye (Small Portion)	**12.5**	1/2	cup	Vegetable
Beans, Green, Cut, No Salt Added, Canned, Del Monte	**13.5**	1	cup	Vegetable
Beans, Green, French Cut, In Butter, Green Giant	**3.0**	1/2	cup	Vegetable
Beans, Green, French Style Cut, Canned, Green Giant	**3.5**	1	cup	Vegetable
Beans, Green, Kitchen Cut, Canned, Green Giant	**4.5**	1	cup	Vegetable
Beans, Green, Whole, Canned, Del Monte	**13.0**	1	cup	Vegetable
Beans, Home Style, Campbell's	**1.0**	1/2	cup	Legume/Nut/Seed
Beans, Kidney, Best Light, Canned, Bush's	**4.0**	1/2	cup	Legume/Nut/Seed
Beans, Kidney, Cooked	**8.5**	1/2	cup	Legume/Nut/Seed
Beans, Lima, Baby, w/Butter, Frozen, Green Giant	**2.0**	1/2	cup	Legume/Nut/Seed
Beans, Lima, Cooked	**9.5**	3/4	cup	Legume/Nut/Seed
Beans, Navy, Cooked	**13.5**	1	cup	Legume/Nut/Seed
Beans, Pinto, Cooked	**6.5**	1/2	cup	Legume/Nut/Seed
Beans, Red w/Southwest Cornbread, Organic, Fzn, Moosewood	**1.5**	1/2	serving	Legume/Nut/Seed
Beans, Refried	**2.0**	1/2	cup	Legume/Nut/Seed
Beans, Refried, Old El Paso	**3.5**	1	cup	Legume/Nut/Seed

Food Name—Alphabetical	Nutripoints	Serving Size		Nutrigroup
Beans, Refried, w/Sausage, Old El Paso	**-1.0**	1/2	cup	Legume/Nut/Seed
Beans, Vegetarian Style, Van Camp's	**2.5**	1/2	cup	Legume/Nut/Seed
Beans, w/Frankfurters Dinner, Frozen, Morton	**2.0**	1/2	portion	Legume/Nut/Seed
Beans, w/Pork	**3.0**	1/2	cup	Legume/Nut/Seed
Beans, w/Pork In Tomato Sauce, Campbell's	**1.5**	1/2	cup	Legume/Nut/Seed
Beans, w/Pork, Showboat, Bush's	**1.5**	1/2	cup	Legume/Nut/Seed
Beans, w/Pork, Van Camp's	**2.0**	1/2	cup	Legume/Nut/Seed
Beans, Yellow Snap, Cooked	**13.5**	1/2	cup	Vegetable
Beef & Broccoli, Uncle Ben's Pasta Bowl	**1.0**	1/2	serving	Grain
Beef Brisket, Lean, Braised	**2.0**	3	wt oz	Meat/Fish/Poultry
Beef Chuck Roast, Lean, Braised	**3.5**	3	wt oz	Meat/Fish/Poultry
Beef Chuck Roast, Medium Fat, Baked	**0.5**	2	wt oz	Meat/Fish/Poultry
Beef Flank Steak, Lean, Broiled	**4.0**	3	wt oz	Meat/Fish/Poultry
Beef Flank Steak, Medium Fat, Choice, Broiled	**1.5**	3	wt oz	Meat/Fish/Poultry
Beef Hart, Braised	**4.0**	3	wt oz	Meat/Fish/Poultry
Beef Jardine, ZonePerfect	**0.5**	1/2	serving	Meat/Fish/Poultry
Beef Jerky	**2.5**	3	pieces	Meat/Fish/Poultry
Beef Liver, Fried	**7.0**	3	wt oz	Meat/Fish/Poultry
Beef Meatloaf Dinner, Frozen, Morton	**0.5**	1/2	portion	Meat/Fish/Poultry
Beef Oriental Pepper Steak, Frozen, Healthy Choice	**1.5**	1	portion	Meat/Fish/Poultry
Beef Oriental, w/Vegetables and Rice, Frozen, Stouffer's	**0.0**	1	portion	Meat/Fish/Poultry
Beef Pepper Oriental, Frozen, Chun King	**3.0**	1/2	portion	Meat/Fish/Poultry
Beef Pie, Frozen, Morton	**-0.5**	1/2	portion	Meat/Fish/Poultry
Beef Pie, Frozen, Stouffer's	**-0.5**	1/2	portion	Meat/Fish/Poultry
Beef Porterhouse Steak, Lean, Broiled	**2.5**	3	wt oz	Meat/Fish/Poultry
Beef Porterhouse Steak, Med. Fat, Choice, Broiled	**0.0**	3	wt oz	Meat/Fish/Poultry
Beef Pot Pie	**0.5**	1/2	pie	Meat/Fish/Poultry
Beef Pot Pie, Frozen, Swanson	**-1.5**	1/2	pie	Meat/Fish/Poultry
Beef Pot Roast, Yankee, Frozen, Budget Gourmet	**0.0**	1/2	portion	Meat/Fish/Poultry
Beef Prime Rib, Baked	**-2.5**	2	wt oz	Meat/Fish/Poultry
Beef Rib Eye, Lean, Broiled	**2.5**	3	wt oz	Meat/Fish/Poultry
Beef Ribs, Baked	**2.0**	3	wt oz	Meat/Fish/Poultry
Beef Round Steak, Lean, Broiled	**4.0**	3	wt oz	Meat/Fish/Poultry
Beef Round Steak, Medium Fat, Broiled	**2.0**	3	wt oz	Meat/Fish/Poultry
Beef Rump Roast, Baked	**0.5**	2	wt oz	Meat/Fish/Poultry
Beef Salisbury Steak Dinner, Frozen, Morton	**0.5**	1/2	portion	Meat/Fish/Poultry
Beef Salisbury Steak, Frozen Dinner	**2.0**	1/2	portion	Meat/Fish/Poultry
Beef Salisbury Steak, Frozen, Le Menu	**0.0**	1	portion	Meat/Fish/Poultry
Beef Salisbury Steak, Homestyle, Frozen, Swanson	**-2.5**	1/2	portion	Meat/Fish/Poultry
Beef Salisbury Steak, In Gravy, Frozen, Stouffer's	**-1.0**	1	portion	Meat/Fish/Poultry

Food Name—Alphabetical	Nutripoints	Serving Size		Nutrigroup
Beef Salisbury Steak, Romana, Frozen, Weight Watchers	**0.0**	1/2	portion	Meat/Fish/Poultry
Beef Salisbury Steak, w/Italian Sauce, Frozen, Stouffer's	**-1.0**	1	portion	Meat/Fish/Poultry
Beef Salisbury Steak, w/Potatoes, Frozen, Morton	**0.0**	1	portion	Meat/Fish/Poultry
Beef Short Ribs, Lean, Braised	**1.0**	3	wt oz	Meat/Fish/Poultry
Beef Short Ribs, Medium Fat, Braised	**-1.0**	2	wt oz	Meat/Fish/Poultry
Beef Sirloin Salisbury Steak, Frozen, Budget Gourmet	**-0.5**	1/2	portion	Meat/Fish/Poultry
Beef Sirloin Salisbury Steak, Slim, Fzn, Budget Gourmet	**1.0**	1	portion	Meat/Fish/Poultry
Beef Sirloin Steak, Broiled	**-2.0**	2	wt oz	Meat/Fish/Poultry
Beef Sirloin Tips w/Country Style Vegetables, Fzn, Budget Gourmet	**-1.0**	1/2	portion	Meat/Fish/Poultry
Beef Sirloin Tips, Frozen, Healthy Choice	**3.0**	1	portion	Meat/Fish/Poultry
Beef Sirloin Tips, w/Burgundy Sauce, Fzn, Budget Gourmet	**0.5**	1/2	portion	Meat/Fish/Poultry
Beef Sirloin, w/Herb Sauce, Slim, Fzn, Budget Gourmet	**1.0**	1	portion	Meat/Fish/Poultry
Beef Steak, Chopped, Fzn, Weight Watchers	**1.5**	1/2	portion	Meat/Fish/Poultry
Beef Stew	**3.5**	1	cup	Meat/Fish/Poultry
Beef Stew, Frozen, Stouffer's	**-0.5**	1	portion	Meat/Fish/Poultry
Beef Stroganoff	**0.0**	1/2	cup	Meat/Fish/Poultry
Beef Stroganoff, Frozen, Weight Watchers	**-1.0**	1/2	portion	Meat/Fish/Poultry
Beef Stroganoff, Fzn, Healthy Choice	**-1.0**	1	serving	Meat/Fish/Poultry
Beef Stroganoff, Slim, Frozen, Budget Gourmet	**0.0**	1	portion	Meat/Fish/Poultry
Beef Stroganoff, w/Parsley Noodles, Fzn, Stouffer's	**-1.5**	1/2	portion	Meat/Fish/Poultry
Beef Swiss Steak	**1.0**	3	wt oz	Meat/Fish/Poultry
Beef Szechuan, Frozen, Chun King	**2.0**	1/2	portion	Meat/Fish/Poultry
Beef Szechwan, w/Noodles and Vegetables, Fzn, Stouffer's	**0.0**	1	portion	Meat/Fish/Poultry
Beef T-Bone Steak, Lean, Choice, Broiled	**2.5**	3	wt oz	Meat/Fish/Poultry
Beef T-Bone Steak, Medium Fat, Broiled	**-0.5**	3	wt oz	Meat/Fish/Poultry
Beef Tenderloin Fillet, Lean, Broiled	**3.5**	3	wt oz	Meat/Fish/Poultry
Beef Tenderloin, Medium Fat, Broiled	**1.0**	3	wt oz	Meat/Fish/Poultry
Beef Teriyaki, Frozen, Chun King	**5.0**	1/2	portion	Meat/Fish/Poultry
Beef Tongue, Simmered	**-0.5**	3	wt oz	Meat/Fish/Poultry
Beef Top Loin, Lean, Broiled	**4.0**	3	wt oz	Meat/Fish/Poultry
Beef Top Loin, Medium Fat, Broiled	**0.5**	3	wt oz	Meat/Fish/Poultry
Beef w/Broccoli & Asian Style Noodles, Fzn, South Beach Diet	**3.5**	1	serving	Meat/Fish/Poultry
Beef w/Cheesy Broccoli, Fzn, South Beach Diet	**3.5**	1	serving	Meat/Fish/Poultry
Beef, Barbecue, Sandwich, w/Bun	**-2.5**	1/2	serving	Meat/Fish/Poultry

Food Name—Alphabetical	Nutripoints	Serving Size		Nutrigroup
Beef, Breakfast Strip, Lean 'n Tasty, Oscar Mayer	**-2.5**	3	pieces	Meat/Fish/Poultry
Beef, Carne Asada, Nutripoint Recipe	**7.0**	1	serving	Meat/Fish/Poultry
Beef, Creamed Chipped	**-1.0**	1/2	cup	Meat/Fish/Poultry
Beef, Frozen Dinner	**3.5**	1/2	portion	Meat/Fish/Poultry
Beef, Land O' Frost	**-2.0**	4	wt oz	Meat/Fish/Poultry
Beef, Light, Rich Meat Service	**0.5**	4	wt oz	Meat/Fish/Poultry
Beef, Macaroni and Tomato Sauce	**3.0**	1	cup	Meat/Fish/Poultry
Beef, Roast, Slices, Frozen, Loma Linda	**6.5**	2	wt oz	Legume/Nut/Seed
Beef, Roasted Sirloin, Michelina's Lean Gourmet	**-0.5**	1	serving	Meat/Fish/Poultry
Beef, Sliced, Frozen, Morton	**4.0**	1	serving	Meat/Fish/Poultry
Beef, Sliced, w/Gravy, Frozen, Morton	**1.5**	1	portion	Meat/Fish/Poultry
Beef, Smoked, Sliced, Buddig	**-2.0**	3	wt oz	Meat/Fish/Poultry
Beefaroni	**2.0**	3/4	cup	Meat/Fish/Poultry
Beer	**-8.0**	12	fl oz	Alcohol
Beer, Alcohol-Free, Clark's	**5.0**	12	fl oz	Alcohol
Beer, Light	**-5.5**	12	fl oz	Alcohol
Beer, Near	**4.0**	12	fl oz	Alcohol
Beer, Nonalcoholic	**1.0**	12	fl oz	Alcohol
Beet Greens, Cooked	**56.5**	1	cup	Vegetable
Beets, Canned, Cooked	**7.5**	1/2	cup	Vegetable
Beets, Cooked	**11.0**	1/2	cup	Vegetable
Beets, Pickled, Canned	**3.5**	1/2	cup	Vegetable
Berries, Fresh, Nutripoint Recipe	**13.0**	1	cup	Fruit
Berries, Fresh, w/Zabaglione Sauce	**-3.5**	1/4	cup	Fruit
Bilberry, Raw	**10.0**	3	wt oz	Fruit
Biscuit	**1.0**	1	biscuit	Grain
Biscuit (mix), Multigrain, Arrowhead Mills	**3.5**	1	biscuit	Grain
Biscuit, Butter, Pillsbury	**2.0**	2	biscuits	Grain
Biscuit, Buttermilk, Big Country, Pillsbury	**1.0**	2	biscuits	Grain
Biscuit, Buttermilk, From Mix	**1.0**	1	biscuit	Grain
Biscuit, Country Style, Pillsbury	**1.5**	2	biscuits	Grain
Biscuit, Extra Rich Buttermilk, Hungry Jack	**3.0**	2	biscuits	Grain
Biscuit, Flaky, Hungry Jack	**0.5**	2	biscuits	Grain
Biscuit, Uneeda	**1.5**	6	biscuits	Grain
Black Russian	**-13.0**	2	fl oz	Alcohol
Blackberries, Fresh	**13.0**	1/2	cup	Fruit
Blackberries, Frozen, Unsweetened	**7.5**	1/2	cup	Fruit
Blackberry Freeze, Nutripoint Recipe	**8.5**	3/4	cup	Fruit
Bloody Mary	**-11.0**	6	fl oz	Alcohol
Blueberries, Fresh	**7.0**	1/2	cup	Fruit
Blueberries, Frozen, Unsweetened	**4.5**	1/2	cup	Fruit
Bok Choy, Raw, Shredded	**72.5**	1	cup	Vegetable
Bologna Slices, Veggie, Yves	**8.0**	4	slices	Legume/Nut/Seed

Food Name—Alphabetical	Nutripoints	Serving Size		Nutrigroup
Bologna, Beef	**-3.5**	2	wt oz	Meat/Fish/Poultry
Bologna, Beef, Armour	**-4.0**	2	slices	Meat/Fish/Poultry
Bologna, Beef, Bryan	**-2.5**	2	slices	Meat/Fish/Poultry
Bologna, Beef, Oscar Mayer	**-3.5**	2	slices	Meat/Fish/Poultry
Bologna, Bryan	**-2.5**	2	slices	Meat/Fish/Poultry
Bologna, Eckrich	**-4.0**	2	slices	Meat/Fish/Poultry
Bologna, Garlic, Eckrich	**-3.5**	2	slices	Meat/Fish/Poultry
Bologna, Oscar Mayer	**-3.5**	2	slices	Meat/Fish/Poultry
Bologna, Pork	**0.5**	2	slices	Meat/Fish/Poultry
Bologna, Slices, Frozen, Loma Linda	**7.0**	2	wt oz	Legume/Nut/Seed
Bologna, Turkey	**-1.5**	2	wt oz	Meat/Fish/Poultry
Bologna, Turkey, Louis Rich	**-2.5**	2	slices	Meat/Fish/Poultry
Bologna, Vegetarian, Bolono, Worthington	**7.0**	3	slices	Legume/Nut/Seed
Bonito, Canned	**1.0**	3	wt oz	Meat/Fish/Poultry
Bouillon Cube	**-1.0**	1	cube	Miscellaneous
Bouillon, Beef, Wyler's, Borden	**-2.0**	1	tsp	Condiment
Bouillon, Chicken, Low-Sodium, Lite-Line, Borden	**0.5**	1	tsp	Condiment
Bouillon, Chicken, Wyler's, Borden	**-2.0**	1	cup	Condiment
Bourbon or Scotch w/Soda	**-17.0**	6	fl oz	Alcohol
Boysenberries, Frozen	**9.0**	1/2	cup	Fruit
BrainSustain Drink (Rice)	**20.0**	8	fl oz	Grain
Bran, Oat, Arrowhead Mills	**9.0**	1/3	cup	Grain
Bran, Rice	**9.0**	2	wt oz	Grain
Bran, Wheat	**26.5**	1/2	cup	Grain
Bran, Wheat, Toasted, Kretschmer	**27.5**	1	wt oz	Grain
Brandy	**-17.0**	3	fl oz	Alcohol
Bratwurst	**-1.0**	2	wt oz	Meat/Fish/Poultry
Braunschweiger	**4.0**	2	wt oz	Meat/Fish/Poultry
Brazil Nuts, Unsalted	**0.0**	6	nuts	Legume/Nut/Seed
Bread Crumbs	**2.0**	1/2	cup	Grain
Bread Crumbs, Plain, Progresso	**1.5**	1/2	cup	Grain
Bread, 100% Whole Wheat, Home Pride	**3.5**	2	slices	Grain
Bread, 100% Whole Wheat, Wonder	**4.0**	2	slices	Grain
Bread, 5 Bran, Home Pride	**5.0**	2	slices	Grain
Bread, 7 Grain, Home Pride	**3.0**	2	slices	Grain
Bread, Banana	**-0.5**	1	slice	Grain
Bread, Bran	**3.5**	2	slices	Grain
Bread, Bran'nola Multi-Bran, Oroweat	**2.5**	2	slices	Grain
Bread, Bran'nola Rice Bran, Oroweat	**3.0**	2	slices	Grain
Bread, Bran'nola, Oroweat	**3.5**	2	slices	Grain
Bread, Carrot, Nut, Pillsbury	**-2.0**	1	slice	Grain
Bread, Cracked Wheat	**4.5**	2	slices	Grain
Bread, Date, Pillsbury	**-1.5**	1	slice	Grain

Food Name—Alphabetical	Nutripoints	Serving Size		Nutrigroup
Bread, Diet 40 Cal/Slice	**5.5**	3	slices	Grain
Bread, Family Style Distinctive, Pepperidge Farm	**2.0**	2	cups	Grain
Bread, French	**3.0**	2	slices	Grain
Bread, Garlic	**0.0**	1	piece	Grain
Bread, Gluten	**1.5**	2	slices	Grain
Bread, Grape-Nuts, Oroweat	**3.0**	2	slices	Grain
Bread, Health Max, Natural Ovens Bakery	**6.5**	2	slices	Grain
Bread, Health Nut, Oroweat	**3.0**	1	slices	Grain
Bread, Hi-Fiber, Wonder	**6.5**	3	slices	Grain
Bread, Honey Nut and Oat Bran, Roman Meal	**3.5**	2	slices	Grain
Bread, Honey Wheat Berry, Arnold	**3.5**	2	slices	Grain
Bread, Honey Wheat Berry, Oroweat	**2.5**	2	slices	Grain
Bread, Honey Wheat Berry, Pepperidge Farm	**3.0**	2	slices	Grain
Bread, Hunger Filler Whole Grain, Natural Ovens Bakery	**10.5**	2	slices	Grain
Bread, Italian	**2.5**	2	slices	Grain
Bread, Less, Mrs. Baird's	**6.0**	3	slices	Grain
Bread, Light Bran & Oat, Oatmeal Goodness	**5.5**	3	slices	Grain
Bread, Low-Sodium	**3.5**	2	slices	Grain
Bread, Mixed Grain	**5.0**	2	slices	Grain
Bread, Oat Bran N' Honey, Light, Roman Meal	**5.5**	3	slices	Grain
Bread, Oat Bran, Honey, Earth Grains	**3.0**	2	slices	Grain
Bread, Oatmeal	**2.0**	2	slices	Grain
Bread, Oatmeal and Bran, Oatmeal Goodness	**3.5**	2	slices	Grain
Bread, Oatmeal and Sunflower Seeds, Oatmeal Goodness	**3.5**	2	slices	Grain
Bread, Oatmeal, Pepperidge Farm	**3.0**	2	slices	Grain
Bread, Oatnut, Oroweat	**2.5**	2	slices	Grain
Bread, Old-Fashioned Buttermilk, Country Hearth	**3.0**	2	slices	Grain
Bread, Original Bran'nola, Arnold	**3.5**	2	slices	Grain
Bread, Pita	**3.5**	1	piece	Grain
Bread, Pita, Whole Wheat	**4.0**	1	piece	Grain
Bread, Potato	**2.0**	2	slices	Grain
Bread, Protogen Protein, Thomas'	**3.5**	2	slices	Grain
Bread, Pumpernickel	**4.5**	2	slices	Grain
Bread, Pumpernickel, Arnold	**2.0**	2	slices	Grain
Bread, Raisin	**4.0**	2	slices	Grain
Bread, Roman Meal	**4.5**	2	slices	Grain
Bread, Rye, Family, Pepperidge Farm	**3.0**	2	slices	Grain
Bread, Rye, Jewish, Real Unseeded, Levy's	**2.5**	2	slices	Grain
Bread, Rye, Light, Earth Grains	**3.0**	2	slices	Grain
Bread, Sandwich, Salt-Free, Earth Grains	**3.5**	2	slices	Grain
Bread, Sourdough	**2.5**	2	slices	Grain

Food Name—Alphabetical	Nutripoints	Serving Size		Nutrigroup
Bread, Sprouted Wheat	**5.0**	2	slices	Grain
Bread, Sprouted Wheat, Pepperidge Farm	**3.0**	2	slices	Grain
Bread, Stuffing	**0.5**	1/2	cup	Grain
Bread, Triticale	**4.5**	2	slices	Grain
Bread, Wheat and Oatmeal, Oatmeal Goodness	**3.0**	2	slices	Grain
Bread, Wheat Berry, Home Pride	**3.0**	2	slices	Grain
Bread, Wheat Berry, Honey, Earth Grains	**4.0**	2	slices	Grain
Bread, Wheat Germ	**4.0**	2	slices	Grain
Bread, Wheat, Fresh Horizons	**5.0**	2	slices	Grain
Bread, Wheat, Lite 35, Earth Grains	**4.5**	2	slices	Grain
Bread, Wheat, Stone-Ground, Earth Grains	**3.5**	2	slices	Grain
Bread, White	**2.5**	2	slices	Grain
Bread, White, Brick Oven, Arnold	**3.0**	2	slices	Grain
Bread, White, Butter-Top, Home Pride	**3.0**	2	slices	Grain
Bread, White, Wonder	**2.5**	2	slices	Grain
Bread, Whole Rye	**4.0**	2	slices	Grain
Bread, Whole Wheat	**6.0**	2	slices	Grain
Bread, Whole Wheat, Brick Oven, Arnold	**2.5**	2	slices	Grain
Bread, Whole Wheat, Stone-Ground, Country Hearth	**4.5**	2	slices	Grain
Bread, Whole Wheat, Stone-Ground, the Sourdough	**6.0**	2	slices	Grain
Bread, Whole Wheat, Thin, Pepperidge Farm	**4.5**	2	slices	Grain
Breadsticks	**3.5**	6	pieces	Grain
Breadsticks, Garlic, Keebler	**1.0**	6	pieces	Grain
Breadsticks, Onion, Keebler	**2.0**	6	pieces	Grain
Breadsticks, Plain, Keebler	**2.5**	6	pieces	Grain
Breadsticks, Sesame, Keebler	**1.5**	6	pieces	Grain
Breakfast Bar	**2.0**	1	bar	Grain
Breakfast Bar, Atkins	**6.0**	1	bar	Legume/Nut/Seed
Breakfast Bar, Chocolate, Carnation	**4.5**	1	bar	Grain
Breakfast Bar, Honey Nut, Carnation	**4.5**	1	bar	Grain
Breakfast Bar, Slim-Fast Optima	**9.5**	1	bar	Grain
Broc/Caul/Car/97% Fat-Free Sauce, Fzn, Green Giant	**5.0**	2/3	cup	Vegetable
Broccoli Florets, Fzn, 365 Organic, Whole Foods	**23.5**	1 1/2	cups	Vegetable
Broccoli Spears, Frozen, Birds Eye	**46.0**	1/2	cup	Vegetable
Broccoli Spears, w/Butter Sauce, Fzn, Green Giant	**6.0**	1/2	cup	Vegetable
Broccoli w/Cheddar Cheese Sauce, Fzn, Stouffer's	**2.0**	1/2	portion	Vegetable
Broccoli, Baby Carrots, & Water Chestnuts, Fzn, Birds Eye	**31.0**	1/2	cup	Vegetable
Broccoli, Carrots, and Cauliflower, Frozen, Pictsweet	**36.0**	1	cup	Vegetable
Broccoli, Carrots, and Red Peppers, Frozen, Birds Eye	**17.0**	3/4	cup	Vegetable

Food Name—Alphabetical	Nutripoints	Serving Size		Nutrigroup
Broccoli, Cauliflower & Carrots w/Cheese Sauce, Fzn, Birds Eye	**13.0**	1/2	cup	Vegetable
Broccoli, Cauliflower & Carrots w/Cheese Sauce, Green Giant	**13.0**	1/2	cup	Vegetable
Broccoli, Cauliflower and Carrots, Frozen, Birds Eye	**30.5**	1	cup	Vegetable
Broccoli, Cauliflower and Carrots, Frozen, Green Giant	**33.0**	1	cup	Vegetable
Broccoli, Cauliflower and Red Peppers, Frozen, Birds Eye	**41.5**	1	cup	Vegetable
Broccoli, Cooked	**38.5**	1	cup	Vegetable
Broccoli, Corn and Red Peppers, Frozen, Birds Eye	**17.0**	1/2	cup	Vegetable
Broccoli, Fried, w/Breading	**1.5**	1/4	cup	Vegetable
Broccoli, Organic, Fzn, Cascadian Farm	**39.0**	1	cup	Vegetable
Broccoli, Raw	**53.0**	1	cup	Vegetable
Broccoli, Sweet Peas, and Carrots, Frozen, Green Giant	**24.5**	1/2	cup	Vegetable
Broth, Beef	**0.0**	1	cup	Condiment
Broth, Chicken	**0.0**	1	cup	Condiment
Broth, Chicken, Organic Free Range, Imagine Foods	**0.0**	1	cup	Condiment
Broth, No-Chicken Organic, Imagine Foods	**0.0**	1	cup	Condiment
Broth, Vegetable Organic, Imagine Foods	**0.5**	1	cup	Vegetable
Brownie, Chocolate, Frozen, Weight Watchers	**-3.0**	1	piece	Grain
Brownie, w/Frosting	**-3.5**	1	piece	Grain
Brownie, w/o Frosting	**-3.5**	1	piece	Grain
Brownie, Walnut, Betty Crocker	**-3.0**	1	piece	Grain
Brownie/Blondie, Fat-Free, Pepperidge Farm	**-3.0**	1	piece	Sugar
Brussels Sprouts w/Butter, Frozen, Green Giant	**12.0**	1/2	cup	Vegetable
Brussels Sprouts, Baby, Frozen, Seabrook Farms	**25.0**	1/2	cup	Vegetable
Brussels Sprouts, Cooked	**40.0**	1/2	cup	Vegetable
Brussels Sprouts, Frozen, Cooked	**27.0**	1/2	cup	Vegetable
Bulgur, Dry	**3.0**	1/4	cup	Grain
Bun, Cinnamon	**0.0**	1	bun	Grain
Bun, Hot Dog, Arnold	**1.5**	1	bun	Grain
Bun, Submarine/Hoagie	**3.0**	1/2	bun	Grain
Bun, White, Hamburger	**2.0**	1	bun	Grain
Burger King Apple Pie	**-1.0**	1/4	pie	Fruit
Burger King Bacon Double Cheeseburger	**-1.0**	1/2	burger	Meat/Fish/Poultry
Burger King Breakfast Croissan'wich w/Bacon	**-4.0**	1/2	serving	Milk/Dairy
Burger King Breakfast Croissan'wich w/Ham	**-3.5**	1/2	serving	Milk/Dairy
Burger King Breakfast Croissan'wich w/Sausage	**-5.5**	1/2	serving	Milk/Dairy
Burger King Cheeseburger	**0.0**	1/2	burger	Meat/Fish/Poultry
Burger King Chicken Specialty Sandwich	**-0.5**	1/2	serving	Meat/Fish/Poultry
Burger King Chicken Tenders	**0.5**	6	pieces	Meat/Fish/Poultry

Food Name—Alphabetical	Nutripoints	Serving Size		Nutrigroup
Burger King Chocolate Shake	**-1.0**	1/2	serving	Milk/Dairy
Burger King Fish Filet Sandwich	**-1.0**	1/2	serving	Meat/Fish/Poultry
Burger King French Toast Sticks	**-1.0**	1/4	serving	Grain
Burger King Great Danish	**-3.0**	1/4	piece	Grain
Burger King Ham and Cheese Specialty Sandwich	**0.5**	1/2	serving	Meat/Fish/Poultry
Burger King Hamburger	**0.5**	1/2	burger	Meat/Fish/Poultry
Burger King Scrambled Egg Platter	**-4.5**	1/2	serving	Milk/Dairy
Burger King Scrambled Egg Platter w/Bacon	**-4.0**	1/2	serving	Milk/Dairy
Burger King Scrambled Egg Platter w/Sausage	**-4.0**	1/4	serving	Milk/Dairy
Burger King Vanilla Shake	**-2.5**	1/2	serving	Milk/Dairy
Burger King Veggie Burger	**1.5**	1/2	serving	Legume/Nut/Seed
Burger King Whopper Jr. Sandwich	**0.0**	1/2	burger	Meat/Fish/Poultry
Burger King Whopper Jr. Sandwich w/Cheese	**-0.5**	1/2	burger	Meat/Fish/Poultry
Burger King Whopper Sandwich w/Cheese	**-1.0**	1/2	burger	Meat/Fish/Poultry
Burrito Dinner, Frozen, Patio	**1.0**	1/4	portion	Legume/Nut/Seed
Burrito, Bean/Beef, Frozen, Patio	**0.0**	1/2	portion	Legume/Nut/Seed
Burrito, Bean/Beef, Green, Frozen, Patio	**0.5**	1/2	serving	Legume/Nut/Seed
Burrito, Bean/Beef, Red Chili, Frozen, Patio	**0.5**	1/2	serving	Legume/Nut/Seed
Burrito, Bean/Cheese	**2.5**	1/2	serving	Legume/Nut/Seed
Burrito, Beans/Rice/Cheese, Lowfat, Cedarlane	**4.5**	1	serving	Legume/Nut/Seed
Burrito, Beef/Bean, Patio	**-1.0**	5	wt oz	Legume/Nut/Seed
Burrito, Beef/Cheese	**0.0**	1/2	serving	Legume/Nut/Seed
Burrito, Beefsteak, Frozen, Weight Watchers	**0.0**	1/2	portion	Legume/Nut/Seed
Burrito, Chicken	**3.5**	1/2	serving	Meat/Fish/Poultry
Burrito, Chicken, Frozen, Weight Watchers	**0.0**	1/2	portion	Legume/Nut/Seed
Burrito, Red Hot, Frozen, Patio	**0.0**	1/2	serving	Legume/Nut/Seed
Butter Beans, Frozen, Pictsweet	**4.0**	1/2	cup	Legume/Nut/Seed
Butter Mix, Imitation, Butter Buds	**-0.5**	2	Tbls	Condiment
Butter, Salted	**-7.5**	1	Tbls	Fat/Oil
Butter, Sweet, Cream, Unsalted, Land O'Lakes	**-6.5**	1	Tbls	Fat/Oil
Butter, Sweet, Light Salt, Land O'Lakes	**-7.0**	1	Tbls	Fat/Oil
Butter, Unsalted	**-6.5**	1	Tbls	Fat/Oil
Buttermilk, Regular	**5.0**	1	cup	Milk/Dairy
Buttermilk, Skim	**9.5**	1	cup	Milk/Dairy
Butternuts	**1.0**	1	wt oz	Legume/Nut/Seed
Cabbage Roll, Frozen Dinner	**1.5**	1/2	portion	Vegetable
Cabbage, Common, Chopped, Cooked	**31.5**	1	cup	Vegetable
Cabbage, Common, Raw, Shredded	**39.0**	1	cup	Vegetable
Cabbage, Red, Raw, Shredded	**29.5**	1	cup	Vegetable
Cabbage, Savoy, Raw, Shredded	**24.5**	1	cup	Vegetable
Cake, Angel Food, Duncan Hines	**-1.5**	1	piece	Grain
Cake, Angel Food, Plain	**-2.5**	1	piece	Grain
Cake, Angel Food, w/Glaze	**-3.5**	1/2	piece	Grain

Food Name—Alphabetical	Nutripoints	Serving Size		Nutrigroup
Cake, Banana, Sara Lee	**-2.0**	1	piece	Grain
Cake, Banana, w/Frosting	**-2.0**	1	piece	Grain
Cake, Black Forest, Frozen, Weight Watchers	**-2.5**	1	piece	Grain
Cake, Boston Cream, Supreme, Pepperidge Farm	**-3.0**	1/2	piece	Grain
Cake, Bundt Pound Supreme, Pillsbury	**-3.0**	1/2	piece	Grain
Cake, Carrot, Frozen, Weight Watchers	**-0.5**	1	piece	Grain
Cake, Carrot, w/Cream Cheese Frosting	**-2.5**	1/2	piece	Grain
Cake, Cheese, Plain	**-3.0**	1/2	piece	Milk/Dairy
Cake, Cheese, w/Fruit Topping	**-2.0**	1/2	piece	Milk/Dairy
Cake, Choco-Bake, Nestle'	**-3.0**	1	piece	Sugar
Cake, Chocolate Fudge Snack, Sara Lee	**-3.5**	1	piece	Grain
Cake, Chocolate Mint Plus, Pillsbury	**-4.0**	1/2	piece	Grain
Cake, Chocolate w/Frosting (12 Pieces/Cake)	**-3.0**	1/2	piece	Grain
Cake, Chocolate w/o Frosting (12 Pieces/Cake)	**-3.0**	1/2	piece	Grain
Cake, Chocolate, Frozen, Weight Watchers	**-2.0**	1	piece	Grain
Cake, Coffee	**-2.0**	1/2	piece	Grain
Cake, Crumb	**-2.0**	1	piece	Grain
Cake, Crumb, Hostess	**-2.0**	1	piece	Grain
Cake, Devil's Food, Deluxe, Duncan Hines	**-3.0**	1/2	piece	Grain
Cake, Dutch Apple, Streusel Swirl, Pillsbury	**-3.0**	1/2	piece	Grain
Cake, Elfin Loaves, Apple Cinnamon, Fzn, Keebler	**0.5**	1	piece	Grain
Cake, Elfin Loaves, Banana, Frozen, Keebler	**0.5**	1	piece	Grain
Cake, Elfin Loaves, Blueberry, Frozen, Keebler	**1.0**	1	piece	Grain
Cake, German Chocolate	**-3.0**	1/2	piece	Grain
Cake, German Chocolate, Frozen, Weight Watchers	**-2.0**	1	piece	Grain
Cake, German Chocolate, Moist, Betty Crocker	**-3.5**	1/2	piece	Grain
Cake, Golden Layer, Pepperidge Farm	**-3.5**	1	piece	Grain
Cake, Pound	**-5.0**	1	piece	Grain
Cake, Pound, Blueberry Topping, Fzn, Weight Watchers	**-2.5**	1	piece	Grain
Cake, Pound, Original, Sara Lee	**-4.0**	1	piece	Grain
Cake, Sponge	**-4.5**	1	piece	Grain
Cake, Sponge, w/Icing	**-3.5**	1/2	piece	Grain
Cake, Sponge, w/Whipped Cream and Fruit	**-2.0**	1/2	piece	Grain
Cake, Torte	**-3.0**	1/2	piece	Grain
Cake, Upside Down, Pineapple	**-0.5**	1/2	piece	Grain
Cake, White	**-0.5**	1	piece	Grain
Candy Bar, $100,000	**-4.0**	1	bar	Sugar
Candy Bar, 3 Musketeers	**-4.0**	1	bar	Sugar
Candy Bar, Baby Ruth	**-2.0**	1/2	bar	Sugar
Candy Bar, Butterfinger	**-2.5**	1	bar	Sugar
Candy Bar, Chocolit	**-4.0**	1	bar	Sugar
Candy Bar, Club Sandwich, Hoffman's	**-1.0**	2	wt oz	Grain

Food Name—Alphabetical	Nutripoints	Serving Size		Nutrigroup
Candy Bar, Coconut Almond Joy	**-4.0**	1/2	bar	Fruit
Candy Bar, Crunchy Nut, Kudos	**-2.5**	1 1/4	wt oz	Grain
Candy Bar, Diet	**-2.0**	1	wt oz	Sugar
Candy Bar, Fruit Nut, Concentrated, Pemmican	**2.0**	1/2	bar	Grain
Candy Bar, Ideal Green Apple, Thompson Foods	**13.5**	2	pieces	Grain
Candy Bar, Kit Kat	**-2.0**	1	bar	Sugar
Candy Bar, Mars Bar	**-3.5**	1/2	bar	Sugar
Candy Bar, Milk Chocolate	**-3.5**	1	wt oz	Milk/Dairy
Candy Bar, Milk Chocolate w/Peanuts	**-3.0**	1	wt oz	Legume/Nut/Seed
Candy Bar, Milky Way	**-4.0**	1/2	bar	Sugar
Candy Bar, Mr. Goodbar	**-3.0**	1/2	bar	Sugar
Candy Bar, Nestle' Crunch	**-4.5**	1.4	wt oz	Sugar
Candy Bar, Peanut, Planters	**0.0**	1	bar	Legume/Nut/Seed
Candy Bar, Rice Krispies, Kellogg's	**0.5**	1	bar	Grain
Candy Bar, Slim-Fast	**16.5**	1	bar	Grain
Candy Bar, Snickers	**-3.0**	1/2	bar	Sugar
Candy Bar, Three Musketeers	**-4.0**	1/2	bar	Sugar
Candy Bar, Tiger's Milk Nutrition	**5.0**	1	bar	Grain
Candy Bar, Twix Caramel	**-4.0**	2	pieces	Sugar
Candy Bar, Twix Peanut Butter	**-1.5**	2	pieces	Legume/Nut/Seed
Candy Bar, Ultra, Wild Cherry, Excel	**-1.0**	1	bar	Grain
Candy, Brach Royals	**-4.0**	1	wt oz	Sugar
Candy, Brach Toffees	**-4.0**	1	wt oz	Sugar
Candy, Caramel w/Nuts, Chocolate-Covered	**-2.5**	1	wt oz	Legume/Nut/Seed
Candy, Caramels	**-3.5**	3	pieces	Sugar
Candy, Chocolate Chips	**-6.0**	1	wt oz	Sugar
Candy, Cracker Jacks	**-3.0**	1	wt oz	Grain
Candy, Gum Drop, Small	**-5.5**	28	pieces	Sugar
Candy, Hard	**-6.0**	1	wt oz	Sugar
Candy, Kisses, Hershey's	**-3.5**	6	pieces	Sugar
Candy, M&M's Chocolate	**-4.5**	1	wt oz	Sugar
Candy, M&M's Peanut	**-2.0**	1	wt oz	Sugar
Candy, Marshmallows (large)	**-5.5**	4	pieces	Sugar
Candy, Milk Chocolate w/Almonds, Hershey's	**-3.5**	1	bar	Sugar
Candy, Peanut Brittle	**-3.0**	1	wt oz	Legume/Nut/Seed
Candy, Peanut Butter Cup	**-3.5**	1	piece	Legume/Nut/Seed
Candy, Peanut Butter Cups, Reese's	**-3.0**	1	piece	Sugar
Candy, Peanut Butter Morsels	**-0.5**	1	wt oz	Legume/Nut/Seed
Candy, Pralines	**-3.0**	1	piece	Sugar
Candy, Reese's Pieces	**-2.0**	1	wt oz	Legume/Nut/Seed
Candy, Rolo	**-4.5**	5	pieces	Sugar
Candy, Semi-Sweet Morsels, Nestle'	**-4.5**	1	wt oz	Sugar
Candy, Spear O Mint, Life Savers	**-6.0**	10	pieces	Sugar

Food Name—Alphabetical	Nutripoints	Serving Size		Nutrigroup
Candy, Taffy, Plain	**-5.5**	1	wt oz	Sugar
Candy, Wild Cherry, Life Savers	**-6.0**	10	pieces	Sugar
Cannelloni, Cheese, Lean Cuisine, Frozen, Stouffer's	**0.5**	1/2	portion	Milk/Dairy
Cannelloni, Florentine, Frozen, Celentano	**5.5**	1/2	portion	Milk/Dairy
Capon, Baked, w/Skin	**1.5**	3	wt oz	Meat/Fish/Poultry
Carambola (starfruit)	**12.5**	1	whole	Fruit
Caraway Seed	**0.5**	1	tsp	Condiment
Carl's Jr. Bacon and Cheese Potato	**-0.5**	1/4	potato	Vegetable
Carl's Jr. Blueberry Muffin	**-1.5**	1/2	muffin	Grain
Carl's Jr. Boston Clam Chowder Soups	**-1.5**	1	cup	Meat/Fish/Poultry
Carl's Jr. Bran Muffin	**-1.0**	1	muffin	Grain
Carl's Jr. Broccoli and Cheese Potato	**2.0**	1/4	potato	Vegetable
Carl's Jr. California Roast Beef 'n Swiss	**1.0**	1/2	serving	Meat/Fish/Poultry
Carl's Jr. Charbroiler Barbeque Chicken Sandwich	**1.5**	1/2	serving	Meat/Fish/Poultry
Carl's Jr. Charbroiler Chicken Club Sandwich	**0.5**	1/2	serving	Meat/Fish/Poultry
Carl's Jr. Cheese Potato	**0.5**	1/4	potato	Vegetable
Carl's Jr. Chef Salad (take-Out)	**4.0**	1/2	serving	Vegetable
Carl's Jr. Chicken Salad (take-Out)	**3.5**	1	serving	Meat/Fish/Poultry
Carl's Jr. Chocolate Cake	**-3.5**	1/2	piece	Grain
Carl's Jr. Chocolate Chip Cookie 2.5 Ounce	**-3.0**	1/2	cookie	Grain
Carl's Jr. Country Fried Steak Sandwich	**-0.5**	1/2	serving	Meat/Fish/Poultry
Carl's Jr. Cream of Broccoli Soup	**1.0**	1/2	cup	Vegetable
Carl's Jr. Danish (all Varieties)	**-0.5**	1/2	piece	Grain
Carl's Jr. Double Western Bacon Cheeseburger	**-1.5**	1/4	burger	Meat/Fish/Poultry
Carl's Jr. English Muffin w/Margarine	**1.0**	1	muffin	Grain
Carl's Jr. Famous Star Hamburger	**-0.5**	1/2	burger	Meat/Fish/Poultry
Carl's Jr. Fiesta Potato	**0.5**	1/4	potato	Vegetable
Carl's Jr. Filet of Fish Sandwich	**-1.0**	1/2	serving	Meat/Fish/Poultry
Carl's Jr. French Toast Dips	**-1.5**	1	serving	Grain
Carl's Jr. Fried Zucchini	**-1.0**	1	serving	Vegetable
Carl's Jr. Garden Salad to Go	**8.5**	1	serving	Vegetable
Carl's Jr. Happy Star Hamburger	**0.0**	1	burger	Meat/Fish/Poultry
Carl's Jr. Hash Browns Nuggets	**-1.5**	2	pieces	Vegetable
Carl's Jr. Hot Cakes w/Margarine	**0.0**	1	serving	Grain
Carl's Jr. Lite Potato	**3.0**	1/2	potato	Vegetable
Carl's Jr. Lumber Jack Mix Vegetable Soup	**2.5**	1	cup	Vegetable
Carl's Jr. Old Fashioned Chicken Noodle Soup	**0.5**	1	cup	Meat/Fish/Poultry
Carl's Jr. Old Time Star Hamburger	**0.0**	1/2	burger	Meat/Fish/Poultry
Carl's Jr. Onion Rings	**-1.0**	1	ring	Vegetable
Carl's Jr. Sausage Patty	**-2.5**	1	patty	Meat/Fish/Poultry
Carl's Jr. Scrambled Eggs	**-11.0**	1	serving	Milk/Dairy
Carl's Jr. Shakes - Reg. Size	**-1.5**	1/2	cup	Milk/Dairy
Carl's Jr. Sour Cream & Chive Potato	**1.0**	1/4	potato	Vegetable

Food Name—Alphabetical	Nutripoints	Serving Size		Nutrigroup
Carl's Jr. Sunrise Sandwich w/Bacon	**-2.0**	1/2	serving	Milk/Dairy
Carl's Jr. Sunrise Sandwich w/Sausage	**-2.5**	1/4	serving	Milk/Dairy
Carl's Jr. Super Star Hamburger	**-1.5**	1/2	burger	Meat/Fish/Poultry
Carl's Jr. Taco Salad to Go	**1.5**	1/4	serving	Vegetable
Carl's Jr. Western Bacon Cheeseburger	**-1.0**	1/2	burger	Meat/Fish/Poultry
Carob Powder	**1.0**	1	Tbls	Miscellaneous
Carp, Baked/Broiled	**0.5**	3	wt oz	Meat/Fish/Poultry
Carp, Floured/Breaded, Fried	**-0.5**	3	wt oz	Meat/Fish/Poultry
Carp, Smoked	**2.5**	3	wt oz	Meat/Fish/Poultry
Carrots, Raw	**35.5**	1	whole	Vegetable
Carrots, Sliced, Cooked	**30.0**	1/2	cup	Vegetable
Cashew Butter, Salted	**0.5**	1	wt oz	Legume/Nut/Seed
Cashews, Dry Roasted, Salted	**0.5**	1	wt oz	Legume/Nut/Seed
Cashews, Dry Roasted, Unsalted	**1.5**	12	nuts	Legume/Nut/Seed
Cashews, Dry Roasted, Unsalted, Planter's	**1.5**	1	wt oz	Legume/Nut/Seed
Cashews, Oil Roasted, Salted	**0.5**	1	wt oz	Legume/Nut/Seed
Cashews, Oil Roasted, Unsalted	**0.5**	1	wt oz	Legume/Nut/Seed
Casserole, Five Cheese, Nutripoint Recipe	**5.5**	1/2	cup	Milk/Dairy
Catfish, Baked	**3.0**	5	wt oz	Meat/Fish/Poultry
Catfish, Fillets, Light, Mrs. Paul's	**0.5**	1	portion	Meat/Fish/Poultry
Catfish, Fried w/Breading	**0.0**	3	wt oz	Meat/Fish/Poultry
Catsup	**1.0**	2	Tbls	Vegetable
Catsup, Low Sodium/Sugar	**0.5**	2	Tbls	Vegetable
Catsup, Tomato, Del Monte	**0.5**	2	Tbls	Vegetable
Cauliflower, Cheddar Cheese Sauce, Fzn, Budget Gourmet	**2.0**	1/2	portion	Vegetable
Cauliflower, Cheese Sauce, Frozen, Green Giant	**6.0**	1/2	cup	Vegetable
Cauliflower, Cooked	**37.0**	1	cup	Vegetable
Cauliflower, Fried w/Breading	**-0.5**	1/4	cup	Vegetable
Cauliflower, Frozen, Birds Eye	**23.0**	1	cup	Vegetable
Cauliflower, Raw	**40.5**	1	cup	Vegetable
Cavatelli, Frozen, Celentano	**3.0**	1/2	portion	Grain
Caviar	**-11.5**	1	Tbls	Miscellaneous
Celeriac, Raw	**8.0**	1/2	cup	Vegetable
Celery Seed	**0.5**	1	tsp	Condiment
Celery, Raw	**20.0**	8	pieces	Vegetable
Cereal, 100% Bran With Oat Bran, Nabisco	**23.5**	1/2	cup	Grain
Cereal, 100% Bran, Nabisco	**31.0**	1/2	cup	Grain
Cereal, 100% Natural, Quaker	**1.0**	1/4	cup	Grain
Cereal, 100% Natural, Raisin & Date, Quaker	**0.0**	1/4	cup	Grain
Cereal, 40+bran Flakes, Kellogg's	**21.0**	2/3	cup	Grain
Cereal, 7 Grain, Stone-Buhr	**4.0**	1	wt oz	Grain
Cereal, All Bran Extra Fiber, Kellogg's	**43.5**	1/2	cup	Grain

Food Name—Alphabetical	Nutripoints	Serving Size		Nutrigroup
Cereal, All-Bran	**40.5**	1/3	cup	Grain
Cereal, Alpen	**3.5**	1/4	cup	Grain
Cereal, Alpha-Bits, Post	**8.5**	1	cup	Grain
Cereal, Apple Cinnamon Cheerios, General Mills	**8.0**	3/4	cup	Grain
Cereal, Apple Jacks, Kellogg's	**9.5**	1	cup	Grain
Cereal, Atkins, All Flavors	**6.0**	2/3	cup	Grain
Cereal, Basic 4, General Mills	**6.0**	1	cup	Grain
Cereal, Benefit w/Raisins, General Mills	**10.0**	1	cup	Grain
Cereal, Benefit, General Mills	**14.5**	3/4	cup	Grain
Cereal, Blueberry Fruit Wheats, Nabisco	**13.0**	1/2	cup	Grain
Cereal, Bran Chex, General Mills	**15.5**	3/4	cup	Grain
Cereal, Bran Flakes, Kellogg's	**21.0**	2/3	cup	Grain
Cereal, C.W. Post, w/Raisins, Post	**7.5**	1/2	cup	Grain
Cereal, Cap'n Crunch, Peanut Butter, Quaker	**9.0**	3/4	cup	Grain
Cereal, Cap'n Crunch, Quaker	**8.5**	3/4	cup	Grain
Cereal, Cheerios, General Mills	**13.0**	1 1/4	cups	Grain
Cereal, Cheerios, Multi-Grain, General Mills	**13.0**	1	cup	Grain
Cereal, Cinnamon Toast Crunch, General Mills	**7.5**	3/4	cup	Grain
Cereal, Cocoa Krispies, Kellogg's	**7.0**	3/4	cup	Grain
Cereal, Cocoa Pebbles, Post	**7.5**	7/8	cup	Grain
Cereal, Cocoa Puffs, General Mills	**6.5**	1	cup	Grain
Cereal, Cocoa Puffs, Reduced Sugar, General Mills	**12.5**	1	cup	Grain
Cereal, Corn Chex, General Mills	**10.0**	1	cup	Grain
Cereal, Corn Flakes, Kellogg's	**18.0**	1	cup	Grain
Cereal, Corn Pops, Kellogg's	**8.0**	1	cup	Grain
Cereal, Country Morning	**0.5**	1/4	cup	Grain
Cereal, Cracklin' Oat Bran, Kellogg's	**14.0**	1/2	cup	Grain
Cereal, Cream of Rice, Cooked	**2.5**	3/4	cup	Grain
Cereal, Cream of Wheat, Quick, Nabisco	**4.5**	1	cup	Grain
Cereal, Crispix, Kellogg's	**10.0**	1	cup	Grain
Cereal, Empower, Health Valley	**19.5**	1	cup	Grain
Cereal, Familia, w/Fruit & Nuts	**2.5**	1/4	cup	Grain
Cereal, Fiber One, General Mills	**31.5**	1/2	cup	Grain
Cereal, Frosted Flakes, Kellogg's	**7.0**	3/4	cup	Grain
Cereal, Frosted Mini-Wheats, Kellogg's	**12.5**	1/2	cup	Grain
Cereal, Frosted Wheat Squares, Nabisco	**11.5**	1/2	cup	Grain
Cereal, Fruit & Fiber w/Dates, Raisins, Walnuts, Post	**15.5**	1/2	cup	Grain
Cereal, Fruit & Fiber w/Raisins, Peaches, Almonds, Post	**15.5**	1/2	cup	Grain
Cereal, Fruit Loops, Kellogg's	**13.0**	1	cup	Grain
Cereal, Fruitful Bran, Kellogg's	**28.5**	2/3	cup	Grain
Cereal, Fruity Pebbles, Post	**7.5**	7/8	cup	Grain
Cereal, Golden Crisp, Post	**8.0**	7/8	cup	Grain
Cereal, Golden Grahams, General Mills	**9.0**	3/4	cup	Grain

Food Name—Alphabetical	Nutripoints	Serving Size		Nutrigroup
Cereal, Grape-Nut Flakes, Post	**18.0**	7/8	cup	Grain
Cereal, Grape-Nuts, Post	**13.5**	1/4	cup	Grain
Cereal, Heart to Heart Hot Oatmeal, Kashi	**13.5**	1	serving	Grain
Cereal, Heart to Heart, Kashi	**23.0**	3/4	cup	Grain
Cereal, Heart Wise, Health Valley	**10.5**	1	cup	Grain
Cereal, H-O Super Bran	**4.5**	1	wt oz	Grain
Cereal, Honey Nut Cheerios, General Mills	**10.0**	3/4	cup	Grain
Cereal, Honey Nut Chex, General Mills	**6.5**	2/3	cup	Grain
Cereal, Honeybunches of Oats w/Almonds, Post	**7.0**	2/3	cup	Grain
Cereal, Honey-Comb, Ralston	**8.5**	1 1/3	cups	Grain
Cereal, Horizon Trail Mix, Post	**10.0**	1/3	cup	Grain
Cereal, Hot, High Fiber, Ralston	**8.5**	1/4	cup	Grain
Cereal, Hot, High Fiber, w/Milk, Ralston	**6.0**	1/4	cup	Grain
Cereal, Instant Cream of Wheat, w/Low-Fat Milk, Nabisco	**4.5**	1/2	cup	Grain
Cereal, Instant Oatmeal w/Apples & Cinnamon, Quaker	**3.5**	1.25	wt oz	Grain
Cereal, Instant Oatmeal w/Maple & Brown Sugar, Quaker	**1.5**	1.25	wt oz	Grain
Cereal, Instant Oatmeal w/Peaches and Cream, Quaker	**5.5**	1	cup	Grain
Cereal, Just Right w/Fruit and Nuts, Kellogg's	**36.5**	3/4	cup	Grain
Cereal, Kashi Medley	**0.0**	3/4	cup	Grain
Cereal, Kellogg's Complete Wheat Bran Flakes	**18.5**	3/4	cup	Grain
Cereal, Kix, General Mills	**10.0**	1 1/2	cups	Grain
Cereal, Life, Cinnamon, Quaker	**11.0**	2/3	cup	Grain
Cereal, Life, Quaker	**9.5**	2/3	cup	Grain
Cereal, Lucky Charms, General Mills	**10.5**	1	cup	Grain
Cereal, Malt O Meal, w/Water, Cooked	**7.5**	1	cup	Grain
Cereal, Malt-O Meal, Quick, w/Whole Milk	**4.5**	1/2	cup	Grain
Cereal, Mueslix, 5 Grain Muesli, Kellogg's	**10.0**	1/2	cup	Grain
Cereal, Mueslix, Bran Muesli, Kellogg's	**12.5**	1/2	cup	Grain
Cereal, Multi-Bran Chex, General Mills	**11.5**	1	cup	Grain
Cereal, Multi-Grain Cheerios, General Mills	**48.5**	1	cup	Grain
Cereal, Multi-Grains/Raisins/Oats, Healthy Choice	**8.5**	1	cup	Grain
Cereal, Natural Bran Flakes, Post	**17.5**	2/3	cup	Grain
Cereal, Oat Bran Prepared w/Low-Fat Milk, Nabisco	**12.0**	1/2	cup	Grain
Cereal, Oat Bran, Instant, w/Skim Milk, 3-Minute Brand	**6.5**	1/2	cup	Grain
Cereal, Oat Bran, Instant, w/Water, 3 Minute Brand	**6.0**	1	wt oz	Grain
Cereal, Oat Bran, Instant, w/Whole Milk, 3-Minute Brand	**5.5**	1	cup	Grain
Cereal, Oat Bran, Quaker	**7.0**	1/2	cup	Grain
Cereal, Oat Squares, Quaker	**17.0**	1/2	cup	Grain
Cereal, Oatbake, Kellogg's	**10.0**	1/3	cup	Grain
Cereal, Oatmeal Crisp Raisin, General Mills	**9.5**	1/2	cup	Grain
Cereal, Oatmeal, Cooked, Prepared w/Water	**2.0**	1	cup	Grain
Cereal, Oatmeal, Dry	**5.5**	1/2	cup	Grain
Cereal, Oatmeal, Fruited Cinnamon, Nutripoint Recipe	**5.0**	1	cup	Grain

Food Name—Alphabetical	Nutripoints	Serving Size		Nutrigroup
Cereal, Oats, Instant, w/Bran, w/Low-Fat Milk, 3-Minute Brand	**9.5**	1/2	cup	Grain
Cereal, Oats, Old Fashioned, Quaker	**4.5**	3/4	cup	Grain
Cereal, Oats, Quick, Prepared w/Low-Fat Milk, Quaker	**3.0**	1/2	cup	Grain
Cereal, Oats, Steel-Cut, Arrowhead Mills	**4.0**	1	wt oz	Grain
Cereal, Orangeola w/Bananas and Hawaiian Fruit, Health Valley	**1.5**	1/4	cup	Grain
Cereal, Product 19, Kellogg's	**56.0**	1	cup	Grain
Cereal, Puffed Rice	**2.0**	2	cups	Grain
Cereal, Puffed Rice, Quaker	**2.5**	1	cup	Grain
Cereal, Puffed Wheat	**4.5**	2	cups	Grain
Cereal, Puffed Wheat, Quaker	**5.5**	1	cup	Grain
Cereal, Puffed, 7 Whole Grains and Sesame, Kashi	**3.0**	2	cup	Grain
Cereal, Puffed, Kashi	**1.5**	2	cups	Grain
Cereal, Quaker Oat Bran	**8.5**	1 1/4	cups	Grain
Cereal, Raisin Bran, Kellogg's	**15.5**	3/4	cup	Grain
Cereal, Raisin Nut Bran, General Mills	**10.0**	1/2	cup	Grain
Cereal, Raspberry Fruit Wheats, Nabisco	**13.0**	1/2	cup	Grain
Cereal, Rice Chex, General Mills	**9.0**	1 1/8	cups	Grain
Cereal, Rice Krispies, Kellogg's	**11.5**	1	cup	Grain
Cereal, Seven in the Morning, Kashi	**2.0**	1/2	cup	Grain
Cereal, Shredded Wheat (large Biscuit), Nabisco	**5.0**	1	piece	Grain
Cereal, Shredded Wheat 'n Bran, Nabisco	**6.0**	1	wt oz	Grain
Cereal, Shredded Wheat, Spoon Size, Nabisco	**5.0**	2/3	cup	Grain
Cereal, Slender, Health Valley	**11.5**	1	cup	Grain
Cereal, Smart Start, Kellogg's	**26.5**	1	cup	Grain
Cereal, Special K, Kellogg's	**14.0**	1	cup	Grain
Cereal, Sun Flakes, Ralston	**10.5**	1	cup	Grain
Cereal, Team Flakes, Nabisco	**11.5**	1	cup	Grain
Cereal, Toasties Corn Flakes, Post	**9.0**	1 1/4	cups	Grain
Cereal, Total Brown Sugar & Oat, General Mills	**55.5**	3/4	cup	Grain
Cereal, Total Corn Flakes, General Mills	**57.5**	1	cup	Grain
Cereal, Total Protein, General Mills	**43.5**	3/4	cup	Grain
Cereal, Total Raisin Bran, General Mills	**40.5**	1/2	cup	Grain
Cereal, Trix, General Mills	**8.0**	1	cup	Grain
Cereal, Trix, Reduced Sugar, General Mills	**12.5**	1	cup	Grain
Cereal, Wheat Chex, General Mills	**13.0**	2/3	cup	Grain
Cereal, Wheaties, General Mills	**12.0**	1	cup	Grain
Cereal, Whole Grain Total, General Mills	**64.5**	1	cup	Grain
Cereal, Whole Wheat, Cooked	**4.5**	1/2	cup	Grain
Cereal, Whole Wheat, Weetabix	**4.0**	2	pieces	Grain
Champagne	**-13.5**	6	fl oz	Alcohol
Cheese Fondue	**-4.5**	1/4	cup	Milk/Dairy

Food Name—Alphabetical	Nutripoints	Serving Size		Nutrigroup
Cheese Food Substitute, Low Cholesterol, Lite-Line	-1.5	1	wt oz	Milk/Dairy
Cheese Puffs, Cheetos	-1.5	25	pieces	Grain
Cheese Spread	-1.5	1	wt oz	Milk/Dairy
Cheese Spread, Cheez Whiz, Kraft	-3.5	1	wt oz	Milk/Dairy
Cheese Spread, Pasteurized Process Slices, Velveeta	-2.5	1	wt oz	Milk/Dairy
Cheese Spread, Pasteurized Process, Velveeta	-3.0	1	wt oz	Milk/Dairy
Cheese Substitute, Pasteurized Process, Formagg	10.5	1	piece	Milk/Dairy
Cheese, American, Light N'Lively, Kraft	-1.0	1	wt oz	Milk/Dairy
Cheese, American, Pasteurized Process, Kraft	-1.5	1	wt oz	Milk/Dairy
Cheese, American, Pasteurized Process, Lite-Line	0.0	2	wt oz	Milk/Dairy
Cheese, American, Process, Borden	-2.5	1	wt oz	Milk/Dairy
Cheese, American, Processed	-3.0	1	wt oz	Milk/Dairy
Cheese, Blue	-2.0	1	wt oz	Milk/Dairy
Cheese, Brick	-1.5	1	wt oz	Milk/Dairy
Cheese, Brie	-2.0	1	wt oz	Milk/Dairy
Cheese, Camembert	-1.0	1	wt oz	Milk/Dairy
Cheese, Cheddar	-2.0	1	wt oz	Milk/Dairy
Cheese, Cheddar, Low Sodium, Tillamook	-3.0	1	wt oz	Milk/Dairy
Cheese, Cheddar, Mild, Reduced Fat, Kraft	-1.0	1	wt oz	Milk/Dairy
Cheese, Cheddar, Natural Mild, Kraft	-3.0	1	wt oz	Milk/Dairy
Cheese, Cheddar, Sharp, Cracker Barrel	-3.5	1	wt oz	Milk/Dairy
Cheese, Cheddar, Tillamook	-3.0	1	wt oz	Milk/Dairy
Cheese, Colby	-2.0	1	wt oz	Milk/Dairy
Cheese, Cottage	1.5	1/2	cup	Milk/Dairy
Cheese, Cottage, Dry	5.5	1/2	cup	Milk/Dairy
Cheese, Cottage, Lowfat (1%)	4.5	1/2	cup	Milk/Dairy
Cheese, Cottage, Lowfat (2%)	3.0	4	wt oz	Milk/Dairy
Cheese, Cottage, Lowfat, Weight Watchers	1.5	1/2	cup	Milk/Dairy
Cheese, Cream	-5.0	2	Tbls	Milk/Dairy
Cheese, Cream, Honey, Nutripoint Recipe	5.5	1/4	cup	Milk/Dairy
Cheese, Edam	-1.0	1	wt oz	Milk/Dairy
Cheese, Feta	-2.5	1	wt oz	Milk/Dairy
Cheese, Gjetost	-0.5	1	wt oz	Milk/Dairy
Cheese, Gouda	-1.5	1	wt oz	Milk/Dairy
Cheese, Gouda, Kraft	-3.5	1	wt oz	Milk/Dairy
Cheese, Grated, Parmesan	0.5	1	wt oz	Milk/Dairy
Cheese, Gruyere	-1.0	1	wt oz	Milk/Dairy
Cheese, Laughing Cow	0.0	2	pieces	Milk/Dairy
Cheese, Limburger	-3.0	1	wt oz	Milk/Dairy
Cheese, Low Cal	3.5	2	wt oz	Milk/Dairy
Cheese, Monterey Jack	-1.5	1	wt oz	Milk/Dairy
Cheese, Monterey Jack, Casino Brand	-3.5	1	wt oz	Milk/Dairy
Cheese, Monterey Jack, Kraft	-3.5	1	wt oz	Milk/Dairy

Food Name—Alphabetical	Nutripoints	Serving Size		Nutrigroup
Cheese, Monterey Jack, Low Fat, Alpine Lace	**-1.5**	2	wt oz	Milk/Dairy
Cheese, Monterey Jack, Reduced Fat, Kraft	**-1.0**	1	wt oz	Milk/Dairy
Cheese, Mozzarella	**-1.5**	1	wt oz	Milk/Dairy
Cheese, Mozzarella, Casino, Kraft	**-3.5**	1	wt oz	Milk/Dairy
Cheese, Mozzarella, Low Fat, Alpine Lace	**-1.0**	2	wt oz	Milk/Dairy
Cheese, Mozzarella, Low-Fat	**0.5**	1	wt oz	Milk/Dairy
Cheese, Mozzarella, Pasteurized Process, Lite-Line	**-0.5**	2	wt oz	Milk/Dairy
Cheese, Mozzarella, Skim, Kraft	**-1.5**	1	wt oz	Milk/Dairy
Cheese, Mozzarella, Skim, Land O'lakes	**0.5**	1	wt oz	Milk/Dairy
Cheese, Muenster	**-1.5**	1	wt oz	Milk/Dairy
Cheese, Muenster, Land O'lakes	**-2.5**	1	wt oz	Milk/Dairy
Cheese, Natural Colby, Kraft	**-3.0**	1	wt oz	Milk/Dairy
Cheese, Neufchatel	**-4.0**	1	wt oz	Milk/Dairy
Cheese, Neufchatel, Philadelphia Brand	**-3.0**	1	wt oz	Milk/Dairy
Cheese, Non-Fat, Processed American or Swiss	**4.0**	2	slices	Milk/Dairy
Cheese, Parmesan, Grated, Kraft	**-1.5**	1	wt oz	Milk/Dairy
Cheese, Parmesan, Imitation, Grated, Formagg	**0.0**	1	wt oz	Milk/Dairy
Cheese, Pasteurized Process, Reduced Sodium, Lite-Line	**-0.5**	1	wt oz	Milk/Dairy
Cheese, Pimento	**-2.0**	1	wt oz	Milk/Dairy
Cheese, Provolone	**-1.0**	1	wt oz	Milk/Dairy
Cheese, Reduced Calorie, Laughing Cow	**2.5**	2	pieces	Milk/Dairy
Cheese, Ricotta	**-2.0**	2	wt oz	Milk/Dairy
Cheese, Ricotta, Low-Fat	**0.5**	3	wt oz	Milk/Dairy
Cheese, Ricotta, Precious Fat Free	**5.5**	1/4	cup	Milk/Dairy
Cheese, Romano	**-2.0**	1	wt oz	Milk/Dairy
Cheese, Roquefort	**-3.0**	1	wt oz	Milk/Dairy
Cheese, Sharp Cheddar, Pasteurized Process, Lite-Line	**-0.5**	1	wt oz	Milk/Dairy
Cheese, Swiss	**-0.5**	1	wt oz	Milk/Dairy
Cheese, Swiss, Light N'Lively, Kraft	**-1.0**	1	wt oz	Milk/Dairy
Cheese, Swiss, Low Fat, Alpine Lace	**-2.0**	1	wt oz	Milk/Dairy
Cheese, Swiss, Low Sodium, Kraft	**-2.5**	1	wt oz	Milk/Dairy
Cheese, Swiss, Natural, Kraft	**-2.0**	1	wt oz	Milk/Dairy
Cheese, Swiss, Pasteurized Process, Kraft	**-4.0**	1	wt oz	Milk/Dairy
Cheese, Swiss, Pasteurized Process, Lite-Line	**-0.5**	2	slices	Milk/Dairy
Cheese, Swiss, Process, Borden	**-2.5**	1	wt oz	Milk/Dairy
Cheese, Swiss, Processed	**-2.5**	1	wt oz	Milk/Dairy
Cheese, Swiss, Reduced Fat, Kraft	**0.5**	1	wt oz	Milk/Dairy
Cheese, Swiss, Sargento	**-2.5**	1	wt oz	Milk/Dairy
Cheeseburger w/Bun, Fast Food, Small Plain	**0.0**	1/2	burger	Meat/Fish/Poultry
Cheeseburger, Vegetarian, Boca Burger	**1.0**	1	burger	Legume/Nut/Seed
Cheesecake, Classic Snack, Sara Lee	**-5.5**	1/2	piece	Grain
Cheesecake, Frozen, Weight Watchers	**-2.0**	1/2	serving	Milk/Dairy

Food Name—Alphabetical	Nutripoints	Serving Size		Nutrigroup
Cheesecake, Strawberry, Fzn, Weight Watchers	**-2.0**	1/2	portion	Milk/Dairy
Cherries, Chocolate Covered	**-3.5**	2	pieces	Fruit
Cherries, Sour, Canned, Heavy Syrup	**1.0**	1/2	cup	Fruit
Cherries, Sour, Canned, Unsweetened	**7.5**	1/2	cup	Fruit
Cherries, Sour, Raw	**7.5**	10	cherries	Fruit
Cherries, Sweet, Canned, Heavy Syrup	**0.0**	1/2	cup	Fruit
Cherries, Sweet, Canned, Water	**5.5**	1/2	cup	Fruit
Cherries, Sweet, Fresh	**5.5**	10	cherries	Fruit
Cherries, Sweet, Frozen, Sweetened	**2.0**	1/2	cup	Fruit
Chicken & Egg Noodles, w/Broccoli, Fzn, Budget Gourmet	**-2.0**	1/2	portion	Meat/Fish/Poultry
Chicken & Pasta Divan, Fzn, Healthy Choice	**2.5**	1	portion	Meat/Fish/Poultry
Chicken & Pasta w/Mushroom Sauce, Michelina's, Fzn, Lean Gourmet	**0.5**	1	serving	Meat/Fish/Poultry
Chicken & Penne w/Broccoli, Fzn, South Beach Diet	**2.5**	1	serving	Meat/Fish/Poultry
Chicken A L'orange, w/Almonds and Rice, Fzn, Stouffer's	**1.5**	1	portion	Meat/Fish/Poultry
Chicken Ala King	**0.0**	1/2	cup	Meat/Fish/Poultry
Chicken Ala King w/Rice, Dining Lite	**3.0**	1	cup	Meat/Fish/Poultry
Chicken Ala King, Frozen, Weight Watchers	**0.0**	1	portion	Meat/Fish/Poultry
Chicken Ala King, w/Rice, Frozen, Stouffer's	**0.0**	1	portion	Meat/Fish/Poultry
Chicken Alfredo Florentine, Michelina's Lean Gourmet	**-0.5**	1	serving	Meat/Fish/Poultry
Chicken Au Gratin, Slim, Fzn, Budget Gourmet	**2.0**	1	portion	Meat/Fish/Poultry
Chicken Breast Portions, Fried, Fzn, Swanson	**-2.0**	1/2	portion	Meat/Fish/Poultry
Chicken Breast, Baked w/o Skin	**4.0**	3	wt oz	Meat/Fish/Poultry
Chicken Breast, Fried w/Batter, w/Skin	**1.0**	3	wt oz	Meat/Fish/Poultry
Chicken Breast, Fried w/o Bread, w/Skin	**2.5**	3	wt oz	Meat/Fish/Poultry
Chicken Breast, Fried w/o Skin	**1.5**	3	wt oz	Meat/Fish/Poultry
Chicken Breast, Glazed, Frozen, Le Menu	**1.5**	1	portion	Meat/Fish/Poultry
Chicken Breast, Marsala w/Vegetables, Fzn, Stouffer's	**1.5**	1	portion	Meat/Fish/Poultry
Chicken Breast, Roasted, Fzn, Healthy Choice	**0.0**	1	serving	Meat/Fish/Poultry
Chicken Cacciatore w/Vermicelli, Fzn, Stouffer's	**0.5**	1	portion	Meat/Fish/Poultry
Chicken Cacciatore, Frozen, Budget Gourmet	**1.0**	1/2	portion	Meat/Fish/Poultry
Chicken Chow Mein w/Rice, Dining Lite	**1.5**	1	cup	Meat/Fish/Poultry
Chicken Chow Mein, Frozen, Chun King	**1.5**	1/2	portion	Meat/Fish/Poultry
Chicken Dijon, ZonePerfect	**1.5**	1/2	serving	Meat/Fish/Poultry
Chicken Divan, Frozen, Stouffer's	**-1.0**	1/2	portion	Meat/Fish/Poultry
Chicken Fettucini Alfredo, Uncle Ben's Pasta Bowl	**-2.0**	12	wt oz	Meat/Fish/Poultry
Chicken Fricassee	**2.5**	1/2	cup	Meat/Fish/Poultry
Chicken Fried Steak	**0.0**	2	wt oz	Meat/Fish/Poultry

Food Name—Alphabetical	Nutripoints	Serving Size		Nutrigroup
Chicken Imperial, Frozen, Weight Watchers	**1.5**	1	portion	Meat/Fish/Poultry
Chicken Kiev	**0.0**	1/2	piece	Meat/Fish/Poultry
Chicken La Russe w/Veg, Cm	**9.5**	1	portion	Meat/Fish/Poultry
Chicken Leg, Baked w/o Skin	**2.5**	3	wt oz	Meat/Fish/Poultry
Chicken Leg, Fried w/o Bread, w/Skin	**1.5**	3	wt oz	Meat/Fish/Poultry
Chicken Liver, Stewed	**2.0**	3	wt oz	Meat/Fish/Poultry
Chicken Marsala w/Broccoli, Fzn, Weight Watchers	**1.5**	1	serving	Meat/Fish/Poultry
Chicken Nuggets, Vegetarian, Morningstar Farms	**8.5**	4	pieces	Legume/Nut/Seed
Chicken Oriental, Frozen, Healthy Choice	**3.5**	1	portion	Meat/Fish/Poultry
Chicken Oriental, Frozen, Stouffer's	**0.5**	1	portion	Meat/Fish/Poultry
Chicken Parmigiana Patty, Fzn, Weight Watchers	**-0.5**	1/2	portion	Meat/Fish/Poultry
Chicken Parmigiana, Frozen, Celentano	**2.0**	1/2	portion	Meat/Fish/Poultry
Chicken Parmigiana, Frozen, Healthy Choice	**3.5**	1	portion	Meat/Fish/Poultry
Chicken Patty, Vegetarian, Morningstar Farms	**5.0**	1	patty	Legume/Nut/Seed
Chicken Pecan, Fzn, Lean Cuisine	**1.0**	1	serving	Meat/Fish/Poultry
Chicken Pie, Frozen, Stouffer's	**-0.5**	1/2	portion	Meat/Fish/Poultry
Chicken Pot Pie	**0.5**	1/2	pie	Meat/Fish/Poultry
Chicken Pot Pie, Claim Jumper	**-1.5**	1/2	cup	Meat/Fish/Poultry
Chicken Pot Pie, Frozen, Swanson	**-1.0**	1/2	pie	Meat/Fish/Poultry
Chicken Primavera, Frozen, Celentano	**6.0**	1/2	portion	Meat/Fish/Poultry
Chicken Salad	**2.0**	1/2	cup	Meat/Fish/Poultry
Chicken Salad, Nutripoint Recipe	**6.5**	3/4	cup	Meat/Fish/Poultry
Chicken Stir Fry, Nutripoint Recipe	**8.5**	1	cup	Meat/Fish/Poultry
Chicken Tenderloins In Peanut Sauce, Fzn, Stouffer's	**1.0**	1	portion	Meat/Fish/Poultry
Chicken Tenders, Sweet 'n Sour, Fzn, Weight Watchers	**1.5**	1	portion	Meat/Fish/Poultry
Chicken Teriyaki, Frozen, Budget Gourmet	**0.5**	1/2	portion	Meat/Fish/Poultry
Chicken Teriyaki, Uncle Ben's Rice Bowl	**1.0**	1/2	serving	Meat/Fish/Poultry
Chicken Thigh, Baked w/o Skin	**1.0**	3	wt oz	Meat/Fish/Poultry
Chicken Thigh, Baked w/Out Skin	**1.0**	1	piece	Meat/Fish/Poultry
Chicken Thigh, Fried w/o Breading	**2.0**	3	wt oz	Meat/Fish/Poultry
Chicken Thigh, Meat & Skin, Baked	**0.0**	1	piece	Meat/Fish/Poultry
Chicken Thigh, Meat & Skin, Fried, Batter	**0.0**	1	piece	Meat/Fish/Poultry
Chicken w/Broccoli & Cauliflower, Fzn, South Beach Diet	**2.5**	1	serving	Meat/Fish/Poultry
Chicken w/Cashews & Snap Peas, Fzn, South Beach Diet	**2.5**	1	serving	Meat/Fish/Poultry
Chicken w/Couscous & Vegetables, Fzn, South Beach Diet	**2.0**	1	serving	Meat/Fish/Poultry
Chicken w/Dumplings	**2.0**	3/4	cup	Meat/Fish/Poultry
Chicken w/Green Beans Almondine, Fzn, South Beach Diet	**2.5**	1	serving	Meat/Fish/Poultry

Food Name—Alphabetical	Nutripoints	Serving Size		Nutrigroup
Chicken Wing, Baked w/Out Skin	**2.0**	3	pieces	Meat/Fish/Poultry
Chicken Wing, Fried w/o Breading	**0.0**	2	pieces	Meat/Fish/Poultry
Chicken Wing, Meat & Skin, Baked	**0.0**	2	pieces	Meat/Fish/Poultry
Chicken Wing, Meat & Skin, Fried, Batter	**-0.5**	1	piece	Meat/Fish/Poultry
Chicken, (Vege) Chick Patties, Morningstar Farms	**3.5**	1	patty	Legume/Nut/Seed
Chicken, Buffalo Wings, Vegetarian, Morningstar Farms	**3.5**	5	pieces	Legume/Nut/Seed
Chicken, Cajun, Nutripoint Recipe	**5.5**	3	wt oz	Meat/Fish/Poultry
Chicken, Canned	**1.0**	1/2	cup	Meat/Fish/Poultry
Chicken, Chunk White, Premium, Canned, Swanson	**-0.5**	4	wt oz	Meat/Fish/Poultry
Chicken, Country Herb, Fzn, Healthy Choice	**-1.0**	1	serving	Meat/Fish/Poultry
Chicken, Creamed	**1.5**	1/2	cup	Meat/Fish/Poultry
Chicken, Fried, Dinner, Frozen, Morton	**0.0**	1/2	portion	Meat/Fish/Poultry
Chicken, Fried, Homestyle, Fzn, Swanson	**-1.0**	1/2	piece	Meat/Fish/Poultry
Chicken, Fried, Lowfat, Nutripoint Recipe	**3.0**	4	wt oz	Meat/Fish/Poultry
Chicken, Fried, w/Corn, Frozen, Morton	**0.5**	1/2	portion	Meat/Fish/Poultry
Chicken, Frozen Dinner	**1.5**	1/2	portion	Meat/Fish/Poultry
Chicken, Grilled w/Mango Sauce, Nutripoint Recipe	**4.5**	4	wt oz	Meat/Fish/Poultry
Chicken, Imperial, Frozen, Chun King	**3.0**	1/2	portion	Meat/Fish/Poultry
Chicken, Land O' Frost	**-5.0**	3	wt oz	Meat/Fish/Poultry
Chicken, Lemon, Nutripoint Recipe	**3.5**	4	wt oz	Meat/Fish/Poultry
Chicken, Lemongrass, Fzn, Lean Cuisine	**2.0**	1	serving	Meat/Fish/Poultry
Chicken, Low Cal, Frozen Dinner	**2.5**	1/2	portion	Meat/Fish/Poultry
Chicken, Mandarin, Slim, Fzn, Budget Gourmet	**1.0**	1	portion	Meat/Fish/Poultry
Chicken, Marinated Hawaiian, Nutripoint Recipe	**3.5**	4	wt oz	Meat/Fish/Poultry
Chicken, Parmesan w/Garden Veg, Fzn, Weight Watchers	**0.0**	1	serving	Meat/Fish/Poultry
Chicken, Pie, Frozen, Morton	**-0.5**	1/2	pie	Meat/Fish/Poultry
Chicken, Roasted w/Vegetables, Uncle Ben's	**1.5**	1	serving	Meat/Fish/Poultry
Chicken, Slices, Frozen, Loma Linda Foods	**5.5**	2	wt oz	Legume/Nut/Seed
Chicken, Smoked Sliced, Buddig	**-1.5**	3	wt oz	Meat/Fish/Poultry
Chicken, Southern Fried Patty, Fzn, Weight Watchers	**-2.0**	1/2	portion	Meat/Fish/Poultry
Chicken, Sweet & Sour, Fzn, Healthy Choice	**3.0**	1	portion	Meat/Fish/Poultry
Chicken, Sweet & Sour, w/Rice, Fzn, Budget Gourmet	**0.5**	1/2	portion	Meat/Fish/Poultry
Chicken, Sweet and Sour	**1.0**	1/2	cup	Meat/Fish/Poultry
Chicken, Vegetables w/Vermicelli, Frozen, Stouffer's	**2.0**	1	portion	Meat/Fish/Poultry
Chicken, Veggie, Italian Marinara	**2.0**	1	piece	Legume/Nut/Seed
Chicken, w/Fettucini, Fzn, Budget Gourmet	**-1.0**	1/2	portion	Meat/Fish/Poultry
Chicken, White and Dark, Premium Chunk, Canned, Swanson	**0.0**	4	wt oz	Meat/Fish/Poultry

Food Name—Alphabetical	Nutripoints	Serving Size		Nutrigroup
Chic-ketts, Meatless, Worthington	3.0	2	wt oz	Legume/Nut/Seed
Chicory Greens, Raw	35.5	1	cup	Vegetable
Chik Nuggets, Meatless, Loma Linda	3.5	5	pieces	Legume/Nut/Seed
Chili Powder	2.0	1	tsp	Condiment
Chili Seasoning Mix, McCormick's	0.5	1	tsp	Condiment
Chili w/Beans, Spicy Vegetarian, Health Valley	3.0	1	cup	Legume/Nut/Seed
Chili w/Lentils, Vegetarian, Health Valley	3.0	1/2	cup	Legume/Nut/Seed
Chili, Bean	5.0	1/2	cup	Legume/Nut/Seed
Chili, Bean/Beef	1.0	1/2	cup	Legume/Nut/Seed
Chili, Meatless, Lowfat, Worthington	4.0	1	cup	Legume/Nut/Seed
Chili, South/Border Vegetarian, Nutripoint Recipe	13.0	3/4	cup	Legume/Nut/Seed
Chili, Vegetarian Burrito Flavor, Health Valley	4.5	1	cup	Legume/Nut/Seed
Chili, Vegetarian Low Fat Texas Style, Health Valley	3.0	1/3	cup	Legume/Nut/Seed
Chili, Vegetarian, Canned, Worthington	4.0	1/2	cup	Legume/Nut/Seed
Chili, Vegetarian, Health Valley Fat Free	11.5	1/2	cup	Legume/Nut/Seed
Chili, Vegetarian, Natural Touch	1.5	1	cup	Legume/Nut/Seed
Chili, Vegetarian, Worthington	2.0	1/2	cup	Legume/Nut/Seed
Chili, Vegetarian, ZonePerfect	3.0	1/2	serving	Legume/Nut/Seed
Chives, Raw	1.0	1	tsp	Condiment
Chlorella (powder or w/water -- standard quantity for powder)	14.5	3	wt oz	Miscellaneous
Chocolate Éclair	-2.0	1/2	éclair	Grain
Chocolate Éclair, Good Humor	-3.5	1	piece	Grain
Chocolate, Baking	-4.0	1	wt oz	Sugar
Chocolate, Hot	0.0	1	cup	Milk/Dairy
Chocolate, Semi-Sweet	-4.5	1	wt oz	Sugar
Chocolate, Semi-Sweet, Baker's	-4.5	1	wt oz	Sugar
Chocolate, Sweet or Dark	-4.5	1	wt oz	Sugar
Chocolate, Unsweetened, Baker's	-3.0	1	wt oz	Sugar
Chop Suey, Beef/Pork	0.5	1/2	cup	Meat/Fish/Poultry
Cinnamon	1.0	1	tsp	Condiment
Clams, Breaded, Fried	4.5	3	wt oz	Meat/Fish/Poultry
Clams, Canned	8.0	1	cup	Meat/Fish/Poultry
Clams, Fried, Light Batter, Mrs. Paul's	-1.0	3	wt oz	Meat/Fish/Poultry
Clams, Mixed Species, Raw	13.5	6	wt oz	Meat/Fish/Poultry
Clams, Smoked, Canned In Oil	5.0	3	wt oz	Meat/Fish/Poultry
Clams, Steamed/Boiled	6.0	6	wt oz	Meat/Fish/Poultry
Cloves	0.5	1	tsp	Condiment
Club Soda	0.0	6	fl oz	Miscellaneous
Cocoa Mix, Chocolate, Quik, Nestle	-2.0	1/2	cup	Milk/Dairy
Cocoa Mix, Hot, 70 Calorie, Carnation	1.0	1	cup	Milk/Dairy
Cocoa Mix, Hot, Regular, Swiss Miss	-1.5	1	cup	Milk/Dairy
Cocoa Mix, Hot, Sugar Free, Carnation	3.0	2	cup	Milk/Dairy

Food Name—Alphabetical	Nutripoints	Serving Size		Nutrigroup
Cocoa Mix, Hot, Sugar-Free, Swiss Miss	**4.0**	1	wt oz	Milk/Dairy
Cocoa Mix, Ovaltine, Chocolate Flavor	**4.0**	1/2	cup	Milk/Dairy
Cocoa Mix, Sugar Free, Quik, Nestle	**2.5**	1	cup	Milk/Dairy
Cocoa Powder	**0.5**	1	Tbls	Miscellaneous
Coconut	**-2.0**	1	Tbls	Fruit
Coconut, Chocolate-Covered	**-2.0**	1	piece	Fruit
Coconut, Dried, Sweetened, Shredded	**-4.0**	1	Tbls	Fruit
Coconut, Raw	**-3.5**	1	wt oz	Fruit
Coconut, Shredded Premium, Baker's	**-3.5**	1	Tbls	Fruit
Cod Fillets, Light, Mrs. Paul's	**-0.5**	1	portion	Meat/Fish/Poultry
Cod, Baked	**3.5**	4	wt oz	Meat/Fish/Poultry
Cod, Floured/Breaded, Fried	**-0.5**	3	wt oz	Meat/Fish/Poultry
Cod, Smoked	**2.0**	6	wt oz	Meat/Fish/Poultry
Coffee	**-4.0**	1	cup	Miscellaneous
Coffee, Caffe' Latte, Starbuck's	**-5.0**	12	fl oz	Miscellaneous
Coffee, Caffe' Mocha, Starbuck's	**-5.0**	12	fl oz	Miscellaneous
Coffee, Caffe' Vanilla, Frappuccino Light, Starbuck's	**-4.0**	12	fl oz	Miscellaneous
Coffee, Cappuccino, Starbuck's	**-5.0**	12	fl oz	Miscellaneous
Coffee, Decaffeinated	**0.5**	1	cup	Miscellaneous
Coffee, Frappuccino, Starbuck's	**-4.5**	9.5	fl oz	Miscellaneous
Coffee, International	**-10.0**	1	tsp	Miscellaneous
Coffee, Mocha Frappuccino, Starbuck's	**-5.5**	12	fl oz	Miscellaneous
Coleslaw	**3.0**	1/2	cup	Vegetable
Coleslaw, Bavarian, Nutripoint Recipe	**10.0**	1/2	cup	Vegetable
Collard Greens, Fresh, Cooked	**42.0**	1	cup	Vegetable
Collard Greens, Frozen, Cooked	**40.0**	1/2	cup	Vegetable
Collard Greens, Raw, Chopped	**42.5**	1	cup	Vegetable
Combination Dinner, Frozen, Patio	**-0.5**	1/2	portion	Legume/Nut/Seed
Consommé	**0.5**	1	cup	Miscellaneous
Cookie Dough, Chocolate Chip, Pillsbury	**-3.5**	2	pieces	Grain
Cookies	**-4.0**	2	cookies	Grain
Cookies, Animal, Oat Bran, Health Valley	**4.0**	10	cookies	Grain
Cookies, Applesauce	**-2.0**	2	cookies	Grain
Cookies, Bordeaux, Pepperidge Farm	**-4.0**	3	cookies	Grain
Cookies, Buttercup, Keebler	**-2.0**	4	cookies	Grain
Cookies, Chessmen, Pepperidge Farm	**-4.0**	3	cookies	Grain
Cookies, Chips Deluxe, Keebler	**-3.0**	2	cookies	Grain
Cookies, Chocolate Chip	**-4.0**	2	cookies	Grain
Cookies, Chocolate Chip Oatmeal, Pillsbury	**-3.5**	1	cookies	Grain
Cookies, Chocolate Chip, Duncan Hines	**-3.5**	2	cookies	Grain
Cookies, Chocolate Chip, Pepperidge Farm	**-4.0**	3	cookies	Grain
Cookies, Chocolate Fudge Sandwich, Keebler	**-1.5**	2	cookies	Grain
Cookies, Commodore, Keebler	**0.0**	2	cookies	Grain

Food Name—Alphabetical	Nutripoints	Serving Size		Nutrigroup
Cookies, Fat-Free, Health Valley (all flavors)	**2.5**	3	cookies	Grain
Cookies, French Vanilla Creme, Keebler	**-1.5**	2	cookies	Grain
Cookies, Fruit Chunks, Health Valley	**3.0**	3	cookies	Grain
Cookies, Homeplate, Keebler	**-2.0**	2	cookies	Grain
Cookies, Keebies, Keebler	**-1.5**	2	cookies	Grain
Cookies, Lemon Creme, Keebler	**-1.5**	4	cookies	Grain
Cookies, Macaroon	**-2.0**	2	cookies	Grain
Cookies, Milano Distinctive, Pepperidge Farm	**-3.5**	3	cookies	Grain
Cookies, Molasses	**-2.0**	2	cookies	Grain
Cookies, Nilla Wafers	**-1.5**	7	cookies	Grain
Cookies, O.F. Chocolate Chip, Keebler	**-2.0**	2	cookies	Grain
Cookies, O.F. Double Fudge, Keebler	**-2.0**	2	cookies	Grain
Cookies, O.F. Granola, Large, Pepperidge Farm	**-3.0**	1	cookies	Grain
Cookies, O.F. Oatmeal, Keebler	**-1.5**	2	cookies	Grain
Cookies, O.F. Sugar, Keebler	**-1.5**	2	cookies	Grain
Cookies, Oatmeal	**-1.5**	2	cookies	Grain
Cookies, Oatmeal Cremes Sandwich, Keebler	**-2.5**	2	cookies	Grain
Cookies, Oatmeal Raisin, Pepperidge Farm	**-3.0**	3	cookies	Grain
Cookies, Oreo	**-2.5**	2	cookies	Grain
Cookies, Peanut Butter	**-1.0**	2	cookies	Legume/Nut/Seed
Cookies, Peanut Butter'n Fudge, Duncan Hines	**-3.5**	2	cookies	Grain
Cookies, Pirouettes, Chocolate-Laced, Pepperidge Farm	**-4.5**	3	cookies	Grain
Cookies, Pitter Patter, Keebler	**-1.5**	2	cookies	Grain
Cookies, Sandwich, Chocolate/Vanilla	**-2.5**	2	cookies	Grain
Cookies, Sandwich, Mystic Mint	**-4.0**	2	cookies	Grain
Cookies, Sugar	**-1.0**	1	cookies	Grain
Cookies, Vanilla Wafer	**-3.0**	6	cookies	Grain
Cookies, Vanilla Wafers, Keebler	**-1.5**	5	cookies	Grain
Cordials/liqueurs	**-8.5**	1.5	fl oz	Alcohol
Coriander, Raw	**0.5**	1/2	cup	Condiment
Corn Cakes, Quaker	**2.5**	3	cakes	Grain
Corn Chips	**-0.5**	1	wt oz	Grain
Corn Chips, Fritos	**-1.0**	17	chips	Vegetable
Corn Chips, Pringles	**0.0**	11	chips	Grain
Corn Dog	**-1.0**	1/2	serving	Meat/Fish/Poultry
Corn Meal, Dry	**3.5**	1/4	cup	Grain
Corn Meal, Yellow Enriched, Aunt Jemima	**3.5**	1/4	cup	Grain
Corn On Cob, Fresh, Cooked	**6.0**	1/2	piece	Vegetable
Corn Puffs, Cheese, Cheez Doodles, Borden	**-1.5**	1	wt oz	Grain
Corn w/Red and Green Peppers, Canned	**5.0**	1/2	cup	Vegetable
Corn, 50% Less Salt, Canned, Green Giant	**3.0**	1/2	cup	Vegetable
Corn, Canned	**4.5**	1/2	cup	Vegetable

Food Name—Alphabetical	Nutripoints	Serving Size		Nutrigroup
Corn, Cream Style, Canned, Green Giant	**-0.5**	1/2	cup	Vegetable
Corn, Cream Style, Golden Sweet, Canned, Del Monte	**0.0**	1/2	cup	Vegetable
Corn, Creamed, Canned	**4.5**	1/2	cup	Vegetable
Corn, Fried w/Breading	**-0.5**	1/4	piece	Vegetable
Corn, Frozen, Cooked	**8.0**	1/2	cup	Vegetable
Corn, Golden, Family Style, No Salt, Canned, Del Monte	**6.0**	1/2	cup	Vegetable
Corn, Little Ears, Frozen, Birds Eye	**7.0**	1	piece	Vegetable
Corn, Niblets, In Butter, Frozen, Green Giant	**1.5**	1/2	cup	Vegetable
Corn, Sweet, Butter Sauce, Fzn, Budget Gourmet	**-0.5**	1/3	piece	Vegetable
Corn, Sweet, Frozen, Birds Eye	**6.0**	1/2	cup	Vegetable
Corn, Whole Kernel, Canned, Del Monte	**2.0**	1/2	cup	Vegetable
Corn, Whole Kernel, Canned, Green Giant	**2.5**	1/2	cup	Vegetable
Cornbread	**1.0**	1	piece	Grain
Cornbread, Southern, Nutripoint Recipe	**2.0**	1	piece	Grain
Corned Beef	**-2.5**	3	wt oz	Meat/Fish/Poultry
Corned Beef, Libby's	**-2.0**	3	wt oz	Meat/Fish/Poultry
Corned Beef, Smoked Sliced, Buddig	**-2.0**	3	wt oz	Meat/Fish/Poultry
Cornstarch	**0.0**	1	Tbls	Miscellaneous
Cowpeas, Cooked	**8.0**	1	cup	Legume/Nut/Seed
Crab Cake	**-3.5**	3	wt oz	Meat/Fish/Poultry
Crab Salad	**-1.0**	1/2	cup	Meat/Fish/Poultry
Crab, Canned	**1.0**	6	wt oz	Meat/Fish/Poultry
Crab, Hard-shell, Steamed	**4.5**	6	wt oz	Meat/Fish/Poultry
Crab, Soft Shell, Fried	**-1.0**	3	wt oz	Meat/Fish/Poultry
Cracker Meal, Keebler	**2.5**	1/4	cup	Grain
Cracker, 5-grain, Harvest Crisps, Nabisco	**2.0**	12	crackers	Grain
Cracker, 7 Grain Vegetable, Stoned Wheat, Health Valley	**1.0**	6	crackers	Grain
Cracker, Amaranth Graham, Health Valley	**1.0**	4	crackers	Grain
Cracker, Cheese & Peanut Butter, Keebler	**-0.5**	3	crackers	Grain
Cracker, Crispbread Breakfast, Wasa	**2.5**	2	crackers	Grain
Cracker, Crispbread Dark Rye, Ryvita	**3.0**	4	crackers	Grain
Cracker, Crispbread Dark, Finn	**2.5**	6	crackers	Grain
Cracker, Crispbread Fiber Plus, Wasa	**7.5**	3	crackers	Grain
Cracker, Crispbread Golden Rye, Wasa	**4.0**	3	crackers	Grain
Cracker, Crispbread Hearty Rye, Wasa	**3.5**	3	crackers	Grain
Cracker, Crispbread Light Natural, Krispen	**2.5**	8	crackers	Grain
Cracker, Crispbread Lite Rye, Wasa	**2.0**	4	crackers	Grain
Cracker, Fat Free, Premium Saltine, Nabisco	**2.5**	10	crackers	Grain
Cracker, Graham, Honey Maid	**0.5**	4	crackers	Grain
Cracker, Graham, Plain	**0.0**	2	crackers	Grain

Food Name—Alphabetical	Nutripoints	Serving Size		Nutrigroup
Cracker, Harvest Wheat, Keebler	**0.0**	6	crackers	Grain
Cracker, Hearty Wheat, Pepperidge Farm	**-1.0**	4	crackers	Grain
Cracker, Honey Graham, Health Valley	**1.5**	2	crackers	Grain
Cracker, Low Salt, Ritz	**0.5**	10	crackers	Grain
Cracker, Low Salt, Saltine, Nabisco	**1.5**	10	crackers	Grain
Cracker, Low Salt, Triscuit, Nabisco	**1.0**	6	crackers	Grain
Cracker, Matzo	**2.5**	1	cracker	Grain
Cracker, Melba Toast	**1.0**	4	crackers	Grain
Cracker, Melba Toast, Garlic, Keebler	**1.0**	10	crackers	Grain
Cracker, Melba Toast, Onion, Keebler	**1.0**	10	crackers	Grain
Cracker, Melba Toast, Plain, Keebler	**1.0**	10	crackers	Grain
Cracker, Melba Toast, Sesame, Keebler	**0.5**	10	crackers	Grain
Cracker, Melba Toast, White, Old London	**2.0**	6	crackers	Grain
Cracker, Norwegian Crispbread, Thick Style, Kavli	**2.5**	3	crackers	Grain
Cracker, Oat Bran Graham, Health Valley	**0.5**	7	crackers	Grain
Cracker, Oat Bran Krisp, Ralston	**1.0**	4	crackers	Grain
Cracker, Original Tiny Goldfish, Pepperidge Farm	**-1.0**	45	crackers	Grain
Cracker, Peanut Butter Sandwich	**0.0**	2	crackers	Legume/Nut/Seed
Cracker, Petite Butter Crescents, Pepperidge Farm	**-0.5**	1	cracker	Grain
Cracker, Rice Cake	**1.5**	4	crackers	Grain
Cracker, Rice, Small	**0.5**	10	crackers	Grain
Cracker, Ritz	**-1.0**	8	crackers	Grain
Cracker, Rykrisp, Ralston	**5.0**	6	crackers	Grain
Cracker, Saltine	**1.0**	8	crackers	Grain
Cracker, Saltine, Low Sodium	**1.0**	10	crackers	Grain
Cracker, Saltine, Nabisco	**1.5**	10	crackers	Grain
Cracker, Saltine, Premium	**0.5**	10	crackers	Grain
Cracker, Sea Toast, Keebler	**1.0**	2	crackers	Grain
Cracker, Seasoned, Rykrisp	**3.0**	6	crackers	Grain
Cracker, Snackbread, High Fiber Ryvita	**9.0**	8	crackers	Grain
Cracker, Soda	**0.5**	10	crackers	Grain
Cracker, Toast & Peanut Butter, Keebler	**-1.0**	4	crackers	Grain
Cracker, Triscuit	**-0.5**	6	crackers	Grain
Cracker, Wheat 'n Bran, Triscuit, Nabisco	**1.0**	6	crackers	Grain
Cracker, Wheat Thins	**-0.5**	16	crackers	Grain
Cracker, Wheat Vegetable, Stone ground, Hain	**1.0**	11	crackers	Grain
Cracker, Whole Wheat	**3.0**	8	crackers	Grain
Cracker, Whole Wheat, Ritz	**0.5**	10	crackers	Grain
Cracker, Whole Wheat, Saltine, Nabisco	**1.5**	10	crackers	Grain
Crackers, Animal	**-1.5**	10	crackers	Grain
Crackers, Animal, Barnum's	**-1.5**	10	crackers	Grain
Crackers, Cheese Nips	**0.5**	20	crackers	Grain
Crackers, Oat Thins, Nabisco	**0.5**	12	crackers	Grain

Food Name—Alphabetical	Nutripoints	Serving Size		Nutrigroup
Crackers, Oyster, Large, Keebler	**0.5**	26	crackers	Grain
Crackers, Oyster, Small	**1.0**	50	crackers	Grain
Crackers, Oyster, Small, Keebler	**1.0**	50	crackers	Grain
Crackers, Teddy Grahams, Nabisco	**0.5**	22	crackers	Grain
Crackers, TLC 7 Grain, Kashi	**0.0**	15	crackers	Grain
Crackers, Wheat Thins, Kraft	**-1.0**	1	wt oz	Grain
Crackers, Wheat Thins, Multi-Grain, Kraft	**-0.5**	1	wt oz	Grain
Cranberry, Raw	**10.0**	1	cup	Fruit
Cream, Coffee, Light	**-6.0**	2	Tbls	Milk/Dairy
Cream, Half and Half	**-3.0**	1/4	cup	Milk/Dairy
Cream, Heavy	**-7.0**	2	Tbls	Milk/Dairy
Cream, Non-Dairy, Coffee Mate, Carnation	**-3.5**	2	Tbls	Milk/Dairy
Cream, Non-Dairy, Cremora	**-4.5**	2	Tbls	Milk/Dairy
Cream, Non-Dairy, Imitation, Liquid	**-4.0**	2	Tbls	Milk/Dairy
Cream, Non-Dairy, Imitation, Liquid, Vegetable Oil	**-1.5**	2	Tbls	Milk/Dairy
Cream, Non-Dairy, Imitation, Powder	**-3.0**	2	Tbls	Milk/Dairy
Cream, Non-Dairy, Mocha Mix	**-2.0**	1/4	cup	Milk/Dairy
Cream, Sour	**-3.5**	1/4	cup	Milk/Dairy
Cream, Sour, Blend, Weight Watchers	**1.0**	1/4	cup	Milk/Dairy
Cream, Sour, Imitation	**-5.5**	2	Tbls	Milk/Dairy
Cream, Sour, Light, Dairy Blend, Land O'Lakes	**-1.5**	1/4	cup	Milk/Dairy
Cream, Sour, New Way, Nutripoint Recipe	**6.5**	1/4	cup	Milk/Dairy
Cream, Sour, Slender Choice	**-1.0**	1/4	cup	Milk/Dairy
Cream, Soy, Solait, Miller Farms	**-1.0**	4	fl oz	Legume/Nut/Seed
Cream, Whipped	**-6.5**	1/4	cup	Milk/Dairy
Cream, Whipping, Light	**-6.5**	2	Tbls	Milk/Dairy
Creamer, Non-Dairy, Fat-Free, Mocha Mix	**0.5**	2	Tbls	Miscellaneous
Cress, Garden, Cooked	**39.5**	1	cup	Vegetable
Crisco, Butter Flavored	**-3.0**	1	Tbls	Fat/Oil
Croissant	**-2.5**	1	whole	Grain
Croutons	**2.0**	1/2	cup	Grain
Croutons, Cheddar and Romano Cheese, Pepperidge Farm	**1.0**	1/2	cup	Grain
Cucumber, Raw	**20.0**	1	whole	Vegetable
Cupcake, Chocolate, Hostess	**-3.0**	1	piece	Grain
Cupcake, w/Frosting	**-4.0**	1	piece	Grain
Cupcake, w/o Frosting	**-3.5**	1	piece	Grain
Currants, Black	**19.0**	3/4	cup	Fruit
Currants, Red, Raw	**14.5**	3	wt oz	Fruit
Currants, Zante	**4.5**	1/4	cup	Fruit
Currants, Zante, Sun-Maid	**3.5**	1/4	cup	Fruit
Curry Powder	**0.5**	1	tsp	Condiment
Custard	**-4.0**	1/2	cup	Milk/Dairy

Food Name—Alphabetical	Nutripoints	Serving Size		Nutrigroup
Daiquiri	**-14.5**	3	fl oz	Alcohol
Dairy Queen All White Chicken Nuggets	**-0.5**	1	serving	Meat/Fish/Poultry
Dairy Queen Buster Bar	**-3.5**	1/4	bar	Milk/Dairy
Dairy Queen Chicken Breast Fillet	**0.0**	1/2	serving	Meat/Fish/Poultry
Dairy Queen Chicken Breast Fillet w/Cheese	**0.0**	1/2	serving	Meat/Fish/Poultry
Dairy Queen Chipper Sandwich	**-1.5**	1/4	serving	Milk/Dairy
Dairy Queen Cone - Medium	**-1.0**	1/2	serving	Milk/Dairy
Dairy Queen Dilly Bar	**-3.5**	1/2	bar	Milk/Dairy
Dairy Queen Dipped Cone - Medium	**-3.5**	1/2	serving	Milk/Dairy
Dairy Queen Double Hamburger	**0.5**	1/2	burger	Meat/Fish/Poultry
Dairy Queen Double Hamburger w/Cheese	**0.5**	1/2	burger	Meat/Fish/Poultry
Dairy Queen DQ Sandwich	**-2.5**	1	serving	Milk/Dairy
Dairy Queen Fish Fillet	**1.0**	1/2	serving	Meat/Fish/Poultry
Dairy Queen Fish Fillet w/Cheese	**1.0**	1/2	serving	Meat/Fish/Poultry
Dairy Queen Float	**-4.0**	1/2	cup	Milk/Dairy
Dairy Queen Freeze (1 Cup)	**-1.5**	1/4	serving	Milk/Dairy
Dairy Queen Frozen Dessert	**0.0**	4	wt oz	Milk/Dairy
Dairy Queen Fudge Nut Bar	**-2.0**	1/4	bar	Grain
Dairy Queen Heath Blizzard	**-1.5**	1/4	serving	Milk/Dairy
Dairy Queen Hot Dog	**-1.0**	1	serving	Meat/Fish/Poultry
Dairy Queen Hot Dog w/Cheese	**-1.5**	1/2	serving	Meat/Fish/Poultry
Dairy Queen Hot Dog w/Chili	**-1.0**	1/2	serving	Meat/Fish/Poultry
Dairy Queen Hounder	**-2.0**	1/2	serving	Meat/Fish/Poultry
Dairy Queen Hounder w/Cheese	**-2.0**	1/2	serving	Meat/Fish/Poultry
Dairy Queen Hounder w/Chili	**-1.5**	1/2	serving	Meat/Fish/Poultry
Dairy Queen Malt - Medium	**-1.5**	1/4	serving	Milk/Dairy
Dairy Queen Mr. Misty - Medium (1 Cup)	**-5.5**	1/2	cup	Sugar
Dairy Queen Mr. Misty Float	**-3.5**	1/2	serving	Milk/Dairy
Dairy Queen Mr. Misty Freeze	**-3.5**	1/4	serving	Milk/Dairy
Dairy Queen Mr. Misty Kiss (1/2 Cup)	**-5.5**	1	cup	Sugar
Dairy Queen Parfait	**-1.5**	1/4	serving	Milk/Dairy
Dairy Queen Peanut Buster Parfait	**-3.5**	1/4	serving	Milk/Dairy
Dairy Queen Shake - Medium	**-2.5**	1/4	serving	Milk/Dairy
Dairy Queen Single Hamburger	**0.5**	1/2	burger	Meat/Fish/Poultry
Dairy Queen Single Hamburger w/Cheese	**0.5**	1/2	burger	Meat/Fish/Poultry
Dairy Queen Sundae - Medium	**-2.5**	1/2	serving	Milk/Dairy
Dairy Queen Triple Hamburger	**0.0**	1/4	serving	Meat/Fish/Poultry
Dairy Queen Triple Hamburger w/Cheese	**0.0**	1/4	burger	Meat/Fish/Poultry
Dandelion Greens, Cooked	**40.0**	3/4	cup	Vegetable
Dandelion Greens, Raw	**44.5**	1	cup	Vegetable
Danish Pastry	**-2.5**	1/2	piece	Grain
Danish, Apple, Pillsbury	**-1.5**	1/2	piece	Grain
Dates	**4.0**	5	pieces	Fruit

Food Name—Alphabetical	Nutripoints	Serving Size		Nutrigroup
Del Taco Big Fat Chicken Taco	**3.0**	1	taco	Meat/Fish/Poultry
Del Taco Big Fat Steak Taco	**2.0**	1	taco	Meat/Fish/Poultry
Del Taco Big Fat Taco	**2.0**	1/2	taco	Legume/Nut/Seed
Del Taco Carnitas Burrito	**1.5**	1/2	serving	Meat/Fish/Poultry
Del Taco Carnitas Taco	**2.0**	1	taco	Legume/Nut/Seed
Del Taco Cheddar Quesadilla	**0.5**	1/2	serving	Milk/Dairy
Del Taco Chicken Cheddar Quesadilla	**0.0**	1/2	serving	Meat/Fish/Poultry
Del Taco Chicken Soft Taco	**3.5**	1	taco	Meat/Fish/Poultry
Del Taco Chicken Works Burrito	**1.5**	1/2	serving	Meat/Fish/Poultry
Del Taco Crispy Fish Taco	**1.0**	1	taco	Meat/Fish/Poultry
Del Taco Del Beef Burrito	**0.5**	1/2	serving	Meat/Fish/Poultry
Del Taco Del Classic Chicken Burrito	**1.0**	1/2	serving	Meat/Fish/Poultry
Del Taco Del Combo Burrito	**2.0**	1/2	serving	Meat/Fish/Poultry
Del Taco Deluxe Chicken Salad	**3.0**	1/4	serving	Meat/Fish/Poultry
Del Taco Deluxe Del Beef Burrito	**1.0**	1/2	serving	Meat/Fish/Poultry
Del Taco Deluxe Taco Salad	**2.0**	1/4	serving	Legume/Nut/Seed
Del Taco Half Pound Red or Green Burrito	**3.5**	1/2	serving	Legume/Nut/Seed
Del Taco Macho Beef Burrito	**1.0**	1/4	serving	Meat/Fish/Poultry
Del Taco Macho Chicken Burrito	**2.5**	1/3	serving	Meat/Fish/Poultry
Del Taco Macho Combo Burrito	**2.0**	1/4	serving	Meat/Fish/Poultry
Del Taco Macho Nachos	**0.5**	1/4	serving	Grain
Del Taco Red or Green Bean/Cheese Burrito	**3.0**	1	serving	Legume/Nut/Seed
Del Taco Regular Taco	**2.0**	1	taco	Legume/Nut/Seed
Del Taco Regular Taco Salad	**0.5**	1/2	serving	Legume/Nut/Seed
Del Taco Soft Taco	**2.5**	1	taco	Legume/Nut/Seed
Del Taco Spicy Chicken Burrito	**2.0**	1/2	serving	Meat/Fish/Poultry
Del Taco Steak Del Carbon Taco	**1.5**	1	taco	Meat/Fish/Poultry
Del Taco Steak Works Burrito	**1.0**	1/2	serving	Meat/Fish/Poultry
Del Taco Ultimate Taco	**0.5**	1	taco	Legume/Nut/Seed
Del Taco Veggie Works Burrito	**3.0**	1/2	serving	Legume/Nut/Seed
Dill Weed	**0.5**	1	tsp	Condiment
Dip, Bean	**3.5**	2	Tbls	Legume/Nut/Seed
Dip, Bean, Black, Nutripoint Recipe	**8.0**	1/4	cup	Legume/Nut/Seed
Dip, Clam	**-0.5**	2	Tbls	Fat/Oil
Dip, Onion	**-5.0**	1	Tbls	Fat/Oil
Dip, Slim Guacamole, Nutripoint Recipe	**7.5**	1/4	cup	Fat/Oil
Domino's Large 16" Cheese Pizza	**1.5**	1	piece	Grain
Domino's Large 16" Deluxe Pizza	**0.5**	1/2	piece	Grain
Domino's Large 16" Double Cheese/Pepperoni Pizza	**0.5**	1/2	piece	Grain
Domino's Large 16" Ham Pizza	**1.0**	1/2	piece	Grain
Domino's Large 16" Pepperoni Pizza	**1.0**	1/2	piece	Grain
Domino's Large 16" Sausage/Mushroom Pizza	**1.5**	1/2	piece	Grain

Food Name—Alphabetical	Nutripoints	Serving Size		Nutrigroup
Domino's Large 16" Veggie Pizza	**1.0**	1/2	piece	Grain
Doughnut, Cake w/Frosting	**-2.5**	1	piece	Grain
Doughnut, Cake w/o Frosting	**-2.0**	1	piece	Grain
Doughnut, Chocolate Creme Filled	**-3.0**	1/2	piece	Grain
Doughnut, Chocolate Iced Kreme Filled, Krispy Kreme	**-3.0**	1	whole	Grain
Doughnut, Chocolate, w/ Chocolate Icing	**-2.5**	1/2	piece	Grain
Doughnut, Custard Filled	**-3.0**	1/2	piece	Grain
Doughnut, Devil's Food, Earth Grains	**-3.0**	1/2	piece	Grain
Doughnut, Glazed	**-2.5**	1	whole	Grain
Doughnut, Jelly	**-3.0**	1/2	piece	Grain
Doughnut, Old Fashioned, Glazed, Earth Grains	**-3.0**	1/2	piece	Grain
Doughnut, Original Glazed, Krispy Kreme	**-2.5**	1	whole	Grain
Doughnut, Powdered Strawberry Filled, Krispy Kreme	**-2.0**	1	whole	Grain
Doughnut, Traditional Cake, Krispy Kreme	**-2.5**	1	whole	Grain
Doughnut, Whole Wheat	**-1.5**	1	whole	Grain
Dressing, Blue Cheese	**-3.0**	2	Tbls	Fat/Oil
Dressing, Blue Cheese, Nutripoint Recipe	**8.0**	1/4	cup	Fat/Oil
Dressing, Caper, Nutripoint Recipe	**2.0**	2	Tbls	Fat/Oil
Dressing, French	**-3.0**	2	Tbls	Fat/Oil
Dressing, French, Catalina, Kraft	**-2.0**	1	Tbls	Fat/Oil
Dressing, French, Free, Kraft	**-1.0**	2	Tbls	Condiment
Dressing, French, Home Recipe	**-3.0**	1	Tbls	Fat/Oil
Dressing, French, Kraft	**-2.5**	1	Tbls	Fat/Oil
Dressing, Green Goddess	**-3.0**	2	Tbls	Fat/Oil
Dressing, Honey Yogurt, Nutripoint Recipe	**2.0**	1/4	cup	Milk/Dairy
Dressing, Italian	**-2.5**	2	Tbls	Fat/Oil
Dressing, Italian, Free, Kraft	**-0.5**	2	Tbls	Condiment
Dressing, Italian, Light, Bernstein's	**-0.5**	1	Tbls	Condiment
Dressing, Lite Italian, Wish-Bone	**-0.5**	1	Tbls	Fat/Oil
Dressing, Lite Red French, Wish-Bone	**0.0**	1	Tbls	Fat/Oil
Dressing, Lite, 16 Island, Nutripoint Recipe	**2.5**	1/4	cup	Fat/Oil
Dressing, Lite, Ranch, Nutripoint Recipe	**3.5**	1/4	cup	Fat/Oil
Dressing, Lite, Zero, Nutripoint Recipe	**1.0**	2	Tbls	Condiment
Dressing, Low Cal, Blue Cheese	**-4.5**	2	Tbls	Fat/Oil
Dressing, Low Cal, French	**-1.5**	2	Tbls	Fat/Oil
Dressing, Mayonnaise Type	**-2.5**	1	Tbls	Fat/Oil
Dressing, Mustard, Spicy, Nutripoint Recipe	**0.5**	1	Tbls	Condiment
Dressing, Non-Fat, Healthy Sensation (all flavors)	**0.0**	1	Tbls	Fat/Oil
Dressing, Non-Fat, Kraft Free (all flavors)	**-0.5**	1	Tbls	Fat/Oil
Dressing, Non-Fat, Take Heart, Hidden Valley (all flavors)	**-0.5**	1	Tbls	Fat/Oil

Food Name—Alphabetical	Nutripoints	Serving Size		Nutrigroup
Dressing, Oil & Vinegar	**-3.0**	1	Tbls	Fat/Oil
Dressing, Oil & Vinegar, Kraft	**-3.5**	1	Tbls	Fat/Oil
Dressing, Ranch, Free, Kraft	**-0.5**	2	Tbls	Condiment
Dressing, Ranch, Take Heart, Hidden Valley	**-1.0**	2	Tbls	Condiment
Dressing, Ranch/Buttermilk	**-3.0**	2	Tbls	Fat/Oil
Dressing, Russian	**-2.5**	2	Tbls	Fat/Oil
Dressing, Russian, Low Cal	**-0.5**	2	Tbls	Fat/Oil
Dressing, Salad	**-3.5**	2	Tbls	Fat/Oil
Dressing, Salad, Low Cal	**-1.0**	2	Tbls	Fat/Oil
Dressing, Salad, Miracle Whip, Kraft	**-3.0**	1	Tbls	Fat/Oil
Dressing, Salad, Reduced Cal, Miracle Whip	**-3.5**	1	Tbls	Fat/Oil
Dressing, Thousand Island	**-3.0**	2	Tbls	Fat/Oil
Dressing, Thousand Island, Low Cal	**-2.5**	2	Tbls	Fat/Oil
Dressing, Vinaigrette, Lite, Nutripoint Recipe	**-1.5**	2	Tbls	Fat/Oil
Dressing, Vinaigrette, Orange, Nutripoint Recipe	**2.5**	2	Tbls	Fat/Oil
Dressing, Yogurt	**0.5**	2	Tbls	Milk/Dairy
Drink Mix, Grape, Sugar-Free, Kool-Aid	**2.0**	8	fl oz	Miscellaneous
Drink Mix, Orange, Sugar Free, Crystal Light	**1.0**	8	fl oz	Miscellaneous
Drink Mix, Rainbow Punch, Sweetened, Kool-Aid	**-4.0**	8	fl oz	Sugar
Drink Mix, Strawberry, Sweetened, Kool-Aid	**-5.0**	8	fl oz	Sugar
Drink Mix, Tropical Punch, Sugar Free, Kool-Aid	**1.5**	8	fl oz	Miscellaneous
Duck, Baked, w/o Skin	**1.5**	3	wt oz	Meat/Fish/Poultry
Duck, Meat and Skin, Baked	**-1.0**	3	wt oz	Meat/Fish/Poultry
Eel	**1.5**	3	wt oz	Meat/Fish/Poultry
Eel, Smoked	**1.5**	3	wt oz	Meat/Fish/Poultry
Egg Foo Young	**-7.0**	1/2	cup	Milk/Dairy
Egg Noodles, Cooked (1.125 C=2 wt oz Dry)	**1.5**	1/2	cup	Grain
Egg Noodles, Creamette, Borden	**-2.0**	1/2	cup	Grain
Egg Roll	**-1.5**	1/2	piece	Grain
Egg Rolls, Chicken, Frozen, Chun King	**0.0**	1	portion	Meat/Fish/Poultry
Egg Rolls, Restaurant, Frozen, Chun King	**2.0**	1	portion	Meat/Fish/Poultry
Egg Rolls, Shrimp, Frozen, Chun King	**0.0**	1	portion	Meat/Fish/Poultry
Egg Rolls, Shrimp/Meat, Frozen, Chun King	**-0.5**	1	portion	Meat/Fish/Poultry
Egg Salad	**-9.0**	1/4	cup	Milk/Dairy
Egg Substitute, Better 'n Eggs	**23.5**	1/4	cup	Milk/Dairy
Egg Substitute, Egg Beaters, Cheez, Fleischmann's	**6.0**	4	wt oz	Milk/Dairy
Egg Substitute, Egg Beaters, Fleischmann's	**17.5**	1/2	cup	Milk/Dairy
Egg Substitute, Egg Beaters, Vegetable Omelette Mix, Fleischmann's	**13.5**	1/2	cup	Milk/Dairy
Egg Substitute, Egg Watchers, Tofutti	**10.0**	1/2	cup	Milk/Dairy
Egg Substitute, Scramblers	**10.0**	1/2	cup	Milk/Dairy
Egg Substitute, Second Nature	**4.5**	1/2	cup	Milk/Dairy
Egg Whites	**6.0**	6	eggs	Milk/Dairy

Food Name—Alphabetical	Nutripoints	Serving Size		Nutrigroup
Egg Yolk	**-15.0**	2	eggs	Milk/Dairy
Egg, Boiled	**-11.5**	2	eggs	Milk/Dairy
Egg, Devilled	**-10.5**	1	piece	Milk/Dairy
Egg, Fried	**-12.5**	1	egg	Milk/Dairy
Egg, Hard	**-11.5**	2	eggs	Milk/Dairy
Egg, Omelet, w/Ham/Cheese (1 Pc=3 Eggs)	**-8.0**	1/2	egg	Milk/Dairy
Egg, Poached	**-11.5**	2	eggs	Milk/Dairy
Egg, Scrambled	**-13.5**	1	egg	Milk/Dairy
Egg, Scrambled, Garden, Egg Beaters, Nutripoint Recipe	**23.5**	3/4	cup	Milk/Dairy
Egg, Scrambled, Garden, Nutripoint Recipe	**5.5**	3/4	cup	Milk/Dairy
Eggnog	**-2.0**	1/2	cup	Milk/Dairy
Eggplant Parmigiana, Frozen, Celentano	**3.0**	1/4	portion	Vegetable
Eggplant Rollettes, Frozen, Celentano	**4.0**	1/4	portion	Vegetable
Eggplant, Cooked	**17.0**	1/2	cup	Vegetable
Elderberry, Raw	**12.0**	3	wt oz	Fruit
Enchiladas Ranchero, Cheese, Fzn, Weight Watchers	**-1.0**	1/2	portion	Milk/Dairy
Enchiladas Suiza, Chicken, Van de Kamp's	**-1.0**	1	portion	Meat/Fish/Poultry
Enchiladas, Bean/Cheese	**0.0**	1/2	serving	Legume/Nut/Seed
Enchiladas, Beef Dinner, Frozen, Patio	**-0.5**	1/2	portion	Meat/Fish/Poultry
Enchiladas, Beef Ranchero, Fzn, Weight Watchers	**0.0**	1/2	portion	Meat/Fish/Poultry
Enchiladas, Beef, Shredded, Van de Kamp's	**-2.5**	1	portion	Meat/Fish/Poultry
Enchiladas, Beef/Cheese	**4.0**	1/2	serving	Legume/Nut/Seed
Enchiladas, Cheese Dinner, Frozen, Patio	**1.0**	1/2	portion	Milk/Dairy
Enchiladas, Cheese Ranchero, Fzn, Weight Watchers	**-0.5**	1/2	portion	Milk/Dairy
Enchiladas, Cheese Ranchero, Van de Kamp's	**-1.0**	1/3	portion	Legume/Nut/Seed
Enchiladas, Chicken w/Sour Cream Sauce	**0.5**	1/2	serving	Legume/Nut/Seed
Enchiladas, Chicken, Nutripoint Recipe	**5.0**	2	pieces	Meat/Fish/Poultry
Enchiladas, Chicken, Suiza, Fzn, Weight Watchers	**-0.5**	1/2	portion	Meat/Fish/Poultry
Enchiladas, Chicken, Suiza, Slim, Budget Gourmet	**0.5**	1	portion	Meat/Fish/Poultry
Enchiladas, Mexican, Legume	**5.5**	1/2	portion	Legume/Nut/Seed
Enchiladas, Sirloin, Ranchero, Slim, Budget Gourmet	**1.0**	1	portion	Meat/Fish/Poultry
Endive, Raw	**1.0**	1/4	cup	Condiment
Energy Bites, Power Bar	**21.0**	1	serving	Grain
Energy Drink, AMP, Pepsi	**-4.5**	8	fl oz	Fruit
Energy Drink, Red Bull	**10.0**	8	fl oz	Sugar
Energy Drink, SoBe No Fear	**8.5**	8	fl oz	Sugar
Energy Gel, GU	**5.5**	1	serving	Sugar
Fajita, Beef	**1.5**	1	serving	Meat/Fish/Poultry
Fajita, Beef, Weight Watchers	**0.5**	1/2	portion	Meat/Fish/Poultry

Food Name—Alphabetical	Nutripoints	Serving Size		Nutrigroup
Fajita, Chicken	1.0	1	serving	Meat/Fish/Poultry
Fajita, Chicken, Frozen, Weight Watchers	0.5	1	portion	Meat/Fish/Poultry
Farina, Cooked	2.5	1	cup	Grain
Fat, Beef Tallow	-6.5	1	Tbls	Fat/Oil
Fat, Chicken	-4.0	1	Tbls	Fat/Oil
Fat, Duck	-4.5	1	Tbls	Fat/Oil
Fat, Goose	-4.0	1	Tbls	Fat/Oil
Fat, Mutton Tallow	-5.5	1	Tbls	Fat/Oil
Fat, Turkey	-4.5	1	Tbls	Fat/Oil
Fettuccini Primavera, Frozen, Stouffer's	-2.0	1/2	portion	Grain
Fettuccini, Chicken, Frozen, Weight Watchers	-1.0	1/2	serving	Grain
Fettuccini, Cooked (1 C=2 wt oz Dry)	1.0	1/2	cup	Grain
Fettuccini, Garden Gourmet, Fzn, Green Giant	2.5	1/2	cup	Grain
Fettucini, w/Meat Sauce, Slim, Fzn, Budget Gourmet	1.5	1/2	portion	Grain
Fiesta Dinner, Frozen, Patio	0.0	1/2	portion	Legume/Nut/Seed
Fig Newton	-2.0	2	pieces	Grain
Figs, Calimyrna, Sun-Maid	4.0	2	whole	Fruit
Figs, Dried	5.0	2	whole	Fruit
Figs, Fresh	4.0	1	whole	Fruit
Figs, Mission, Sun-Maid	4.5	2	whole	Fruit
Filberts, Dry Roasted, Salted	-1.0	1	wt oz	Legume/Nut/Seed
Filberts, Oil Roasted, Salted	0.5	1	wt oz	Legume/Nut/Seed
Fish Almondine, Frozen Dinner	-1.5	1	serving	Meat/Fish/Poultry
Fish Dinner, Frozen, Morton	2.0	1/2	portion	Meat/Fish/Poultry
Fish Fillet, Au Gratin, Fzn, Weight Watchers	0.5	1	portion	Meat/Fish/Poultry
Fish Fillet, Batter Dipped, Fzn, Mrs. Paul's	-1.0	1	portion	Meat/Fish/Poultry
Fish Fillet, Crispy Crunchy, Fzn, Mrs. Paul's	-1.5	1	whole	Meat/Fish/Poultry
Fish Fillet, Divan, Frozen, Stouffer's	1.5	1	portion	Meat/Fish/Poultry
Fish Fillet, Florentine, Frozen, Stouffer's	-0.5	1	whole	Meat/Fish/Poultry
Fish Fillet, Light Recipe, Frozen, Gorton's	-1.0	4	wt oz	Meat/Fish/Poultry
Fish Sticks	0.5	4	pieces	Meat/Fish/Poultry
Fish Sticks, Crispy Crunchy, Mrs. Paul's	-1.5	3.75	wt oz	Meat/Fish/Poultry
Fish Sticks, Crunchy, Frozen, Mrs. Paul's	-1.0	4	wt oz	Meat/Fish/Poultry
Fish, Crunchy, Nutripoint Recipe	6.5	3	wt oz	Meat/Fish/Poultry
Fish, Fried	0.5	3	wt oz	Meat/Fish/Poultry
Fish, Herb Baked, Fzn, Healthy Choice	-0.5	1	serving	Meat/Fish/Poultry
Fish, Sandwich, Fast Food	1.0	1/2	whole	Meat/Fish/Poultry
Fish, Smoked	3.5	3	wt oz	Meat/Fish/Poultry
Fish, w/Chips, Frozen, Morton	2.0	1/2	portion	Meat/Fish/Poultry
Flounder Fillet, Light, Mrs. Paul's	-1.0	1	whole	Meat/Fish/Poultry
Flounder, Baked	3.5	3	wt oz	Meat/Fish/Poultry
Flounder, Fillet, Breaded, Fried	-0.5	3	wt oz	Meat/Fish/Poultry
Flour, All-Purpose Enriched, Pillsbury	3.0	1/4	cup	Grain
Flour, All-Purpose, Gold Medal	3.0	1/4	cup	Grain

Food Name—Alphabetical	Nutripoints	Serving Size		Nutrigroup
Flour, Ezekiel, Arrowhead Mills	**4.0**	1/4	cup	Grain
Flour, Potato	**5.5**	1/4	cup	Vegetable
Flour, Rye, Medium, Pillsbury	**2.5**	1/4	cup	Grain
Flour, Rye, Whole Grain	**4.0**	1/4	cup	Grain
Flour, Soybean	**2.5**	1/4	cup	Grain
Flour, Triticale, Whole, Arrowhead Mills	**3.5**	1/4	cup	Grain
Flour, White	**3.0**	1/4	cup	Grain
Flour, White, All-Purpose Plain, Martha	**3.0**	1/4	cup	Grain
Flour, Whole Buckwheat	**3.5**	1/4	cup	Grain
Flour, Whole Wheat	**6.0**	1/4	cup	Grain
Flour, Whole Wheat, Gold Medal	**5.5**	1/4	cup	Grain
Flour, Whole Wheat, Pillsbury	**3.5**	1/4	cup	Grain
Frankfurter, Ball Park	**-4.0**	1	serving	Meat/Fish/Poultry
Frankfurter, Beef	**-2.5**	1	serving	Meat/Fish/Poultry
Frankfurter, Beef, Armour	**-4.0**	1	serving	Meat/Fish/Poultry
Frankfurter, Beef, Ball Park	**-4.0**	2	wt oz	Meat/Fish/Poultry
Frankfurter, Beef, Eckrich	**-3.5**	1	serving	Meat/Fish/Poultry
Frankfurter, Beef, Oscar Mayer	**-3.5**	1	serving	Meat/Fish/Poultry
Frankfurter, Bryan	**-2.5**	1	serving	Meat/Fish/Poultry
Frankfurter, Chicken, Tyson	**-3.5**	1	serving	Meat/Fish/Poultry
Frankfurter, Chicken, w/Bun	**-1.0**	1	serving	Meat/Fish/Poultry
Frankfurter, Eckrich	**-3.5**	1	serving	Meat/Fish/Poultry
Frankfurter, Linketts, Loma Linda Foods	**14.0**	1	serving	Legume/Nut/Seed
Frankfurter, Original Brown & Serve, Beef, Swift	**-2.5**	1	serving	Meat/Fish/Poultry
Frankfurter, Original Brown & Serve, Pork, Swift	**-3.5**	1	serving	Meat/Fish/Poultry
Frankfurter, Oscar Mayer	**-3.0**	1	serving	Meat/Fish/Poultry
Frankfurter, Pork & Beef	**-3.5**	1	serving	Meat/Fish/Poultry
Frankfurter, Pork & Beef, w/Bun	**-0.5**	1/2	serving	Meat/Fish/Poultry
Frankfurter, Turkey	**-3.5**	1	serving	Meat/Fish/Poultry
Frankfurter, Vegetarian, Big Franks, Loma Linda	**3.5**	1	serving	Legume/Nut/Seed
Frankfurter, Vegetarian, Lowfat, Big Franks, Loma Linda	**4.5**	1	serving	Legume/Nut/Seed
Frankfurter, Vegetarian, Worthington	**1.0**	1	serving	Legume/Nut/Seed
Frankfurter, With Cheese, Oscar Mayer	**-3.0**	1	serving	Meat/Fish/Poultry
French Fries (18 Pc=.5 C)	**1.0**	4	pieces	Vegetable
French Toast	**-2.5**	1	piece	Grain
French Toast, Nutripoint Recipe	**0.5**	1 1/2	pieces	Grain
Fried Cheese Sticks	**-4.5**	4	pieces	Milk/Dairy
Frog Legs, Fried	**-2.0**	2	pieces	Meat/Fish/Poultry
Frosting	**-4.5**	2	Tbls	Sugar
Frosting, Chocolate	**-4.5**	2	Tbls	Sugar
Frozen Dessert, Banana, Creamy, Frozfruit	**-1.5**	1/2	cup	Fruit
Frozen Dessert, Banana, Pudding Pops, Jello	**-3.0**	1	bar	Fruit
Frozen Dessert, Chocolate, Pudding Pops, Jello	**-1.5**	1	bar	Milk/Dairy
Frozen Dessert, Creamsicle	**-4.0**	1	bar	Sugar
Frozen Dessert, Fruit Bar	**1.0**	1	bar	Fruit
Frozen Dessert, Fudgesicle	**0.5**	1	bar	Fruit

Food Name—Alphabetical	Nutripoints	Serving Size		Nutrigroup
Frozen Dessert, Fudgesicle, Sugar-Free, Good Humor	**2.0**	2	bars	Miscellaneous
Frozen Dessert, Lowfat, Tofutti	**-2.0**	1/2	cup	Legume/Nut/Seed
Frozen Dessert, Orange, Vitari Soft Serve	**4.5**	1/2	cup	Fruit
Frozen Dessert, Peach, Vitari Soft Serve	**6.5**	1/2	cup	Fruit
Frozen Dessert, Pineapple, Frozfruit	**-0.5**	1	bar	Fruit
Frozen Dessert, Popsicle	**-5.0**	2	pieces	Sugar
Frozen Dessert, Popsicle, Sugar-Free, Good Humor	**0.5**	2	bars	Miscellaneous
Frozen Dessert, Strawberry, Chunky, Frozfruit	**1.0**	1/2	cup	Fruit
Frozen Dessert, Strawberry, Vitari Soft Serve	**3.0**	1/2	cup	Fruit
Frozen Dessert, Vanilla, Lite Bar, Dove	**-2.0**	1	piece	Milk/Dairy
Frozen Dessert, Wild Berry, Vitari Soft Serve	**3.5**	1/2	cup	Fruit
Fruit and Nut Muffins	**3.5**	1	muffin	Grain
Fruit Bits, Dried, Sun-Maid	**3.5**	1	wt oz	Fruit
Fruit Cocktail, Canned, Heavy Syrup	**1.0**	1/2	cup	Fruit
Fruit Cocktail, Canned, Unsweetened	**10.0**	1/2	cup	Fruit
Fruit Cocktail, Hot, Nutripoint Recipe	**5.0**	1/2	cup	Fruit
Fruit Cocktail, Light Syrup, Del Monte	**2.5**	1/2	cup	Fruit
Fruit Cocktail, Light Syrup, Libby's	**2.5**	1/2	cup	Fruit
Fruit Drink Mix, Crystal Light (all flavors)	**2.0**	8	fl oz	Miscellaneous
Fruit Drink Mix, Wild Grape, Sugar Free, Wyler's	**1.0**	8	fl oz	Miscellaneous
Fruit Drink, Citrus Punch, Sunny Delite	**3.5**	6	fl oz	Fruit
Fruit Drink, Crangrape, Ocean Spray	**2.5**	6	fl oz	Fruit
Fruit Drink, Cranicot, Ocean Spray	**-1.5**	6	fl oz	Fruit
Fruit Drink, Five Alive, Minute Maid	**-2.0**	8	fl oz	Fruit
Fruit Drink, Fruit Juicy Red, Hawaiian Punch	**1.5**	6	fl oz	Fruit
Fruit Drink, Fuze Energize	**5.0**	8	fl oz	Fruit
Fruit Drink, Fuze Focus	**9.5**	8	fl oz	Fruit
Fruit Drink, Fuze Green Tea	**22.0**	8	fl oz	Fruit
Fruit Drink, Fuze Lemon AID	**6.5**	8	fl oz	Fruit
Fruit Drink, Fuze Refresh	**15.0**	8	fl oz	Fruit
Fruit Drink, Fuze Replenish	**18.0**	8	fl oz	Fruit
Fruit Drink, Fuze Vitaboost	**11.0**	8	fl oz	Fruit
Fruit Drink, Fuze White Tea	**26.5**	8	fl oz	Fruit
Fruit Drink, Grape, Frozen, Welchade	**0.0**	6	fl oz	Fruit
Fruit Drink, Grape, Hi-C	**1.5**	6	fl oz	Fruit
Fruit Drink, Guava, Ocean Spray	**3.0**	6	fl oz	Fruit
Fruit Drink, Hawaiian Punch	**-1.5**	6	fl oz	Fruit
Fruit Drink, Hawaiian Punch, Low Cal	**4.5**	8	fl oz	Fruit
Fruit Drink, Lemonade	**-4.5**	6	fl oz	Fruit
Fruit Drink, Limeade	**-3.0**	1	cup	Fruit
Fruit Drink, Orange, Capri Sun	**-5.5**	6	fl oz	Fruit
Fruit Drink, Punch, Capri Sun	**-5.5**	6	fl oz	Fruit
Fruit Drink, Snapple-A-Day Meal Replacement	**11.0**	6	fl oz	Fruit
Fruit Drink, SoBe Elixir 3C, Orange Carrot	**6.5**	8	fl oz	Fruit
Fruit Drink, SoBe Elixir 3C, Pomegranate Cranberry	**0.0**	8	fl oz	Fruit

Food Name—Alphabetical	Nutripoints	Serving Size		Nutrigroup
Fruit Drink, SoBe Lean	**5.5**	16	fl oz	Fruit
Fruit Drink, Strawberry Smoothie, Nutripoint Recipe	**13.0**	1	cup	Fruit
Fruit Drink, Sugar Added	**-1.5**	6	fl oz	Fruit
Fruit Drink, Sunrise Cooler, Nutripoint Recipe	**15.5**	1/2	cup	Fruit
Fruit Drink, Tang	**3.0**	6	fl oz	Sugar
Fruit Leather	**2.0**	1	wt oz	Fruit
Fruit Leather, With Sugar	**-2.0**	1	piece	Fruit
Fruit Platter, Fresh, Nutripoint Recipe	**16.5**	1/2	cup	Fruit
Fruit Salad Plate, Nutripoint Recipe	**14.5**	1/2	cup	Fruit
Fruit Salad, Fresh	**13.0**	1/2	cup	Fruit
Fruit Shake, Melaleuca Sustain	**4.0**	8	fl oz	Fruit
Fruit Slices, Fresh, Nutripoint Recipe	**20.0**	1	cup	Fruit
Fruit, Rainbow Compote, Nutripoint Recipe	**18.0**	1/2	cup	Fruit
Fruitcake	**-1.0**	1	piece	Grain
Fudge, Chocolate	**-5.5**	1	wt oz	Sugar
Fudge, Chocolate w/Nuts	**-3.5**	1	piece	Sugar
Fudge, Divinity	**-3.5**	1	piece	Sugar
Fudge, Peanut Butter	**-2.5**	1	piece	Sugar
Fudge, Vanilla	**-4.0**	1	piece	Sugar
Fudge, Vanilla, w/Nuts	**-3.5**	1	piece	Sugar
Garlic Powder	**0.5**	1	tsp	Condiment
Garlic, Raw	**0.5**	1	piece	Condiment
Gatorade	**-6.5**	2	cups	Sugar
Gazpacho	**1.5**	1	cup	Vegetable
Gelatin, Cherry Flavor, Jell-O	**-5.0**	1/2	cup	Fruit
Gelatin, Cherry, Sugar-Free, Jell-O	**1.0**	1	cup	Fruit
Gelatin, Holiday Dessert	**11.0**	1	cup	Fruit
Gelatin, Strawberry-Banana, Royal	**-4.0**	1/2	cup	Fruit
Gin	**-17.5**	2	fl oz	Alcohol
Gin and Tonic	**-11.0**	8	fl oz	Alcohol
Gin Rickey	**-15.5**	6	fl oz	Alcohol
Ginger	**0.5**	1	tsp	Condiment
Ginger Chicken Dinner, Cm	**6.0**	1	portion	Meat/Fish/Poultry
Ginger Snaps	**-1.0**	6	pieces	Sugar
Gingerbread	**0.0**	1	piece	Grain
Goat	**0.5**	3	wt oz	Meat/Fish/Poultry
Gold Cadillac	**-9.5**	2	fl oz	Alcohol
Goose, Meat and Skin, Baked	**0.0**	3	wt oz	Meat/Fish/Poultry
Goulash	**1.5**	1/2	cup	Vegetable
Graham Crumbs, Keebler	**-0.5**	1/4	cup	Grain
Granola	**0.0**	1/4	cup	Grain
Granola Bar	**-0.5**	1	bar	Grain
Granola Bar, Chewy Chocolate Chip, Quaker	**0.5**	1	bar	Grain
Granola Bar, Chewy Fruit & Nut, Jack La Lanne	**4.0**	1	bar	Grain
Granola Bar, Chewy Fruit, Quaker	**-1.5**	1	bar	Grain
Granola Bar, Chewy Honey & Oats, Quaker	**-1.0**	1	bar	Grain
Granola Bar, Chewy, Low-Fat, Quaker (all flavors)	**-1.5**	1	bar	Grain

Food Name—Alphabetical	Nutripoints	Serving Size		Nutrigroup
Granola Bar, Oats 'n Honey, Nature Valley	**-2.0**	1	bar	Grain
Granola Bar, w/Roasted Almonds, Nature Valley	**-1.5**	1	bar	Grain
Granola, Heartland	**1.0**	1/4	cup	Grain
Granola, Maple Nut, Arrowhead Mills	**1.5**	1/4	cup	Grain
Granola, No Sugar	**1.5**	1/4	cup	Grain
Grapefruit, Fresh	**13.0**	1/2	fruit	Fruit
Grapes, Raw	**4.5**	20	grapes	Fruit
Grasshopper	**-8.5**	2	fl oz	Alcohol
Gravy	**-2.5**	1/4	cup	Fat/Oil
Gravy Mix, Brown, French's	**-4.0**	1/4	cup	Fat/Oil
Gravy Mix, Chicken, McCormick's	**-4.5**	1/4	cup	Fat/Oil
Gravy Mix, Chicken, Prepared	**0.0**	1/4	cup	Fat/Oil
Gravy Mix, Chicken, Prepared w/Milk/Butter	**-2.5**	1/4	cup	Fat/Oil
Gravy Mix, Mushroom, French's	**-4.0**	1/4	cup	Fat/Oil
Gravy Mix, Mushroom, Prepared	**-0.5**	1/4	cup	Fat/Oil
Gravy Mix, Turkey, Prep w/Milk & Butter	**-2.5**	1/4	cup	Fat/Oil
Gravy Mix, Turkey, Prepared	**-0.5**	1/4	cup	Fat/Oil
Gravy, Beef, Canned	**1.0**	1/4	cup	Fat/Oil
Gravy, Chicken, Canned	**-1.5**	1/4	cup	Fat/Oil
Gravy, Chicken, Franco-American	**-4.0**	1/4	cup	Fat/Oil
Gravy, Dehydrated	**-3.0**	1	Tbls	Miscellaneous
Gravy, Mix, Pork, Prepared	**-2.0**	1/4	cup	Fat/Oil
Gravy, Mushroom, Canned	**0.0**	1/4	cup	Fat/Oil
Gravy, Mushroom, Franco-American	**-3.5**	1/4	cup	Fat/Oil
Gravy, Turkey, Canned	**0.0**	1/4	cup	Fat/Oil
Green Pepper, Raw	**37.5**	2	whole	Vegetable
Green Pepper, Stuffed w/Meat	**2.5**	1	whole	Meat/Fish/Poultry
Green Pepper, Stuffed, w/Beef & Tomato Sauce, Fzn, Stouffer's	**-0.5**	1	portion	Meat/Fish/Poultry
Grits, Cooked	**3.0**	1	cup	Grain
Grouper, Baked	**3.0**	5	wt oz	Meat/Fish/Poultry
Guacamole	**4.5**	1/4	cup	Fruit
Guava	**21.0**	1	whole	Fruit
Gum	**-3.0**	10	pieces	Sugar
Gum, Bubble, Original, Hubba Bubba	**-6.0**	5	pieces	Sugar
Gum, Doublemint, Wrigley's	**-4.5**	10	pieces	Sugar
Gummies, Juice Plus+®, Fruit	**34.0**	6	pieces	Fruit
Gummies, Juice Plus+®, Veggie	**29.0**	6	pieces	Vegetable
Gummy Bear	**-3.0**	17	pieces	Sugar
Gummy Bear, Fruit Juice	**-2.5**	17	pieces	Fruit
Haddock Fillet, Light, Mrs. Paul's	**0.0**	1	portion	Meat/Fish/Poultry
Haddock, Baked	**2.5**	4	wt oz	Meat/Fish/Poultry
Haddock, Floured/Breaded, Fried	**-1.0**	3	wt oz	Meat/Fish/Poultry
Haddock, Smoked	**2.0**	6	wt oz	Meat/Fish/Poultry
Halibut Fillet, Batter-Fried	**3.5**	3	wt oz	Meat/Fish/Poultry
Halibut, Baked	**7.5**	4	wt oz	Meat/Fish/Poultry
Halibut, Smoked	**-1.5**	3	wt oz	Meat/Fish/Poultry

Food Name—Alphabetical	Nutripoints	Serving Size		Nutrigroup
Halibut, w/Yellow Bell Pepper Sauce, Nutripoint Recipe	**7.0**	4	wt oz	Meat/Fish/Poultry
Halvah, Plain	**-2.0**	1	wt oz	Sugar
Ham and Cheese Loaf/Roll	**0.0**	2	slices	Meat/Fish/Poultry
Ham Dinner, Frozen, Morton	**5.0**	1	portion	Meat/Fish/Poultry
Ham Salad	**1.0**	1/2	cup	Meat/Fish/Poultry
Ham, Asparagus Au Gratin, Slim, Frozen, Budget Gourmet	**0.0**	1	portion	Meat/Fish/Poultry
Ham, Baked, Canned, 13% Fat	**2.0**	3	wt oz	Meat/Fish/Poultry
Ham, Canned, Armour Golden Star	**1.0**	4	wt oz	Meat/Fish/Poultry
Ham, Chopped	**0.5**	2	wt oz	Meat/Fish/Poultry
Ham, Deviled, Underwood	**-3.5**	2	wt oz	Meat/Fish/Poultry
Ham, Frozen Dinner	**2.5**	1/2	portion	Meat/Fish/Poultry
Ham, Land O' Frost	**-3.5**	3	wt oz	Meat/Fish/Poultry
Ham, Lean, Baked, Canned, 4% Fat	**5.0**	4	wt oz	Meat/Fish/Poultry
Ham, Meatless, Wham, Worthington	**8.0**	3	slices	Legume/Nut/Seed
Ham, Minced	**0.0**	2	wt oz	Meat/Fish/Poultry
Ham, Slices, Jubilee, Oscar Mayer	**5.5**	4	slices	Meat/Fish/Poultry
Ham, Turkey, Mr. Turkey	**-2.0**	4	wt oz	Meat/Fish/Poultry
Hamburger Crumbles, Vegetarian, Morningstar Farms	**6.0**	1/2	cup	Legume/Nut/Seed
Hamburger Helper, Prepared	**1.0**	1/4	cup	Meat/Fish/Poultry
Hamburger Patty, Broiled	**0.0**	3	wt oz	Meat/Fish/Poultry
Hamburger Patty, Lean, Broiled	**3.0**	3	wt oz	Meat/Fish/Poultry
Hamburger Patty, Lean, Fried	**1.5**	3	wt oz	Meat/Fish/Poultry
Hamburger w/Bun, Fast Food Small Plain	**1.5**	1/2	burger	Meat/Fish/Poultry
Hamburger w/Bun/Lettuce/Tomato, Fast Food	**3.0**	1/2	burger	Meat/Fish/Poultry
Hamburger, (Vege) Harvest Burger, Green Giant	**7.5**	1	patty	Legume/Nut/Seed
Hamburger, Aerobics, Nutripoint Recipe	**5.0**	1	burger	Meat/Fish/Poultry
Hamburger, Garden Veggie Patties, Morningstar Farms	**5.5**	1	patty	Vegetable
Hamburger, Vegan, Natural Touch	**15.5**	1	burger	Legume/Nut/Seed
Hamburger, Vegetarian, Better 'N Burgers, Worthington	**15.0**	1	burger	Legume/Nut/Seed
Hamburger, Vegetarian, Boca Burger	**5.5**	1	burger	Legume/Nut/Seed
Hamburger, Vegetarian, Dr. Praeger's	**5.5**	1	burger	Legume/Nut/Seed
Hamburger, Vegetarian, Fzn, Gardenburger	**0.0**	1	burger	Grain
Hamburger, Vegetarian, Grillers Prime, Fzn, Morningstar Farms	**0.0**	1	burger	Legume/Nut/Seed
Hamburger, Vegetarian, Grillers, Fzn, Morningstar Farms	**8.0**	1	burger	Legume/Nut/Seed
Hamburger, Vegetarian, Spicy Black Bean, Worthington	**14.5**	1	burger	Legume/Nut/Seed
Hash	**-0.5**	1/2	cup	Meat/Fish/Poultry
Herring, Canned	**1.5**	1/2	cup	Meat/Fish/Poultry
Herring, Pickled	**0.5**	2	pieces	Meat/Fish/Poultry
Honey	**-5.5**	2	Tbls	Sugar
Horseradish	**0.0**	1	Tbls	Condiment
Hot Dog, Veggie Dogs, Yves	**12.5**	2	servings	Legume/Nut/Seed

Food Name—Alphabetical	Nutripoints	Serving Size		Nutrigroup
Hush Puppies	**-1.0**	2	pieces	Grain
Ice Cream Bar, Chocolate Peanut Butter, Haagen-Dazs	**-3.0**	1/2	bar	Milk/Dairy
Ice Cream Bar, Eskimo Pie	**-3.5**	1	bar	Milk/Dairy
Ice Cream Bar, Non-Dairy, Chocolate Covered, Mocha Mix	**-2.5**	1/2	bar	Milk/Dairy
Ice Cream Bar, Vanilla/Almonds, Haagen-Dazs	**-4.0**	1/2	bar	Milk/Dairy
Ice Cream Bar, Vanilla/Milk Chocolate, Haagen-Dazs	**-4.0**	1/2	bar	Milk/Dairy
Ice Cream Butter Pecan, Meadow Gold	**-5.0**	1/2	cup	Milk/Dairy
Ice Cream Cone, Vanilla	**-1.5**	1/2	serving	Milk/Dairy
Ice Cream Sandwich	**-2.5**	1	serving	Milk/Dairy
Ice Cream Sandwich, Good Humor	**-2.5**	1/2	serving	Milk/Dairy
Ice Cream Soda	**-3.5**	6	fl oz	Milk/Dairy
Ice Cream Sundae, Caramel	**-2.0**	1/2	serving	Milk/Dairy
Ice Cream Sundae, Hot Fudge	**-1.0**	1/2	serving	Milk/Dairy
Ice Cream Sundae, Strawberry	**0.0**	1/2	serving	Milk/Dairy
Ice Cream, Buttered Pecan, Borden's	**-4.0**	1/2	cup	Milk/Dairy
Ice Cream, Choc/Choc Chip, Haagen-Dazs	**-3.5**	1/4	cup	Milk/Dairy
Ice Cream, Chocolate, Schrafft's	**-4.0**	1/4	cup	Milk/Dairy
Ice Cream, Coffee, Haagen-Dazs	**-3.5**	1/4	cup	Milk/Dairy
Ice Cream, Dutch Chocolate, Borden	**-2.0**	1/2	cup	Milk/Dairy
Ice Cream, Extra Light, Blue Bell	**1.5**	1	cup	Milk/Dairy
Ice Cream, French Vanilla, Meadow Gold	**-4.0**	1/2	cup	Milk/Dairy
Ice Cream, Non-Dairy, Vanilla, Mocha Mix	**-2.5**	1/2	cup	Milk/Dairy
Ice Cream, Regular Fat, Vanilla	**-2.0**	1/2	cup	Milk/Dairy
Ice Cream, Simple Pleasures, (w/Simplesse)	**-0.5**	4	fl oz	Milk/Dairy
Ice Cream, Simple Pleasures, Coffee	**-0.5**	4	wt oz	Milk/Dairy
Ice Cream, Sorbet & Cream, Key Lime, Haagen-Dazs	**-3.5**	1/2	cup	Milk/Dairy
Ice Cream, Strawberry, Borden	**-3.5**	1/2	cup	Milk/Dairy
Ice Cream, Vanilla Swiss Almond, Haagen-Dazs	**-4.0**	1/4	cup	Milk/Dairy
Ice Cream, Vanilla, Haagen-Dazs	**-4.0**	1/4	cup	Milk/Dairy
Ice Cream, Vanilla, Louis Sherry	**-3.5**	1/2	cup	Milk/Dairy
Ice Cream, Vanilla, Party Time, Knudsen	**-4.0**	1/2	cup	Milk/Dairy
Ice Cream, Vanilla, Rich	**-2.0**	1/4	cup	Milk/Dairy
Ice Cream, Vanilla, Soft Serve	**-3.5**	1/2	cup	Milk/Dairy
Ice Milk, Chocolate, Borden	**-2.0**	1/2	cup	Milk/Dairy
Ice Milk, Strawberry, Borden	**-2.0**	1/2	cup	Milk/Dairy
Ice Milk, Vanilla	**-1.0**	1/2	cup	Milk/Dairy
Ice Milk, Vanilla, Borden	**-2.0**	1/2	cup	Milk/Dairy
Iced Tea Mix, Sugar & Lemonade Flavor, Nestea	**-6.5**	8	fl oz	Sugar
Instant Breakfast, Chocolate, Carnation	**6.0**	1/2	cup	Milk/Dairy
Instant Breakfast, Vanilla, Carnation	**6.0**	1/2	cup	Milk/Dairy
Instant Breakfast, w/Low-Fat Milk, No Sugar, Carnation	**12.0**	1	cup	Milk/Dairy

Food Name—Alphabetical	Nutripoints	Serving Size		Nutrigroup
Jack In the Box Bacon Cheeseburger	**-1.0**	1/2	burger	Meat/Fish/Poultry
Jack In the Box Beef Fajita Pita	**1.5**	1/2	serving	Meat/Fish/Poultry
Jack In the Box Bleu Cheese Dressing	**-3.0**	1	Tbls	Fat/Oil
Jack In the Box Breakfast Jack	**-2.5**	1/2	serving	Meat/Fish/Poultry
Jack In the Box Buttermilk House Dressing	**-3.0**	1	Tbls	Fat/Oil
Jack In the Box Canadian Crescent Breakfast	**-3.0**	1/2	serving	Meat/Fish/Poultry
Jack In the Box Cheeseburger	**0.0**	1/2	burger	Meat/Fish/Poultry
Jack In the Box Cheesecake	**-3.0**	1/2	piece	Milk/Dairy
Jack In the Box Chef Salad	**-2.5**	1/4	serving	Vegetable
Jack In the Box Chicken Fajita Pita	**2.0**	1/2	serving	Meat/Fish/Poultry
Jack In the Box Chicken Strips-4 Piece	**-1.0**	2	pieces	Meat/Fish/Poultry
Jack In the Box Chicken Strips-6 Piece	**-1.0**	3	pieces	Meat/Fish/Poultry
Jack In the Box Chicken Supreme	**-1.5**	1/2	serving	Meat/Fish/Poultry
Jack In the Box Club Pita	**2.5**	1/2	serving	Meat/Fish/Poultry
Jack In the Box Double Cheeseburger	**-1.0**	1/2	burger	Meat/Fish/Poultry
Jack In the Box Egg Rolls- 3 Piece	**-1.0**	2	pieces	Meat/Fish/Poultry
Jack In the Box Egg Rolls-5 Piece	**-0.5**	2	pieces	Meat/Fish/Poultry
Jack In the Box Fish Supreme	**-1.0**	1/2	serving	Meat/Fish/Poultry
Jack In the Box Grilled Chicken Fillet	**1.0**	1/2	serving	Meat/Fish/Poultry
Jack In the Box Hamburger	**0.0**	1	burger	Meat/Fish/Poultry
Jack In the Box Hash Browns	**-2.0**	1	piece	Vegetable
Jack In the Box Hot Apple Turnover	**-2.5**	1/4	serving	Fruit
Jack In the Box Hot Club Supreme	**-0.5**	1/2	serving	Meat/Fish/Poultry
Jack In the Box Jumbo Jack	**0.0**	1/2	burger	Meat/Fish/Poultry
Jack In the Box Jumbo Jack w/Cheese	**-1.5**	1/2	burger	Meat/Fish/Poultry
Jack In the Box Mexican Chicken Salad	**-0.5**	1/4	serving	Vegetable
Jack In the Box Pancake Platter	**-0.5**	1/2	serving	Grain
Jack In the Box Reduced Calorie French Dressing	**-4.5**	2	Tbls	Fat/Oil
Jack In the Box Sausage Crescent Breakfast	**-3.0**	1/2	serving	Meat/Fish/Poultry
Jack In the Box Scrambled Egg Platter	**-3.5**	1/4	serving	Milk/Dairy
Jack In the Box Shrimp - 10 Piece	**-2.5**	7	pieces	Meat/Fish/Poultry
Jack In the Box Shrimp - 15 Piece	**-2.5**	7	pieces	Meat/Fish/Poultry
Jack In the Box Side Salad	**-0.5**	1	cup	Vegetable
Jack In the Box Super Taco	**-2.0**	1/2	piece	Legume/Nut/Seed
Jack In the Box Supreme Crescent Breakfast	**-2.5**	1/2	serving	Meat/Fish/Poultry
Jack In the Box Swiss & Bacon Burger	**-2.5**	1/2	burger	Meat/Fish/Poultry
Jack In the Box Taco	**-1.5**	1	taco	Legume/Nut/Seed
Jack In the Box Taco Salad	**-1.0**	1/4	serving	Vegetable
Jack In the Box Taquitos (7 Pieces)	**-0.5**	1/2	serving	Meat/Fish/Poultry
Jack In the Box Thousand Island Dressing	**-3.5**	1	Tbls	Fat/Oil
Jack In the Box Ultimate Cheeseburger	**-2.0**	1/4	burger	Meat/Fish/Poultry
Jam, Grape, Welch's	**-5.5**	1	Tbls	Fruit
Jam, Low Cal	**-0.5**	2	Tbls	Fruit

Food Name—Alphabetical	Nutripoints	Serving Size		Nutrigroup
Jam, Preserves, All Flavors	**-3.0**	1	Tbls	Fruit
Jam, Strawberry, Smucker's	**-6.0**	1	Tbls	Fruit
Jambalaya, Nutripoint Recipe	**7.5**	1	cup	Grain
Jelly Beans	**-5.5**	15	pieces	Sugar
Jelly, All Flavors	**-3.5**	2	Tbls	Sugar
Jelly, Blackberry Spread, Smucker's	**-5.5**	2	Tbls	Fruit
Jelly, Cranberry	**-5.5**	2	Tbls	Fruit
Jelly, Fruit Butters, All Flavors	**0.0**	1	Tbls	Fruit
Jelly, Grape, Concord, Smucker's	**-6.0**	1	Tbls	Fruit
Jelly, Grape, Imitation, Smucker's	**0.5**	2	Tbls	Fruit
Jelly, Grape, Welch's	**-5.5**	1	Tbls	Fruit
Jelly, Low Cal, All Flavors	**-1.0**	4	Tbls	Sugar
Juice, Apple	**2.5**	6	fl oz	Fruit
Juice, Apple, From Concentrate, Fzn, Tree Top	**1.0**	6	fl oz	Fruit
Juice, Apple, From Concentrate, Tree Top	**1.5**	6	fl oz	Fruit
Juice, Apple, Frozen, Seneca	**4.5**	6	fl oz	Fruit
Juice, Apple, Lucky Leaf	**1.0**	6	fl oz	Fruit
Juice, Apple, Mott's	**2.5**	6	fl oz	Fruit
Juice, Blue Machine, Naked Juice	**22.5**	6	fl oz	Fruit
Juice, Carrot	**15.0**	6	fl oz	Vegetable
Juice, Cranapple, Low Cal, Ocean Spray	**12.5**	8	fl oz	Fruit
Juice, Cranapple, Ocean Spray	**1.5**	6	fl oz	Fruit
Juice, Cranberry Cocktail, Frozen, Welch's	**0.0**	6	fl oz	Fruit
Juice, Cranberry Cocktail, Ocean Spray	**7.0**	6	fl oz	Fruit
Juice, Cranberry, Low Cal	**12.5**	1	cup	Fruit
Juice, Cranberry, Low Cal, Ocean Spray	**10.5**	8	fl oz	Fruit
Juice, Cranberry, Sweetened	**3.5**	6	fl oz	Fruit
Juice, Grape, Purple, Welch's	**3.5**	6	fl oz	Fruit
Juice, Grape, Red, Welch's	**3.5**	6	fl oz	Fruit
Juice, Grape, Sweetened, Frozen, Welch's	**2.0**	6	fl oz	Fruit
Juice, Grape, Unsweetened	**5.5**	6	fl oz	Fruit
Juice, Grape, Unsweetened, Frozen, Welch's	**5.5**	6	fl oz	Fruit
Juice, Grape, White, Welch's	**2.0**	6	fl oz	Fruit
Juice, Grapefruit, Ocean Spray	**8.0**	6	fl oz	Fruit
Juice, Grapefruit, Pink, Ocean Spray	**6.0**	6	fl oz	Fruit
Juice, Grapefruit, Sweetened	**7.0**	6	fl oz	Fruit
Juice, Grapefruit, Unsweetened	**11.0**	6	fl oz	Fruit
Juice, Green, Machine, Naked Juice	**11.0**	6	fl oz	Fruit
Juice, Guava Nectar, Kern's	**3.0**	6	fl oz	Fruit
Juice, Just Apple, Naked Juice	**13.0**	6	fl oz	Fruit
Juice, Just Carrot, Naked Juice	**16.0**	6	fl oz	Vegetable
Juice, Just Fresh O-J, Naked Juice	**11.5**	6	fl oz	Fruit
Juice, Just Grapefruit, Naked Juice	**12.0**	6	fl oz	Fruit

Food Name—Alphabetical	Nutripoints	Serving Size		Nutrigroup
Juice, Just O-J, Naked Juice	**11.0**	6	fl oz	Fruit
Juice, Kiwi, Sweetened, Kiwi Island	**4.5**	6	fl oz	Fruit
Juice, Kombucha Organic	**22.0**	16	wt oz	Fruit
Juice, Lemon	**1.0**	1	Tbls	Condiment
Juice, Lemon, ReaLemon	**1.0**	1	Tbls	Condiment
Juice, Lime	**0.5**	1	Tbls	Condiment
Juice, Mango Nectar, Kern's	**3.5**	6	fl oz	Fruit
Juice, Mango-Mango, Ocean Spray	**2.0**	6	fl oz	Fruit
Juice, Mighty Mango, Naked Juice	**7.0**	6	fl oz	Fruit
Juice, Orange Light, Minute Maid	**17.5**	8	fl oz	Fruit
Juice, Orange Passion, Minute Maid	**9.0**	6	fl oz	Fruit
Juice, Orange Tangerine, Minute Maid	**11.0**	6	fl oz	Fruit
Juice, Orange w/C, E, Zinc, Minute Maid	**15.0**	6	fl oz	Fruit
Juice, Orange, Calcium Fortified, Minute Maid	**11.0**	6	fl oz	Fruit
Juice, Orange, Fresh Squeezed	**11.5**	6	fl oz	Fruit
Juice, Orange, Frozen, Minute Maid	**10.0**	6	fl oz	Fruit
Juice, Orange, Frozen, Reconstituted	**11.0**	6	fl oz	Fruit
Juice, Orange, Healthy Heart, Tropicana	**13.0**	6	fl oz	Fruit
Juice, Orange, Healthy Kids, Tropicana	**12.0**	6	fl oz	Fruit
Juice, Orange, Heartwise, Minute Maid	**11.5**	6	fl oz	Fruit
Juice, Orange, Home Squeezed + Calcium & D, Minute Maid	**11.5**	6	fl oz	Fruit
Juice, Orange, Home Squeezed, Minute Maid	**9.5**	6	fl oz	Fruit
Juice, Orange, Immunity Defense, Tropicana	**12.5**	6	fl oz	Fruit
Juice, Orange, Kids+, Minute Maid	**12.0**	6	fl oz	Fruit
Juice, Orange, Light 'n Healthy, Tropicana	**22.0**	8	fl oz	Fruit
Juice, Orange, Low Acid, Minute Maid	**9.5**	6	fl oz	Fruit
Juice, Orange, Low Acid, Tropicana	**11.0**	6	fl oz	Fruit
Juice, Orange, Tropicana	**11.0**	6	fl oz	Fruit
Juice, Orange, w/Calcium, Citrus Hill	**10.5**	6	fl oz	Fruit
Juice, Orange-Grapefruit, Unsweetened, Canned	**10.0**	6	fl oz	Fruit
Juice, Orange-Pineapple	**9.5**	6	fl oz	Fruit
Juice, Pineapple, Dole	**5.0**	6	fl oz	Fruit
Juice, Pineapple, Unsweetened, Canned	**6.0**	6	fl oz	Fruit
Juice, Protein Zone, Naked Juice	**6.0**	4	fl oz	Fruit
Juice, Prune, Canned	**5.0**	4	fl oz	Fruit
Juice, Prune, Sunsweet	**4.0**	4	fl oz	Fruit
Juice, Red Machine, Naked Juice	**13.0**	6	fl oz	Fruit
Juice, SoBe Synergy	**6.5**	8	fl oz	Fruit
Juice, Strawberry/Banana Nectar, Kern's	**3.5**	6	fl oz	Fruit
Juice, Synergy Organic Elixir	**22.0**	16	wt oz	Fruit
Juice, Tomato	**24.5**	6	fl oz	Vegetable
Juice, Tomato, Campbell's	**12.0**	3/4	cup	Vegetable

Food Name—Alphabetical	Nutripoints	Serving Size		Nutrigroup
Juice, Tomato, Low Sodium	**26.0**	6	fl oz	Vegetable
Juice, Tropical Blend, Vruit	**11.5**	6	fl oz	Fruit
Juice, Tropical Orange, Tropicana	**7.0**	6	fl oz	Fruit
Juice, V8 Splash	**7.0**	8	fl oz	Vegetable
Juice, V8 Splash Smoothies, All Flavors	**9.5**	8	fl oz	Fruit
Juice, V8 Splash, Diet, All Flavors	**24.5**	16	fl oz	Fruit
Juice, V8 Splash, Mango Peach	**11.5**	8	fl oz	Fruit
Juice, V8 Splash, Tropical Blend	**11.0**	8	fl oz	Fruit
Juice, V8 Vegetable	**24.5**	6	fl oz	Vegetable
Juice, V8 Vegetable, No Salt Added	**28.5**	6	fl oz	Vegetable
Juice, V8 Vegetable, Spicy	**26.0**	6	fl oz	Vegetable
Juice, V8, Bone Health	**27.0**	8	fl oz	Vegetable
Juice, V8, Essential Antioxidants	**30.0**	6	fl oz	Vegetable
Juice, Verry Pro-Berry, Naked Juice	**7.5**	4	fl oz	Fruit
Kale, Chopped, Cooked	**38.5**	1	cup	Vegetable
Kelp	**18.0**	1/2	cup	Vegetable
Kentucky Fried Chicken	**-1.0**	1	piece	Meat/Fish/Poultry
Kentucky Fried Chicken, Chicken Keel	**-1.0**	1	piece	Meat/Fish/Poultry
Kentucky Fried Chicken, Chicken Keel, Extra Crispy	**-0.5**	1	piece	Meat/Fish/Poultry
Kentucky Fried Chicken, Chicken Wing	**-2.5**	1	piece	Meat/Fish/Poultry
Kentucky Fried Chicken, Cole Slaw	**1.5**	1/2	cup	Vegetable
Kentucky Fried Chicken, Corn	**2.5**	1/2	cup	Vegetable
Kentucky Fried Chicken, Drumstick	**-1.5**	1	piece	Meat/Fish/Poultry
Kentucky Fried Chicken, Drumstick, Extra Crispy	**-1.5**	1	piece	Meat/Fish/Poultry
Kentucky Fried Chicken, Gravy	**-1.5**	1/4	cup	Fat/Oil
Kentucky Fried Chicken, Mashed Potatoes	**-2.5**	1/2	cup	Vegetable
Kentucky Fried Chicken, Roll	**2.0**	2	rolls	Grain
Kentucky Fried Chicken, Side Breast	**-1.5**	1	piece	Meat/Fish/Poultry
Kentucky Fried Chicken, Side Breast, Extra Crispy	**-1.0**	1	piece	Meat/Fish/Poultry
Kentucky Fried Chicken, Thigh	**-2.5**	1	piece	Meat/Fish/Poultry
Kentucky Fried Chicken, Thigh, Extra Crispy	**-2.0**	1	piece	Meat/Fish/Poultry
Kentucky Fried Chicken, Wing, Extra Crispy	**-2.0**	1	piece	Meat/Fish/Poultry
Ketchup, Heinz	**-0.5**	2	Tbls	Condiment
Ketchup, Low Sodium, Heinz	**0.5**	2	Tbls	Condiment
Kielbasa	**-1.5**	3	wt oz	Meat/Fish/Poultry
Kiwi Fruit	**17.0**	1	whole	Fruit
Knockwurst	**-2.0**	2	wt oz	Meat/Fish/Poultry
Kohlrabi, Raw	**24.5**	2	cups	Vegetable
Kumquats	**10.0**	6	whole	Fruit
Lamb Chop, Loin, Med. Fat, Baked	**-0.5**	2	wt oz	Meat/Fish/Poultry

Food Name—Alphabetical	Nutripoints	Serving Size		Nutrigroup
Lamb Roast, Leg, Baked	**3.5**	3	wt oz	Meat/Fish/Poultry
Lamb Roast, Leg, Med. Fat, Baked	**0.5**	3	wt oz	Meat/Fish/Poultry
Lamb Shoulder, Lean, Baked	**3.0**	3	wt oz	Meat/Fish/Poultry
Lamb Shoulder, Med. Fat, Baked	**-1.0**	3	wt oz	Meat/Fish/Poultry
Lard	**-5.0**	1	Tbls	Fat/Oil
Lasagna	**2.5**	1/2	cup	Grain
Lasagna Florentine, Weight Watchers Smart Ones	**1.0**	1	serving	Grain
Lasagna, Frozen, Celentano	**1.5**	1/2	portion	Grain
Lasagna, Italian Cheese, Fzn, Weight Watchers	**1.0**	1/2	portion	Grain
Lasagna, Italian Sausage, Fzn, Budget Gourmet	**0.5**	1/4	portion	Grain
Lasagna, Low Cal Frozen Meal	**4.0**	1/2	serving	Grain
Lasagna, Meat Sauce, Frozen, Stouffer's	**0.5**	1/2	portion	Grain
Lasagna, Meat Sauce, Fzn, Weight Watchers	**1.0**	1/2	portion	Grain
Lasagna, Primavera, Frozen, Celentano	**2.5**	1/2	portion	Grain
Lasagna, Single Serving, Frozen, Stouffer's	**0.0**	1/2	serving	Grain
Lasagna, Spinach, Nutripoint Recipe	**9.0**	1	cup	Grain
Lasagna, Three Cheese, Fzn, Budget Gourmet	**1.5**	1/3	portion	Grain
Lasagna, Tuna, Spinach Noodles & Vegetables, Fzn, Stouffer's	**2.0**	1	portion	Meat/Fish/Poultry
Lasagna, Vegetable, 365 Organic, Whole Foods	**-0.5**	1/2	serving	Grain
Lasagna, Vegetable, Single Serving, Fzn, Stouffer's	**0.5**	1/2	portion	Grain
Lasagna, Vegetarian, Boca	**0.5**	1/2	serving	Grain
Lasagna, w/Bread, Frozen, Morton	**1.5**	1/2	portion	Grain
Lasagna, w/Meat Sauce, Slim, Fzn, Budget Gourmet	**0.0**	1/2	serving	Grain
Lasagna, Zucchini, Lean Cuisine, Stouffer's	**2.0**	1/2	portion	Grain
Leeks, Cooked	**7.5**	1	cup	Vegetable
Leeks, Raw	**16.0**	2	whole	Vegetable
Lemon	**2.5**	1/4	lemon	Condiment
Lemonade Mix, Sugar Free, Country Time	**1.0**	8	fl oz	Miscellaneous
Lemonade, Minute Maid	**-5.0**	6	fl oz	Fruit
Lentils and Rice, Herbed, Nutripoint Recipe	**6.5**	1	cup	Legume/Nut/Seed
Lentils, Cooked	**8.0**	1	cup	Legume/Nut/Seed
Lettuce and Tomato	**18.5**	1	cup	Vegetable
Lettuce, Butterhead/Boston/Bibb, chopped	**34.0**	2	cups	Vegetable
Lettuce, Iceberg	**18.0**	10	pieces	Vegetable
Lettuce, Loose leaf	**30.5**	10	pieces	Vegetable
Lettuce, Romaine	**47.5**	2	cups	Vegetable
Lime	**1.0**	1/4	lime	Condiment
Linguine, Buitoni, (2oz Dry=3/4c Cooked)	**3.0**	2	wt oz	Grain
Linguine, San Georgio,(2oz Dry=3/4c Cooked)	**2.5**	2	wt oz	Grain

Food Name—Alphabetical	Nutripoints	Serving Size		Nutrigroup
Linguine, Spinach High-Protein, Buitoni	**3.5**	1/2	cup	Grain
Linguine, Thin, Ronzoni (2 Oz Dry = 3/4 C Cooked)	**2.5**	2	wt oz	Grain
Linguini, Clam Sauce, Frozen, Stouffer's	**-0.5**	1/2	portion	Grain
Linguini, Seafood, Frozen, Weight Watchers	**2.0**	1	portion	Grain
Linguini, w/Scallops & Clams, Slim, Fzn, Budget Gourmet	**-0.5**	1/2	serving	Grain
Linguini, w/Shrimp, Frozen, Budget Gourmet	**0.5**	1/2	portion	Grain
Litchi, Fresh	**16.0**	6	whole	Fruit
Liverwurst	**4.5**	2	wt oz	Meat/Fish/Poultry
Liverwurst, Original, Jones	**-3.0**	2	wt oz	Meat/Fish/Poultry
Lobster Newburg, Frozen Dinner	**1.0**	1/2	portion	Meat/Fish/Poultry
Lobster, Baked/Broiled w/Butter	**-1.0**	4	wt oz	Meat/Fish/Poultry
Lobster, Floured/Breaded, Fried	**-0.5**	3	wt oz	Meat/Fish/Poultry
Lobster, Steamed/Boiled	**2.5**	6	wt oz	Meat/Fish/Poultry
Loquat, Fresh	**10.0**	5	whole	Fruit
Luncheon Meat, Beef	**-1.5**	2	wt oz	Meat/Fish/Poultry
Luncheon Meat, Head Cheese	**-1.5**	2	slices	Meat/Fish/Poultry
Luncheon Meat, Honeyloaf	**3.5**	3	slices	Meat/Fish/Poultry
Luncheon Meat, Olive Loaf	**-0.5**	1	slice	Fruit
Luncheon Meat, Olive Loaf, Eckrich	**-2.5**	2	wt oz	Meat/Fish/Poultry
Luncheon Meat, Olive Loaf, Oscar Mayer	**-2.0**	2	slices	Meat/Fish/Poultry
Luncheon Meat, Oscar Mayer	**-3.5**	2	slices	Meat/Fish/Poultry
Luncheon Meat, Pickle and Pimiento Loaf	**-1.0**	2	slices	Meat/Fish/Poultry
Luncheon Meat, Picnic Loaf, Oscar Mayer	**-1.0**	2	slices	Meat/Fish/Poultry
Luncheon Meat, Pimento Loaf	**-1.0**	2	wt oz	Meat/Fish/Poultry
Luncheon Meat, Turkey Ham	**2.0**	4	wt oz	Meat/Fish/Poultry
Macadamia Nuts, Oil Roasted, Salted	**0.5**	8	nuts	Legume/Nut/Seed
Macaroni & Cheese	**0.0**	1/4	cup	Grain
Macaroni & Cheese Dinner, Deluxe, Kraft	**0.0**	1/2	cup	Grain
Macaroni & Cheese, Casserole, Frozen, Morton	**-1.5**	1/2	portion	Grain
Macaroni & Cheese, Frozen, Budget Gourmet	**0.0**	1/2	portion	Grain
Macaroni & Cheese, Frozen, Stouffer's	**-1.5**	1/2	portion	Grain
Macaroni & Cheese, Weight Watchers 99% Fat Free	**0.0**	1	serving	Grain
Macaroni & Spaghetti, Enriched, Prince	**4.0**	1/2	cup	Grain
Macaroni Ribbons, Spinach, Creamette, Borden	**3.0**	1/2	cup	Grain
Macaroni Salad	**0.0**	1/2	cup	Grain
Macaroni, Cooked, All Shapes, Mueller's	**3.5**	1/2	cup	Grain
Macaroni, Cooked, No Salt (2 wt oz dry = 1 c cooked)	**3.5**	1/2	cup	Grain
Macaroni, Dry (2 wt oz = 1 c Cooked)	**3.5**	1	wt oz	Grain
Macaroni, Elbow, Creamette, Borden	**2.5**	1/2	cup	Grain
Macaroni, Superoni, Prince	**3.0**	1/2	cup	Grain
Mackerel, Baked	**4.0**	3	wt oz	Meat/Fish/Poultry

Food Name—Alphabetical	Nutripoints	Serving Size		Nutrigroup
Mai Tai	-11.5	2	fl oz	Alcohol
Malted Milk Powder	1.0	1	Tbls	Milk/Dairy
Mandarin Oranges, Canned	5.0	1/2	cup	Fruit
Mandarin Oranges, Canned, Unsweetened	15.5	1/2	cup	Fruit
Mango	17.5	1/2	mango	Fruit
Manhattan	-13.5	3	fl oz	Alcohol
Manicotti, 3 Cheese, Tomato Sauce, Le Menu	0.5	1/2	portion	Milk/Dairy
Manicotti, Cheese, Frozen, Weight Watchers	0.0	1/2	portion	Milk/Dairy
Manicotti, Cheese, w/Meat Sauce, Fzn, Budget Gourmet	0.5	1/3	portion	Milk/Dairy
Manicotti, Frozen, Celentano	2.0	1/2	portion	Milk/Dairy
Margarine	-3.0	1	Tbls	Fat/Oil
Margarine, 20% Corn Oil, Smart Beat	1.0	1	fl oz	Fat/Oil
Margarine, 37% Light, Smart Balance	-2.5	1	Tbls	Fat/Oil
Margarine, 67% Light, Smart Balance	-3.0	1	Tbls	Fat/Oil
Margarine, Benecol	-1.5	1	Tbls	Fat/Oil
Margarine, Benecol Light	0.0	1	Tbls	Fat/Oil
Margarine, Brummel & Brown Spread	-2.5	2	Tbls	Fat/Oil
Margarine, Cookery, Parkay	-2.5	1	Tbls	Fat/Oil
Margarine, Corn Oil	-2.5	1	Tbls	Fat/Oil
Margarine, Corn Oil Spread, Light, Mazola	-2.5	2	Tbls	Fat/Oil
Margarine, Country Crock Spread, Shedd's	-3.0	1	Tbls	Fat/Oil
Margarine, Diet Imitation, Mazola	-2.5	2	Tbls	Fat/Oil
Margarine, Diet, Fleischmann's	-2.5	2	Tbls	Fat/Oil
Margarine, Diet, Soft, Parkay	-2.5	2	Tbls	Fat/Oil
Margarine, Extra Light, Promise	-2.5	2	Tbls	Fat/Oil
Margarine, Family Spread, Mrs. Filbert's	-2.0	1	Tbls	Fat/Oil
Margarine, Hard, Coconut, Safflower and Palm	-2.5	1	Tbls	Fat/Oil
Margarine, Heart Beat	-3.0	4	Tbls	Fat/Oil
Margarine, I Can't Believe It's Not Butter	-2.5	1	Tbls	Fat/Oil
Margarine, Liquid, Soybean & Cottonseed	-3.0	1	Tbls	Fat/Oil
Margarine, Low Cal	-1.0	1	Tbls	Fat/Oil
Margarine, Mazola	-2.5	1	Tbls	Fat/Oil
Margarine, Omega Plus w/Flax, Smart Balance	-2.5	1	Tbls	Fat/Oil
Margarine, Parkay	-2.5	1	Tbls	Fat/Oil
Margarine, Promise	-2.0	1	Tbls	Fat/Oil
Margarine, Reduced Cal Spread, Blue Bonnet	-2.5	2	Tbls	Fat/Oil
Margarine, Reduced Cal, Diet, Mazola	-2.5	2	Tbls	Fat/Oil
Margarine, Reduced Cal, Unsalted, Weight Watchers	-2.0	2	Tbls	Fat/Oil
Margarine, Reduced Cal, Weight Watchers	-2.5	2	Tbls	Fat/Oil
Margarine, Safflower, Hain	-2.5	1	Tbls	Fat/Oil
Margarine, Soft Imperial	-3.0	1	Tbls	Fat/Oil
Margarine, Soft, Blue Bonnet	-3.0	1	Tbls	Fat/Oil
Margarine, Soft, Chiffon	-3.0	1	Tbls	Fat/Oil
Margarine, Soft, Corn Oil, Mrs. Filbert's	-2.5	1	Tbls	Fat/Oil

Food Name—Alphabetical	Nutripoints	Serving Size		Nutrigroup
Margarine, Soft, Low Salt, Country Morning Blend, Land O'Lakes	**-4.0**	1	Tbls	Fat/Oil
Margarine, Soft, Spread, Touch of Butter, Kraft	**-2.5**	2	Tbls	Fat/Oil
Margarine, Soybean, Willow Run (Shedd's)	**-3.0**	1	Tbls	Fat/Oil
Margarine, Squeeze, Parkay	**-2.5**	1	Tbls	Fat/Oil
Margarine, Stick, Blue Bonnet	**-3.0**	1	Tbls	Fat/Oil
Margarine, Stick, Fleischmann's	**-3.0**	1	Tbls	Fat/Oil
Margarine, Stick, Imperial	**-3.0**	1	Tbls	Fat/Oil
Margarine, Stick, Land O'lakes	**-2.5**	1	Tbls	Fat/Oil
Margarine, Stick, Unsalted, Fleischmann	**-2.5**	1	Tbls	Fat/Oil
Margarine, Sweet Unsalted, Heart Beat	**-2.0**	4	Tbls	Fat/Oil
Margarine, Take Control	**-1.0**	1	Tbls	Fat/Oil
Margarine, Take Control Light	**0.0**	1	Tbls	Fat/Oil
Margarine, Unsalted, Mazola	**-2.5**	1	Tbls	Fat/Oil
Margarine, Whipped Spread, Parkay	**-2.5**	1	Tbls	Fat/Oil
Margarine, Whipped, Imperial	**-2.5**	2	Tbls	Fat/Oil
Margarine-like Spread, Smart Beat Squeeze	**1.0**	2	Tbls	Fat/Oil
Margarita	**-13.5**	3	fl oz	Alcohol
Marjoram	**0.5**	1	tsp	Condiment
Marmalade	**-5.0**	2	Tbls	Sugar
Marmalade, Orange, Smucker's	**-6.0**	1	Tbls	Fruit
Marshmallows, Jet-Puffed (large), Kraft	**-5.5**	4	pieces	Sugar
Martini	**-15.5**	3	fl oz	Alcohol
Mayo Mix, Lite, Nutripoint Recipe	**1.5**	1/4	cup	Fat/Oil
Mayonnaise	**-2.5**	1	Tbls	Fat/Oil
Mayonnaise, Blue Plate	**-3.0**	1	Tbls	Fat/Oil
Mayonnaise, Canola Oil, Smart Beat	**-2.5**	1	Tbls	Fat/Oil
Mayonnaise, Cholesterol Free, Kraft	**-2.5**	1	Tbls	Fat/Oil
Mayonnaise, Cholesterol Free, Miracle Whip	**-2.5**	1	Tbls	Fat/Oil
Mayonnaise, Imitation, Milk Cream	**-3.5**	1	Tbls	Fat/Oil
Mayonnaise, Imitation, Soybean	**-3.0**	1	Tbls	Fat/Oil
Mayonnaise, Light Reduced Cal, Hellman's	**-3.0**	2	Tbls	Fat/Oil
Mayonnaise, Light Reduced Cal, Kraft	**-2.5**	2	Tbls	Fat/Oil
Mayonnaise, Light, Kraft	**0.0**	2	Tbls	Fat/Oil
Mayonnaise, Light, Miracle Whip	**-3.0**	2	Tbls	Fat/Oil
Mayonnaise, Low Cal	**-2.5**	2	Tbls	Fat/Oil
Mayonnaise, Non-Fat, Kraft Free	**0.0**	1	Tbls	Fat/Oil
Mayonnaise, Real, Best Foods	**-3.0**	1	Tbls	Fat/Oil
Mayonnaise, Real, Hellmann's	**-3.5**	1	Tbls	Fat/Oil
Mayonnaise, Real, Kraft	**-3.5**	1	Tbls	Fat/Oil
Mayonnaise, Reduced Cal, Light N' Lively	**0.5**	1	Tbls	Condiment
McDonald's 1000 Island Dressing	**-3.0**	2	Tbls	Fat/Oil
McDonald's Apple Pie	**-2.0**	1/4	serving	Fruit
McDonald's Bacon Bits	**-1.5**	1	Tbls	Meat/Fish/Poultry
McDonald's Barbeque Sauce	**0.0**	1	Tbls	Condiment
McDonald's Big Mac	**-1.0**	1/2	burger	Meat/Fish/Poultry
McDonald's Biscuit w/Bacon, Egg & Cheese	**-4.5**	1/2	serving	Milk/Dairy

Food Name—Alphabetical	Nutripoints	Serving Size		Nutrigroup
McDonald's Biscuit w/Biscuit Spread	**-0.5**	1/2	serving	Grain
McDonald's Biscuit w/Sausage	**-1.5**	1/2	serving	Meat/Fish/Poultry
McDonald's Biscuit w/Sausage & Egg	**-4.5**	1/2	serving	Meat/Fish/Poultry
McDonald's Bleu Cheese Dressing	**-3.5**	1	Tbls	Fat/Oil
McDonald's Caesar Salad w/Grilled Chicken	**7.0**	1	serving	Meat/Fish/Poultry
McDonald's California Cobb Salad w/Grilled Chicken	**3.0**	1	serving	Meat/Fish/Poultry
McDonald's Cheeseburger	**0.0**	1/2	burger	Meat/Fish/Poultry
McDonald's Chef Salad	**-0.5**	1/4	serving	Vegetable
McDonald's Chicken McGrill Sandwich	**2.0**	1/2	serving	Meat/Fish/Poultry
McDonald's Chicken McNuggets	**-1.5**	1	serving	Meat/Fish/Poultry
McDonald's Chicken Salad Oriental	**5.0**	1	serving	Meat/Fish/Poultry
McDonald's Chocolate Milk Shake	**-3.0**	1/2	serving	Milk/Dairy
McDonald's Chocolaty Chip Cookies	**-2.5**	1	cookie	Grain
McDonald's Chow Mein Noodles	**0.0**	2	Tbls	Grain
McDonald's Croutons	**5.0**	2	Tbls	Grain
McDonald's Egg McMuffin	**-4.0**	1/2	muffin	Milk/Dairy
McDonald's English Muffin w/Butter	**1.0**	1	muffin	Grain
McDonald's Filet-O-Fish Sandwich	**-1.0**	1/2	serving	Meat/Fish/Poultry
McDonald's French Dressing	**-2.5**	2	Tbls	Fat/Oil
McDonald's Garden Salad	**0.5**	1/2	serving	Vegetable
McDonald's Hamburger	**0.5**	1	burger	Meat/Fish/Poultry
McDonald's Hashbrown Potatoes	**-2.0**	1/2	serving	Vegetable
McDonald's Hot Caramel Sundae	**-1.5**	1/2	serving	Milk/Dairy
McDonald's Hot Fudge Sundae	**-1.5**	1/2	serving	Milk/Dairy
McDonald's Hot Mustard Sauce	**-0.5**	1	Tbls	Condiment
McDonald's Hotcakes w/Butter & Syrup	**-0.5**	1/2	serving	Grain
McDonald's Lite Vinaigrette Dressing	**0.0**	1	Tbls	Condiment
McDonald's Lowfat Milk Jug	**8.0**	1	serving	Milk/Dairy
McDonald's McChicken Sandwich	**0.5**	1/2	serving	Meat/Fish/Poultry
McDonald's McDonaldland Cookies	**-2.0**	1	cookie	Grain
McDonald's McLean Deluxe Hamburger	**1.5**	1	burger	Meat/Fish/Poultry
McDonald's Newman's Own Lowfat Balsamic Vinaigrette Dressing	**-3.5**	4	Tbls	Fat/Oil
McDonald's Oriental Dressing	**0.0**	1	Tbls	Condiment
McDonald's Pork Sausage	**-3.5**	1	piece	Meat/Fish/Poultry
McDonald's Quarter Pounder	**-0.5**	1/2	burger	Meat/Fish/Poultry
McDonald's Quarter Pounder w/Cheese	**-1.0**	1/2	burger	Meat/Fish/Poultry
McDonald's Ranch Dressing	**-3.0**	2	Tbls	Fat/Oil
McDonald's Regular French Fries	**-0.5**	1/4	serving	Vegetable
McDonald's Sausage McMuffin	**-0.5**	1/2	muffin	Meat/Fish/Poultry
McDonald's Sausage McMuffin w/ Egg	**-4.0**	1/2	muffin	Meat/Fish/Poultry
McDonald's Scrambled Eggs	**-19.5**	1	serving	Milk/Dairy
McDonald's Side Salad	**1.0**	1	serving	Vegetable
McDonald's Soft Serve Cone	**-1.0**	1	serving	Milk/Dairy
McDonald's Strawberry Milk Shake	**-3.0**	1/2	serving	Milk/Dairy
McDonald's Strawberry Sundae	**-1.5**	1/2	serving	Milk/Dairy

Food Name—Alphabetical	Nutripoints	Serving Size		Nutrigroup
McDonald's Sweet & Sour Sauce	**0.0**	1	Tbls	Condiment
McDonald's Vanilla Milk Shake	**-3.0**	1/2	serving	Milk/Dairy
McDonald's Vanilla Reduced Fat Ice Cream Cone	**-1.5**	1	serving	Milk/Dairy
Meal Bar, All Flavors, South Beach Diet	**5.5**	1	bar	Legume/Nut/Seed
Meal Bar, Glucerna	**12.5**	1	bar	Grain
Meal Bar, Slim-Fast Optima	**8.5**	1	bar	Grain
Meatballs	**-0.5**	2	pieces	Meat/Fish/Poultry
Meatballs, Italian, w/Noodles/Peppers, Fzn, Budget Gourmet	**0.0**	1/2	portion	Meat/Fish/Poultry
Meatballs, Swedish, w/Noodles, Frozen, Budget Gourmet	**-2.5**	1/3	portion	Meat/Fish/Poultry
Meatloaf	**-0.5**	3	wt oz	Meat/Fish/Poultry
Meatloaf, Frozen Dinner	**1.5**	1/2	portion	Meat/Fish/Poultry
Melon, Cantaloupe	**29.0**	1/4	melon	Fruit
Melon, Casaba	**11.0**	1/4	melon	Fruit
Melon, Honeydew	**14.0**	1/4	melon	Fruit
Mexican Combination Dinner, Frozen, Swanson	**-1.0**	1/3	portion	Legume/Nut/Seed
Mexican Dinner, Frozen, Patio	**0.0**	1/4	portion	Legume/Nut/Seed
Mexican Style Combo Dinner, Frozen, Patio	**0.0**	1/3	portion	Legume/Nut/Seed
Mexican Style Dinner, Frozen, Morton	**4.5**	1/2	portion	Legume/Nut/Seed
Milk Drink Mix, Non-Fat, Hot Cocoa, Swiss Miss	**-2.0**	1	cup	Milk/Dairy
Milk Drink Mix, Strawberry, Quik, Nestle	**-2.0**	1/2	cup	Milk/Dairy
Milk Drink, Alba	**4.0**	16	fl oz	Milk/Dairy
Milk Drink, Atkins Ready to Drink Shakes	**13.5**	11	fl oz	Milk/Dairy
Milk Drink, Balance 40-30-30 (mixed w/water)	**11.0**	1	serving	Milk/Dairy
Milk Drink, Boost Breeze	**7.5**	8	fl oz	Milk/Dairy
Milk Drink, Boost High Protein	**10.0**	8	fl oz	Milk/Dairy
Milk Drink, Carnation Instant Breakfast	**8.0**	10	fl oz	Milk/Dairy
Milk Drink, Diet, Lite, Sego	**13.5**	10	fl oz	Milk/Dairy
Milk Drink, Diet, Sego	**7.5**	6	fl oz	Milk/Dairy
Milk Drink, Ensure	**8.0**	8	fl oz	Milk/Dairy
Milk Drink, Ensure High Protein	**8.5**	8	fl oz	Milk/Dairy
Milk Drink, Ensure Light	**9.5**	8	fl oz	Milk/Dairy
Milk Drink, Ensure Plus	**5.0**	8	fl oz	Milk/Dairy
Milk Drink, Ensure w/Fiber	**8.0**	8	fl oz	Milk/Dairy
Milk Drink, Gatorade Nutrition Shake	**4.0**	1/2	serving	Milk/Dairy
Milk Drink, Glucerna	**12.5**	1	cup	Milk/Dairy
Milk Drink, Juice Plus+ Complete® (w/water)	**31.0**	8	fl oz	Legume/Nut/Seed
Milk Drink, MET-Rx Carb Count RTD	**8.0**	11	fl oz	Milk/Dairy
Milk Drink, MET-Rx Protein Plus Powder (w/water)	**6.0**	12	fl oz	Milk/Dairy
Milk Drink, MET-Rx RTD Lite	**6.5**	11	fl oz	Milk/Dairy
Milk Drink, MET-Rx RTD-40	**12.0**	15	fl oz	Milk/Dairy
Milk Drink, MET-Rx RTD-51	**18.5**	12	fl oz	Milk/Dairy
Milk Drink, MET-Rx Total Nutrition Drink Powder (w/water)	**22.5**	12	fl oz	Milk/Dairy

Food Name—Alphabetical	Nutripoints	Serving Size		Nutrigroup
Milk Drink, MET-Rx White Box Protein Powder (w/water)	**23.0**	16	fl oz	Milk/Dairy
Milk Drink, Muscle Milk, Cytomax	**6.0**	4	fl oz	Milk/Dairy
Milk Drink, Nestle Sweet Success	**13.0**	10	fl oz	Milk/Dairy
Milk Drink, Nutrament	**4.5**	12	fl oz	Milk/Dairy
Milk Drink, NutraStart	**5.5**	8	fl oz	Milk/Dairy
Milk Drink, Ready to Drink, ZonePerfect	**15.0**	8	fl oz	Milk/Dairy
Milk Drink, Resource	**7.0**	8	fl oz	Milk/Dairy
Milk Drink, Resource Plus	**6.5**	8	fl oz	Milk/Dairy
Milk Drink, Shake Mix, Slim-Fast Optima	**20.5**	8	fl oz	Milk/Dairy
Milk Drink, Shake Mix, ZonePerfect	**22.5**	8	fl oz	Milk/Dairy
Milk Drink, Slim Fast	**13.0**	8	fl oz	Milk/Dairy
Milk Drink, Slim-Fast Optima	**16.0**	12	fl oz	Milk/Dairy
Milk Drink, Smart Fuel Protein Anytime Mix	**17.5**	1	serving	Milk/Dairy
Milk Drink, Soy Protein, Health Source	**12.5**	8	fl oz	Legume/Nut/Seed
Milk Drink, Spiru-Tein (w/skim milk)	**34.0**	8	fl oz	Milk/Dairy
Milk Drink, Sustical High Protein	**5.5**	8	fl oz	Milk/Dairy
Milk Drink, Sustical Plus	**4.5**	8	fl oz	Milk/Dairy
Milk Drink, Ultra Slim Fast	**11.5**	8	fl oz	Milk/Dairy
Milk Substitute, Non-Dairy, Vitamite	**4.0**	1	cup	Milk/Dairy
Milk, Canned, Evaporated, Unsweetened	**1.0**	1/2	cup	Milk/Dairy
Milk, Canned, Skim, Evaporated	**9.5**	1/2	cup	Milk/Dairy
Milk, Chocolate	**-0.5**	1/2	cup	Milk/Dairy
Milk, Chocolate, Lowfat (1%)	**2.5**	1	cup	Milk/Dairy
Milk, Chocolate, Lowfat (2%)	**2.5**	6	fl oz	Milk/Dairy
Milk, Condensed, Sweetened, Eagle Brand	**-3.0**	1/4	cup	Milk/Dairy
Milk, Evaporated Skimmed, Carnation	**9.0**	3/4	cup	Milk/Dairy
Milk, Evaporated, Carnation	**1.0**	1/2	cup	Milk/Dairy
Milk, Goat	**1.5**	1	cup	Milk/Dairy
Milk, Instant Natural Malted, Carnation	**-0.5**	1/2	cup	Milk/Dairy
Milk, Instant Nonfat Dry, Carnation	**11.5**	2	cup	Milk/Dairy
Milk, Lowfat (1%)	**8.0**	1	cup	Milk/Dairy
Milk, Lowfat (2%), Hi-Calcium, Borden	**7.5**	1	cup	Milk/Dairy
Milk, Lowfat (2%), Protein Fortified	**6.0**	1	cup	Milk/Dairy
Milk, Non-Dairy, Soy, West Soy	**0.5**	1	cup	Legume/Nut/Seed
Milk, Nonfat Dry	**10.5**	1/4	cup	Milk/Dairy
Milk, Skim	**9.5**	1	cup	Milk/Dairy
Milk, Soy Dream, Vanilla, Imagine Foods	**5.5**	8	fl oz	Legume/Nut/Seed
Milk, Soy, Chocolate, 8th Continent	**1.5**	8	fl oz	Legume/Nut/Seed
Milk, Soy, Light Chocolate, 8th Continent	**4.0**	8	fl oz	Legume/Nut/Seed
Milk, Soy, Light Original, 8th Continent	**9.0**	2	cup	Legume/Nut/Seed
Milk, Soy, Light Vanilla, 8th Continent	**7.0**	2	cup	Legume/Nut/Seed
Milk, Soy, Natural Creamy Original, Vitasoy	**1.0**	1	cup	Legume/Nut/Seed
Milk, Soy, Natural, Edensoy	**2.0**	1	cup	Legume/Nut/Seed
Milk, Soy, Original Flavor, 8th Continent	**4.5**	8	fl oz	Legume/Nut/Seed
Milk, Soy, Power Dream, Imagine Foods	**7.5**	8	fl oz	Legume/Nut/Seed
Milk, Soy, Silk Chocolate Organic	**4.5**	8	fl oz	Legume/Nut/Seed

Food Name—Alphabetical	Nutripoints	Serving Size		Nutrigroup
Milk, Soy, Silk Light Organic	**9.5**	8	fl oz	Legume/Nut/Seed
Milk, Soy, Silk Organic	**6.5**	8	fl oz	Legume/Nut/Seed
Milk, Soy, Solait, Miller Farms	**0.5**	8	fl oz	Legume/Nut/Seed
Milk, Soy, Soyamel, Worthington	**7.5**	8	fl oz	Legume/Nut/Seed
Milk, Soy, Soymoo, Health Valley	**0.0**	1	cup	Legume/Nut/Seed
Milk, Soy, Vanilla, 8th Continent	**3.5**	8	fl oz	Legume/Nut/Seed
Milk, Sweetened Condensed, Canned	**-2.0**	2	fl oz	Milk/Dairy
Milk, Sweetened Condensed, Carnation	**-2.0**	1/4	cup	Milk/Dairy
Milk, Whole (3.3%)	**2.5**	1	cup	Milk/Dairy
Milk, Whole (3.7%)	**2.0**	1	cup	Milk/Dairy
Milkshake, Chocolate	**-1.0**	1/2	cup	Milk/Dairy
Milkshake, Vanilla	**-1.0**	1/2	cup	Milk/Dairy
Mint Julep	**-15.0**	2	fl oz	Alcohol
Mixed Fruits, Dried, Sun-Maid	**3.5**	2	wt oz	Fruit
Mixed Nuts, Dry Roast, Unsalted	**1.0**	1	wt oz	Legume/Nut/Seed
Mixed Nuts, Oil Roasted, Salted	**1.0**	1	wt oz	Legume/Nut/Seed
Mixed Vegetables, Frozen, Veg-All	**21.0**	1/2	cup	Vegetable
Mixed Vegetables, Fzn, 365 Organic, Whole Foods	**11.5**	2/3	cup	Vegetable
Mixed Vegetables, Natural Pack, Canned, Libby's	**18.5**	1/2	cup	Vegetable
Mixed Vegetables, Organic, Fzn, Cascadian Farm	**16.0**	1	cup	Vegetable
Mixed Vegetables, w/Butter, Frozen, Green Giant	**7.5**	1/2	cup	Vegetable
Molasses	**-3.0**	2	Tbls	Sugar
Molasses, Blackstrap	**3.5**	2	Tbls	Sugar
Moose	**5.5**	3	wt oz	Meat/Fish/Poultry
Moroccan Stew, Organic, Fzn, Moosewood	**2.5**	1/2	serving	Vegetable
Mousse, Cheesecake, Sans Sucre de Paris	**3.5**	1/2	cup	Milk/Dairy
Mousse, Chocolate	**-5.5**	1/2	cup	Sugar
Mousse, Chocolate, Frozen, Weight Watchers	**-1.5**	1	piece	Milk/Dairy
Mousse, Chocolate, Light, Sara Lee	**-4.0**	1/2	serving	Grain
Mousse, Key Lime, Nutripoint Recipe	**5.5**	1/2	cup	Milk/Dairy
Mousse, Raspberry, Frozen, Weight Watchers	**-2.5**	1/2	serving	Fruit
Muffin	**0.5**	1	muffin	Grain
Muffin Mix, Blueberry, Wild, Betty Crocker	**-1.5**	1	muffin	Grain
Muffin Mix, Blueberry, Wild, Duncan Hines	**-1.5**	1	muffin	Grain
Muffin Mix, Bran Date, Jiffy	**-1.0**	1	muffin	Grain
Muffin Mix, Bran, Original Wheat, Arrowhead Mills	**2.0**	1	muffin	Grain
Muffin Mix, Corn, Betty Crocker	**-1.0**	1	muffin	Grain
Muffin Mix, Corn, Jiffy	**-1.0**	1	muffin	Grain
Muffin Mix, Corn, Old Fashioned, Frozen, Pepperidge Farm	**-1.0**	1	muffin	Grain
Muffin Mix, Oat Bran, Wheat Free, Arrowhead Mills	**2.5**	1	muffin	Grain
Muffin, Blueberry	**0.0**	1	muffin	Grain
Muffin, Bran	**3.0**	1	muffin	Grain
Muffin, Bran, w/Raisin & Nuts	**3.5**	1	muffin	Grain
Muffin, Cornbread	**0.5**	1	muffin	Grain
Muffin, English	**4.0**	1	whole	Grain

Food Name—Alphabetical	Nutripoints	Serving Size		Nutrigroup
Muffin, English, Cracked Wheat	**3.5**	1	whole	Grain
Muffin, English, Health Nut, Oroweat	**3.0**	1	whole	Grain
Muffin, English, Honey Wheat, Thomas'	**2.0**	1	whole	Grain
Muffin, English, Pepperidge Farm	**4.0**	1	whole	Grain
Muffin, English, Regular, Thomas'	**2.5**	1	whole	Grain
Muffin, English, Roman Meal	**4.5**	1	whole	Grain
Muffin, English, w/Raisins	**4.5**	1	whole	Grain
Muffin, English, Whole Wheat	**6.0**	1	whole	Grain
Muffin, Extra Crisp, Arnold	**3.5**	1	muffin	Grain
Muffin, Nutripoint Recipe	**10.5**	1	muffin	Grain
Muffin, Oat Bran, Nutripoint Recipe	**3.5**	1	muffin	Grain
Muffin, Oatmeal	**1.0**	1	muffin	Grain
Muffin, Raisin Oat Bran, Health Valley	**5.0**	1	muffin	Grain
Muffin, w/Fruit And/Or Nuts	**-0.5**	1	muffin	Grain
Mushrooms, Canned, Green Giant	**13.0**	1	cup	Vegetable
Mushrooms, Cooked	**19.0**	1	cup	Vegetable
Mushrooms, Fresh	**32.5**	1	cup	Vegetable
Mushrooms, Fried w/Breading	**-1.0**	1/4	cup	Vegetable
Mussels, Cooked	**2.0**	6	wt oz	Meat/Fish/Poultry
Mustard	**0.0**	1	tsp	Condiment
Mustard Greens, Cooked	**61.5**	1	cup	Vegetable
Mustard Greens, Frozen, Cooked	**48.0**	1	cup	Vegetable
Mustard, Bold 'n Spice, French's	**-0.5**	1	Tbls	Condiment
Mustard, Dry	**0.5**	1	tsp	Condiment
Mustard, w/Horseradish, French's	**-0.5**	1	Tbls	Condiment
Mustard, Yellow, Prepared, French's	**-0.5**	1	Tbls	Condiment
Nachos, Cheese/Hot Peppers	**1.0**	5	pieces	Grain
Nectarine, Fresh	**10.0**	1	whole	Fruit
Noodles & Cheese Dinner, Deboles	**1.0**	1/4	cup	Grain
Noodles, Chow Mein	**1.0**	1/4	cup	Grain
Noodles, Egg, Cholesterol Free, No Yolks	**3.0**	1	wt oz	Grain
Noodles, Egg, Cooked, Mueller's	**2.0**	1/2	cup	Grain
Noodles, Egg, Ronzoni	**0.0**	1/2	cup	Grain
Noodles, Egg, Veggie, Hodgson Mill	**2.5**	1	wt oz	Grain
Noodles, Egg, Whole Wheat, Hodgson Mill	**2.0**	1	wt oz	Grain
Noodles, Spaghetti, Whole Wheat, Hodgson Mill	**2.5**	1	wt oz	Grain
Noodles, Spinach	**3.5**	1/2	cup	Grain
Noodles, Spinach, Whole Wheat, Hodgson Mill	**2.0**	1	wt oz	Grain
Noodles, Whole Wheat	**4.0**	1/2	cup	Grain
Nut Meat, Nuteena, Loma Linda Foods	**2.0**	2	wt oz	Legume/Nut/Seed
Nutmeg	**0.0**	1	tsp	Condiment
Nuts, Mixed, w/Peanuts, Planter's	**-1.5**	1	wt oz	Legume/Nut/Seed
Ocean Perch Fillet, Frozen, Gorton's	**2.5**	4	wt oz	Meat/Fish/Poultry
Ocean Perch Fillet, Light, Mrs. Paul's	**-1.0**	1	serving	Meat/Fish/Poultry
Ocean Perch, Baked	**4.5**	4	wt oz	Meat/Fish/Poultry
Octopus, Fried	**2.0**	3	wt oz	Meat/Fish/Poultry
Oil	**-3.0**	1	Tbls	Fat/Oil

Food Name—Alphabetical	Nutripoints	Serving Size		Nutrigroup
Oil, Almond	**-2.5**	1	Tbls	Fat/Oil
Oil, Canola, Puritan	**-2.5**	1	Tbls	Fat/Oil
Oil, Cocoa Butter	**-5.5**	1	Tbls	Fat/Oil
Oil, Coconut	**-7.0**	1	Tbls	Fat/Oil
Oil, Corn, Crisco	**-3.0**	1	Tbls	Fat/Oil
Oil, Corn, Mazola	**-3.0**	1	Tbls	Fat/Oil
Oil, Cottonseed	**-3.5**	1	Tbls	Fat/Oil
Oil, Crisco	**-3.0**	1	Tbls	Fat/Oil
Oil, Hazelnut	**-2.5**	1	Tbls	Fat/Oil
Oil, Linseed	**-2.5**	1	Tbls	Fat/Oil
Oil, Olive	**-3.0**	1	Tbls	Fat/Oil
Oil, Olive, Bertolli	**-3.0**	1	Tbls	Fat/Oil
Oil, Palm	**-5.0**	1	Tbls	Fat/Oil
Oil, Palm Kernel	**-6.5**	1	Tbls	Fat/Oil
Oil, Pam Spray	**-0.5**	1/3	gram	Condiment
Oil, Peanut	**-3.0**	1	Tbls	Fat/Oil
Oil, Puritan	**-2.5**	1	Tbls	Fat/Oil
Oil, Safflower	**-2.5**	1	Tbls	Fat/Oil
Oil, Safflower, Hollywood	**-2.5**	1	Tbls	Fat/Oil
Oil, Sesame	**-3.0**	1	Tbls	Fat/Oil
Oil, Soybean	**-3.0**	1	Tbls	Fat/Oil
Oil, Sunflower	**-2.5**	1	Tbls	Fat/Oil
Oil, Sunlite	**-2.5**	1	Tbls	Fat/Oil
Oil, Vegetable, Puritan	**-2.5**	1	Tbls	Fat/Oil
Oil, Walnut	**-2.5**	1	Tbls	Fat/Oil
Oil, Wesson	**-3.0**	1	Tbls	Fat/Oil
Oil, Wheat Germ	**-3.0**	1	Tbls	Fat/Oil
Okra, Cooked	**31.0**	1/2	cup	Vegetable
Okra, Fried w/Breading	**1.0**	1/4	cup	Vegetable
Okra, Raw	**26.0**	1	cup	Vegetable
Old Fashioned	**-15.5**	2	fl oz	Alcohol
Olives, Black	**-2.0**	8	olives	Fruit
Olives, Green	**-4.0**	8	olives	Fruit
Olives, Medium, Mammoth Queen, S&W	**-3.0**	8	olives	Fruit
Olives, Ripe, Lindsay	**0.0**	4	olives	Fruit
Onion Powder	**0.5**	1	tsp	Condiment
Onion Rings, Fried	**0.0**	2	pieces	Vegetable
Onion, Green	**1.0**	2	pieces	Condiment
Onion, Raw (1 T=1 Tsp Dry Onion Flakes)	**8.5**	1/2	cup	Vegetable
Orange Roughy, Raw	**4.0**	5	wt oz	Meat/Fish/Poultry
Orange, Fresh	**13.5**	1	whole	Fruit
Oregano	**1.0**	1	tsp	Condiment
Oyster Stew	**3.0**	1	cup	Meat/Fish/Poultry
Oysters, Broiled w/Butter	**6.5**	3	wt oz	Meat/Fish/Poultry
Oysters, Eastern, Raw	**13.0**	12	whole	Meat/Fish/Poultry
Oysters, Fried	**1.5**	3	whole	Meat/Fish/Poultry
Oysters, Pacific, Raw	**8.0**	4	whole	Meat/Fish/Poultry

Food Name—Alphabetical	Nutripoints	Serving Size		Nutrigroup
Pancake & Waffle Mix, Blue Corn	**-1.0**	1	cake	Grain
Pancake & Waffle Mix, Buttermilk, Hungry Jack	**-1.5**	2	cakes	Grain
Pancake & Waffle Mix, Extra Light, Hungry Jack	**-1.0**	2	cakes	Grain
Pancake Mix, Complete Buttermilk, Aunt Jemima	**3.5**	2	cakes	Grain
Pancake Mix, Original Complete, Aunt Jemima	**2.5**	2	cakes	Grain
Pancake, Buckwheat	**1.0**	1	cake	Grain
Pancake, Cornmeal	**1.0**	1	cake	Grain
Pancake, Plain	**0.5**	1	cake	Grain
Pancake, w/Fruit	**0.5**	1	cake	Grain
Pancake, Whole Wheat	**0.5**	1	cake	Grain
Pancake, Whole Wheat, Orange, Nutripoint Recipe	**5.5**	4	cakes	Grain
Pancakes, Buckwheat, Aunt Jemima (from mix)	**6.0**	3	small	Grain
Pancakes, Lite Buttermilk, Aunt Jemima (from mix)	**8.0**	3	small	Grain
Pancakes, Lite, Buttermilk, Aunt Jemima	**7.0**	3	cakes	Grain
Pancakes, Whole Wheat, Aunt Jemima (from mix)	**8.5**	3	small	Grain
Papaya	**20.5**	1/2	fruit	Fruit
Papaya Nectar, Canned	**4.0**	6	fl oz	Fruit
Paprika	**2.5**	1	tsp	Condiment
Parsley, Dried	**1.5**	1	tsp	Condiment
Parsley, Fresh	**54.5**	1	cup	Vegetable
Parsnips, Cooked	**8.5**	1/2	cup	Vegetable
Parsnips, Raw	**11.5**	1/2	cup	Vegetable
Passion Fruit, Purple, Fresh	**9.0**	2	whole	Fruit
Pasta & Cheese, Baked, Frozen, Celentano	**0.0**	1/2	portion	Grain
Pasta & Sauce, Marinara, Hain	**1.0**	1/4	cup	Grain
Pasta & Sauce, Swiss, Creamy, Hain	**-1.5**	1/4	cup	Grain
Pasta Accents, Cheddar Cheese, Green Giant	**4.0**	1/2	cup	Grain
Pasta Accents, Garlic Seasoning, Green Giant	**3.5**	1/2	cup	Grain
Pasta Alfredo, w/Broccoli, Fzn, Budget Gourmet	**0.0**	1/2	piece	Grain
Pasta Carbonara, Frozen, Stouffer's	**-1.5**	1/4	portion	Grain
Pasta Casino, Frozen, Stouffer's	**1.0**	1/2	portion	Grain
Pasta e Fagioli, Organic, Fzn, Moosewood	**4.0**	1	serving	Grain
Pasta Mexicali, Frozen, Stouffer's	**-1.0**	1/2	serving	Grain
Pasta Oriental, Frozen, Stouffer's	**0.5**	1/2	serving	Grain
Pasta Primavera, Frozen, Weight Watchers	**2.5**	1/2	serving	Grain
Pasta Salad, Fresh, Nutripoint Recipe	**4.5**	1/2	cup	Grain
Pasta Salad, Home Recipe	**-1.0**	1/4	cup	Grain
Pasta Salad, Italian, Cool Side, Lipton	**0.5**	1/2	cup	Grain
Pasta Shells & Beef, Frozen, Budget Gourmet	**1.5**	1/2	portion	Grain
Pasta Shells, Cheese Stuffed, w/Meat Sauce, Stouffer's	**-0.5**	1/2	portion	Milk/Dairy
Pasta Shells, Stuffed, Fzn, Healthy Choice	**0.5**	1	serving	Grain
Pasta, Angel Hair, w/Sunshine Sauce, Nutripoint Recipe	**10.0**	1 1/2	cup	Grain
Pasta, Broccoli and Parmesan, Organic, Fzn, Moosewood	**0.0**	1/2	serving	Grain

Food Name—Alphabetical	Nutripoints	Serving Size		Nutrigroup
Pasta, Farfalle & Spinach Pesto, Organic, Fzn, Moosewood	0.5	1/2	serving	Grain
Pasta, Penne & Ricotta, Weight Watchers	1.0	1	serving	Grain
Pastrami, Beef	-2.5	2	wt oz	Meat/Fish/Poultry
Pastrami, Land O' Frost	-2.0	4	wt oz	Meat/Fish/Poultry
Pastrami, Turkey	1.0	3	slices	Meat/Fish/Poultry
Pate	-3.5	2	wt oz	Meat/Fish/Poultry
Pate, Chicken Liver, Canned	0.5	2	wt oz	Meat/Fish/Poultry
Pate, de Foie Gras, Canned (goose Liver)	-1.0	1	wt oz	Meat/Fish/Poultry
Peach Nectar, Canned	4.0	6	fl oz	Fruit
Peach, Fresh	11.0	1	whole	Fruit
Peaches, Canned In Juice	6.5	1	cup	Fruit
Peaches, Canned, Heavy Syrup	0.0	1/2	cup	Fruit
Peaches, Canned, Unsweetened	10.5	1/2	cup	Fruit
Peaches, Dried, Sulfured, Uncooked	5.0	2	pieces	Fruit
Peaches, Dried, Sun-Maid	5.0	4	pieces	Fruit
Peaches, Light Yellow Cling, Fruit Juice, Canned, Libby's	6.5	1/2	cup	Fruit
Peaches, Yellow Cling, Light Syrup, Canned, Del Monte	4.0	1/2	cup	Fruit
Peanut Butter	0.5	1	Tbls	Legume/Nut/Seed
Peanut Butter, 25% less fat, Laura Scudder's Natural	1.5	2	Tbls	Legume/Nut/Seed
Peanut Butter, 25% less fat, Skippy	1.0	2	Tbls	Legume/Nut/Seed
Peanut Butter, 30% less fat, Peter Pan Smart Choice	1.0	2	Tbls	Legume/Nut/Seed
Peanut Butter, Chunky, Health Valley	1.5	2	Tbls	Legume/Nut/Seed
Peanut Butter, Chunky, No Salt, Health Valley	1.5	2	Tbls	Legume/Nut/Seed
Peanut Butter, Creamy, Jif	0.0	1	Tbls	Legume/Nut/Seed
Peanut Butter, Creamy, Skippy	0.0	1	Tbls	Legume/Nut/Seed
Peanut Butter, Crunchy, Peter Pan	0.0	1	Tbls	Legume/Nut/Seed
Peanut Butter, Low Sodium	1.0	1	Tbls	Legume/Nut/Seed
Peanut Butter, Natural, Smucker's	1.0	1	Tbls	Legume/Nut/Seed
Peanut Butter, No Salt Added, Natural, Smucker's	1.0	1	Tbls	Legume/Nut/Seed
Peanut Butter, Reduced Fat, Jiff	1.0	2	Tbls	Legume/Nut/Seed
Peanut Butter, Skippy Reduced Fat	0.5	2	Tbls	Legume/Nut/Seed
Peanut Butter, Super Chunk, Skippy	0.0	1	Tbls	Legume/Nut/Seed
Peanut Butter, Unsalted	1.0	1	Tbls	Legume/Nut/Seed
Peanuts, Chocolate Covered	-1.0	1	wt oz	Legume/Nut/Seed
Peanuts, Cocktail, Planter's	1.0	1	wt oz	Legume/Nut/Seed
Peanuts, Dry Roasted, Salted, Frito-Lay	1.0	25	nuts	Legume/Nut/Seed
Peanuts, Dry Roasted, Salted, Planter's	1.0	1	wt oz	Legume/Nut/Seed
Peanuts, Dry Roasted, Unsalted, Planter's	1.5	1	wt oz	Legume/Nut/Seed
Peanuts, Honey Roasted	0.5	1	wt oz	Legume/Nut/Seed
Peanuts, Oil Roasted, Salted	1.0	25	nuts	Legume/Nut/Seed
Peanuts, Oil Roasted, Unsalted	1.5	25	nuts	Legume/Nut/Seed
Peanuts, Spanish, Salted, Planter's	1.0	1	wt oz	Legume/Nut/Seed
Peanuts, Yogurt-Covered	-1.0	1	wt oz	Legume/Nut/Seed

Food Name—Alphabetical	Nutripoints	Serving Size		Nutrigroup
Pear Nectar, Canned	**2.5**	6	fl oz	Fruit
Pear, Fresh	**4.5**	1	whole	Fruit
Pear, Poached, Nutripoint Recipe	**4.0**	1/2	serving	Fruit
Pears, Bartlett, Light Syrup, Canned, Del Monte	**1.5**	1/2	cup	Fruit
Pears, Canned No Sugar	**3.5**	1/2	cup	Fruit
Pears, Canned, Heavy Syrup	**-1.0**	1/2	cup	Fruit
Pears, Dried	**3.0**	2	pieces	Fruit
Peas and Carrots, Canned	**25.0**	1/2	cup	Vegetable
Peas and Carrots, Frozen, Cooked	**28.0**	1/2	cup	Vegetable
Peas, Black-Eyed, Canned	**9.0**	1	cup	Legume/Nut/Seed
Peas, Black-Eyed, Cooked	**8.5**	1	cup	Legume/Nut/Seed
Peas, Canned	**7.5**	1	cup	Legume/Nut/Seed
Peas, Early June, Canned, Le Sueur	**4.5**	1	cup	Legume/Nut/Seed
Peas, Frozen, Cooked	**14.0**	1	cup	Legume/Nut/Seed
Peas, Green, Frozen, Birds Eye	**12.0**	1	cup	Legume/Nut/Seed
Peas, Green, No Salt Added, Canned, Del Monte	**14.0**	1	cup	Legume/Nut/Seed
Peas, Split	**8.0**	1/2	cup	Legume/Nut/Seed
Peas, Sweet, 50% Less Salt, Canned, Green Giant	**6.5**	1/2	cup	Legume/Nut/Seed
Peas, Sweet, Canned, Green Giant	**6.5**	1/2	cup	Legume/Nut/Seed
Peas, Sweet, Early Garden, Canned, Del Monte	**6.0**	1/2	cup	Legume/Nut/Seed
Pecans, Oil Roasted, Salted	**-0.5**	1	wt oz	Legume/Nut/Seed
Pecans, Unsalted, Raw	**0.0**	15	nuts	Legume/Nut/Seed
Penne Pasta, Spicy Puttanesca, Organic, Fzn, Moosewood	**1.0**	1/2	serving	Grain
Pepper Steak, w/Rice, Frozen, Budget Gourmet	**0.0**	1/2	portion	Meat/Fish/Poultry
Pepper, Black	**0.5**	1	tsp	Condiment
Pepper, Cayenne/Red	**1.5**	1	tsp	Condiment
Pepper, Jalapeno	**0.5**	1	whole	Condiment
Pepperoni	**-5.0**	1	wt oz	Meat/Fish/Poultry
Pepperoni, Gallo	**-6.0**	1	wt oz	Meat/Fish/Poultry
Pepperoni, Veggie Pizza, Yves	**14.5**	2	servings	Legume/Nut/Seed
Peppers, Green, Hot Chili	**2.5**	1	Tbls	Condiment
Peppers, Sweet, Red, Raw	**42.5**	2	whole	Vegetable
Peppers, Sweet, Stuffed, Frozen, Celentano	**2.0**	1/2	portion	Meat/Fish/Poultry
Perch Fillet, Broiled/Baked	**4.0**	4	wt oz	Meat/Fish/Poultry
Perch, Fried w/ Breading	**1.0**	3	wt oz	Meat/Fish/Poultry
Perrier Mineral Water	**0.0**	8	fl oz	Miscellaneous
Persimmon	**7.5**	1	whole	Fruit
Pheasant, w/o Skin	**5.5**	4	wt oz	Meat/Fish/Poultry
Pickle Relish	**-6.0**	2	Tbls	Vegetable
Pickles, Bread 'n Butter, Cucumber Slices, Heinz	**-1.0**	8	slices	Vegetable
Pickles, Dill	**-3.5**	2	whole	Vegetable
Pickles, Kosher Crunchy Dills, Half/Salt Vlasic	**3.0**	2	whole	Vegetable
Pickles, Kosher Dill Spears, Vlasic	**0.5**	2	whole	Vegetable
Pickles, Kosher, Claussen	**-4.0**	2	whole	Vegetable
Pickles, Sweet	**-5.0**	1	whole	Vegetable

Food Name—Alphabetical	Nutripoints	Serving Size		Nutrigroup
Pickles, Sweet Butter Chips, Vlasic	**-1.0**	1	wt oz	Condiment
Pickles, Sweet Gherkins, Heinz	**-2.5**	1	whole	Vegetable
Pickles, Sweet 'n Sour, Claussen	**2.5**	1	whole	Vegetable
Pie Crust	**-3.0**	1	piece	Grain
Pie Crust Mix, Betty Crocker	**-2.5**	1	piece	Grain
Pie Crust, Pet Ritz	**-2.5**	1	piece	Grain
Pie Filling, Apple, Lite, Thank You	**-1.5**	1/2	cup	Fruit
Pie Filling, Apple, Thank You	**-3.0**	1/2	cup	Fruit
Pie Filling, Cherry, Thank You	**-4.0**	1/2	cup	Fruit
Pie, Apple	**-2.0**	1/4	piece	Fruit
Pie, Apple, Frozen, Weight Watchers	**-2.0**	1/2	piece	Fruit
Pie, Apple, Natural Juice, Mrs. Smith's	**-2.5**	1/4	piece	Fruit
Pie, Banana Cream	**-1.0**	1/2	piece	Fruit
Pie, Berry	**-2.0**	1/2	piece	Fruit
Pie, Blackberry	**-1.5**	1/2	piece	Fruit
Pie, Blueberry	**-2.0**	1/2	piece	Fruit
Pie, Blueberry, Hostess	**-2.0**	1/4	piece	Fruit
Pie, Boston Cream	**-1.0**	1/2	piece	Milk/Dairy
Pie, Boston Cream Classic, Betty Crocker	**-2.5**	1/2	piece	Milk/Dairy
Pie, Boston Cream, Frozen, Weight Watchers	**-2.5**	1	piece	Milk/Dairy
Pie, Cherry	**-5.0**	1/2	piece	Fruit
Pie, Cherry, Hostess	**-2.0**	1/4	piece	Fruit
Pie, Cherry, Natural Juice, Mrs. Smith's	**-2.0**	1/4	piece	Fruit
Pie, Cherry, w/Cream Cheese & Sour Cream	**-3.5**	1/4	piece	Fruit
Pie, Chiffon	**-4.5**	1/2	piece	Sugar
Pie, Chocolate Cream	**-2.5**	1/2	piece	Sugar
Pie, Coconut Cream	**-3.5**	1/2	piece	Fruit
Pie, Custard	**-3.5**	1/2	piece	Milk/Dairy
Pie, Fruit	**-2.0**	1/4	piece	Fruit
Pie, Fruit Yogurt, Nutripoint Recipe	**0.5**	1	piece	Milk/Dairy
Pie, Lemon Meringue	**-4.0**	1/4	piece	Fruit
Pie, Mincemeat	**-1.0**	1/4	piece	Fruit
Pie, Peach	**-2.0**	1/2	piece	Fruit
Pie, Peach, Mrs. Smith's	**-2.5**	1/4	piece	Fruit
Pie, Pecan	**-3.5**	1/2	piece	Legume/Nut/Seed
Pie, Pumpkin Custard, Mrs. Smith's	**-1.5**	1/2	piece	Milk/Dairy
Pie, Pumpkin, Homemade	**-3.0**	1/2	piece	Fruit
Pie, Raspberry	**-1.0**	1/2	piece	Fruit
Pie, Rhubarb, Homemade	**-2.5**	1/4	piece	Vegetable
Pie, Strawberry	**-1.5**	1/2	piece	Fruit
Pie, Vanilla Cream	**-3.0**	1/2	piece	Milk/Dairy
Pie, Yogurt	**-2.5**	1/2	piece	Milk/Dairy
Pigeon Peas, Green, Cooked	**11.0**	1	cup	Legume/Nut/Seed
Pike Fillet, Breaded, Fried	**0.5**	3	wt oz	Meat/Fish/Poultry
Pike, Baked	**7.5**	6	wt oz	Meat/Fish/Poultry
Pilaf, Breakfast, 7 Whole Grains & Sesame, Kashi	**3.5**	1/2	cup	Grain
Pilaf, Couscous, Casbah	**3.0**	1/2	cup	Grain

Food Name—Alphabetical	Nutripoints	Serving Size		Nutrigroup
Pilaf, Kashi	**2.0**	1/2	cup	Grain
Pilaf, Vegetarian Amaranth, Health Valley	**6.5**	4	wt oz	Grain
Pina Colada	**-7.5**	3	fl oz	Alcohol
Pine Nuts, Pignolia	**1.0**	1	wt oz	Legume/Nut/Seed
Pineapple, Canned, Heavy Syrup	**1.0**	1/2	cup	Fruit
Pineapple, Chunks, In Juice, Canned, Del Monte	**4.0**	1/2	cup	Fruit
Pineapple, Fresh	**8.0**	1/2	cup	Fruit
Pineapple, Sliced, Canned, Light Syrup, Dole	**2.0**	1/2	cup	Fruit
Pineapple, Sliced, In Juice, Canned, Del Monte	**4.0**	1/2	cup	Fruit
Pineapple, Sliced, In Juice, Canned, Dole	**4.0**	1/2	cup	Fruit
Pistachios, Dry Roasted, Salted	**0.0**	1/4	cup	Legume/Nut/Seed
Pistachios, Raw	**1.0**	1	wt oz	Legume/Nut/Seed
Pizza Deluxe, Fzn, South Beach Diet	**4.0**	1	serving	Grain
Pizza Hut Cheese Pan Pizza	**2.5**	1/2	piece	Grain
Pizza Hut Cheese Thin 'n Crispy Pizza	**3.0**	1	piece	Grain
Pizza Hut Chicken Supreme Thin 'N Crispy Pizza	**5.0**	1	slice	Meat/Fish/Poultry
Pizza Hut Fit 'N Delicious Pizza (ave. all varieties)	**3.5**	1	slice	Grain
Pizza Hut Hand Tossed Cheese Pizza	**2.0**	1/2	piece	Grain
Pizza Hut Meat Lover's Thin 'N Crispy Pizza	**1.5**	1	slice	Meat/Fish/Poultry
Pizza Hut Pepperoni Hand Tossed Pizza	**1.5**	1/2	piece	Grain
Pizza Hut Pepperoni Pan Pizza	**3.0**	1/2	piece	Grain
Pizza Hut Pepperoni Personal Pan Pizza	**1.5**	1/4	piece	Grain
Pizza Hut Pepperoni Thin 'n Crispy Pizza	**1.5**	1/2	piece	Grain
Pizza Hut Super Supreme Hand Tossed Pizza	**2.0**	1/2	piece	Grain
Pizza Hut Super Supreme Pan Pizza	**2.0**	1/2	piece	Grain
Pizza Hut Super Supreme Thin 'n Crispy Pizza	**2.0**	1/2	piece	Grain
Pizza Hut Supreme Hand Tossed Pizza	**3.5**	1/2	piece	Grain
Pizza Hut Supreme Pan Pizza	**2.0**	1/2	piece	Grain
Pizza Hut Supreme Personal Pan Pizza	**2.0**	1/4	piece	Grain
Pizza Hut Supreme Thin 'n Crispy Pizza	**2.0**	1/2	piece	Grain
Pizza Hut Veggie Lover's Thin 'N Crispy Pizza	**3.5**	1	slices	Grain
Pizza, 9 Slice, Frozen, Celentano	**0.5**	1	slice	Grain
Pizza, BBQ Chicken, California Pizza Kitchen	**-1.5**	1/2	slice	Grain
Pizza, Cheese, Chef Boy-Ar-Dee	**0.5**	4	wt oz	Grain
Pizza, Cheese, Deluxe, Frozen, Totino's	**1.0**	1	piece	Grain
Pizza, Cheese, French Bread, Fzn, Weight Watchers	**0.5**	1/2	piece	Grain
Pizza, Cheese, French Bread, Lean Cuisine, Stouffer's	**2.0**	1/2	portion	Grain
Pizza, Cheese, Frozen, Celeste	**0.0**	1	piece	Grain
Pizza, Cheese, Frozen, Tree Tavern	**0.5**	1/2	piece	Grain
Pizza, Cheese, Frozen, Weight Watchers	**1.5**	1	piece	Grain
Pizza, Cheese, Round Family Style, Elios	**0.0**	1	piece	Grain
Pizza, Chicken & Vegetable, Fzn, South Beach Diet	**5.0**	1	serving	Meat/Fish/Poultry
Pizza, Combo, Deluxe, Frozen, Weight Watchers	**1.5**	1/2	piece	Grain
Pizza, Combos	**0.0**	1	wt oz	Grain

Food Name—Alphabetical	Nutripoints	Serving Size		Nutrigroup
Pizza, Five Cheese & Tomato, California Pizza Kitchen	**-1.5**	1/2	slice	Grain
Pizza, Four Cheese, Fzn, South Beach Diet	**4.0**	1	serving	Grain
Pizza, French Bread Deluxe, Fzn, Weight Watchers	**0.5**	1/2	piece	Grain
Pizza, French Bread Pepperoni, Stouffer	**1.0**	1/2	piece	Grain
Pizza, French Bread, Cheese, Fzn, Stouffer's	**0.5**	1/2	piece	Grain
Pizza, French Bread, Nutripoint Recipe	**6.0**	1	piece	Grain
Pizza, French Bread, Pepperoni & Mushroom, Fzn, Stouffer's	**0.0**	1/2	piece	Grain
Pizza, French Bread, Vegetable Deluxe, Fzn, Stouffer's	**0.5**	1/2	piece	Grain
Pizza, Mushroom & Spinach, Linda McCartney	**0.5**	1/2	serving	Grain
Pizza, Party Cheese, Frozen, Totino's	**0.5**	1	piece	Grain
Pizza, Pepperoni, Chef Boy-Ar-Dee	**-0.5**	4	wt oz	Grain
Pizza, Pepperoni, French Bread, Fzn, Weight Watchers	**0.0**	1/2	piece	Grain
Pizza, Pepperoni, Frozen, Elio's	**0.0**	1/2	piece	Grain
Pizza, Pepperoni, Frozen, Weight Watchers	**1.0**	1/2	piece	Grain
Pizza, Pepperoni, Fzn, South Beach Diet	**3.5**	1	serving	Meat/Fish/Poultry
Pizza, Sausage, Frozen, Weight Watchers	**1.0**	1/2	piece	Grain
Pizza, Thai Recipe Chicken, California Pizza Kitchen	**-0.5**	1/2	slice	Grain
Pizza, Thick Crust, Frozen, Celentano	**0.5**	1	piece	Grain
Pizza, Veggie Supreme, Morningstar Farms	**-0.5**	1	serving	Grain
Pizza, w/Cheese	**1.0**	1	piece	Grain
Pizza, w/Pepperoni	**-2.0**	1/2	piece	Grain
Pizza, w/Sausage	**-1.0**	1/2	piece	Grain
Plantain, Cooked	**5.5**	1/2	cup	Fruit
Plantain, Fresh	**6.0**	1/2	piece	Fruit
Plum, Fresh	**6.0**	2	whole	Fruit
Plums, Canned, Heavy Syrup	**0.0**	1/2	cup	Fruit
Plums, Canned, Unsweetened	**14.0**	1/2	cup	Fruit
Poi	**3.5**	1/2	cup	Vegetable
Pomegranate	**3.5**	1	whole	Fruit
Pompano, Baked/Broiled	**0.0**	3	wt oz	Meat/Fish/Poultry
Pompano, Floured/Breaded, Fried	**-0.5**	3	wt oz	Meat/Fish/Poultry
Popcorn, Air Popped	**2.0**	2	cups	Grain
Popcorn, Caramel	**0.0**	1	cup	Grain
Popcorn, Cooked w/Oil	**0.0**	2	cups	Grain
Popcorn, Gourmet, Microwave, O. Redenbacher	**-0.5**	2	cups	Vegetable
Popcorn, Gourmet, O. Redenbacher	**2.5**	2	cups	Vegetable
Popcorn, Light, Orville Redenbacher's	**3.0**	3	cups	Grain
Popcorn, Natural Salt Free, Orville Redenbacher's	**0.5**	2	cups	Grain
Popcorn, Original Lite	**1.0**	2	cups	Grain
Pop-Tarts, Blueberry, Kellogg's	**0.5**	1	piece	Grain
Pop-Tarts, Frosted Cherry w/Smucker's Fruit, Kellogg's	**0.5**	1	tart	Grain

Food Name—Alphabetical	Nutripoints	Serving Size		Nutrigroup
Pop-Tarts, Frosted Strawberry, Kellogg's	**0.5**	1	tart	Grain
Pop-Tarts, Kellogg's Lowfat	**0.5**	1	tart	Grain
Pork Chop, Broiled	**-0.5**	2	wt oz	Meat/Fish/Poultry
Pork Chop, Loin, Lean, Baked	**3.0**	3	wt oz	Meat/Fish/Poultry
Pork Chop, Pan-Fried	**-0.5**	1	piece	Meat/Fish/Poultry
Pork Feet, Pickled	**-1.0**	3	wt oz	Meat/Fish/Poultry
Pork Roast, Baked	**0.0**	2	wt oz	Meat/Fish/Poultry
Pork Skins	**0.0**	1	wt oz	Meat/Fish/Poultry
Pork Spareribs	**-1.5**	3	pieces	Meat/Fish/Poultry
Pork w/Pecans & Green Beans, Fzn, South Beach Diet	**2.0**	1	serving	Meat/Fish/Poultry
Pork, Frozen Dinner	**2.0**	1/2	portion	Meat/Fish/Poultry
Pork, Light, Rich Meat Service	**3.5**	4	wt oz	Meat/Fish/Poultry
Pork, Sweet and Sour	**0.0**	3/4	cup	Meat/Fish/Poultry
Pork, Sweet and Sour, Frozen, Chun King	**2.0**	1/2	portion	Meat/Fish/Poultry
Portabello Mushroom, Uncle Ben's Pasta Bowl	**0.5**	1	serving	Grain
Postum	**5.5**	6	fl oz	Miscellaneous
Potato Chips	**0.0**	5	chips	Vegetable
Potato Chips, Baked Lay's	**1.5**	12	chips	Vegetable
Potato Chips, Lay's Light, BBQ, Nonfat	**1.0**	20	chips	Vegetable
Potato Chips, Lay's Light, Nonfat	**2.0**	20	chips	Vegetable
Potato Chips, Lay's	**0.0**	8	chips	Vegetable
Potato Chips, Light, Pringle's	**-1.0**	1/2	cup	Vegetable
Potato Chips, Light, Ruffles	**1.0**	9	chips	Vegetable
Potato Chips, Pringle's	**-1.5**	1/2	cup	Vegetable
Potato Chips, Pringles Fat Free	**1.0**	16	chips	Vegetable
Potato Chips, Ruffles	**0.0**	9	chips	Vegetable
Potato Chips, Ruffles Light, Nonfat	**1.5**	17	chips	Vegetable
Potato Chips, Sour Cream 'n Onion, Pringle's	**-1.5**	1/2	cup	Vegetable
Potato Chips, Unsalted, Lay's	**0.0**	8	chips	Vegetable
Potato Chips, Wise	**-1.0**	5	chips	Vegetable
Potato Salad, Home Recipe	**-1.0**	1/4	cup	Vegetable
Potato Salad, Nutripoint Recipe	**9.0**	1/2	cup	Vegetable
Potato Sticks, Shoestring	**0.0**	1/4	cup	Vegetable
Potato, Baked	**8.5**	1/2	potato	Vegetable
Potato, Baked, Broccoli & Cheese, Fzn, Weight Watchers	**1.5**	1/4	portion	Vegetable
Potato, Baked, Chicken Divan, Fzn, Weight Watchers	**1.5**	1/4	portion	Vegetable
Potatoes, Au Gratin	**2.5**	1/4	cup	Vegetable
Potatoes, Au Gratin, Betty Crocker	**-0.5**	1/4	cup	Vegetable
Potatoes, Au Gratin, Frozen, Stouffer's	**-0.5**	1/2	serving	Vegetable

Food Name—Alphabetical	Nutripoints	Serving Size		Nutrigroup
Potatoes, Cheddared, w/Broccoli, Fzn, Budget Gourmet	**1.5**	1/2	portion	Vegetable
Potatoes, Golden Crinkles, Ore-Ida	**0.5**	1/2	cup	Vegetable
Potatoes, Hash Browned	**0.5**	1/4	cup	Vegetable
Potatoes, Homestyle, Nutripoint Recipe	**5.5**	1/2	cup	Vegetable
Potatoes, Instant Mashed, Betty Crocker	**-0.5**	1/4	cup	Vegetable
Potatoes, Instant Mashed, Hungry Jack	**0.0**	1/4	cup	Vegetable
Potatoes, Mashed, From Flakes	**2.0**	1/4	cup	Vegetable
Potatoes, Mashed, Home Recipe	**1.0**	1/4	cup	Vegetable
Potatoes, Scalloped	**2.0**	1/4	cup	Vegetable
Potatoes, Scalloped, Frozen, Stouffer's	**0.5**	1/2	portion	Vegetable
Potatoes, Tater Tots, Ore-Ida	**-0.5**	1/4	cup	Vegetable
Power Gel, Power Bar	**-1.5**	1	serving	Sugar
Preserves, All Varieties, Kraft	**-5.0**	1	Tbls	Fruit
Preserves, Raspberry, Smucker's	**-6.0**	1	Tbls	Fruit
Preserves, Strawberry, Welch's	**-5.5**	1	Tbls	Fruit
Pretzel, Fat Free, Mr. Salty, Nabisco	**1.5**	1	fl oz	Grain
Pretzels, 3 Ring	**0.5**	10	pieces	Grain
Pretzels, Keebler	**1.5**	1/2	cup	Grain
Pretzels, Sticks	**0.5**	50	pieces	Grain
Pretzels, Twists, Rold Gold	**1.0**	1	wt oz	Grain
Prickly pear	**10.0**	1	pear	Fruit
Protein Powder	**2.0**	1	Tbls	Miscellaneous
Prunes, Canned, Heavy Syrup	**4.5**	1/4	cup	Fruit
Prunes, Cooked, Unsweetened	**6.5**	1/2	cup	Fruit
Prunes, Cooked, w/Sugar	**4.0**	1/4	cup	Fruit
Prunes, Dried	**6.0**	4	pieces	Fruit
Prunes, Pitted, Bite Size, Sunsweet	**5.0**	1	wt oz	Fruit
Prunes, Whole, Sunsweet	**6.0**	3	prunes	Fruit
Pudding Mix, Americana Tapioca, Jell-O	**-2.0**	1	cup	Milk/Dairy
Pudding Mix, Vanilla, Jell-O	**-2.5**	1	cup	Milk/Dairy
Pudding Mix, Vanilla, Sugar-Free, Instant, Jell-O	**2.0**	1	cup	Milk/Dairy
Pudding, Banana	**1.0**	1/4	cup	Milk/Dairy
Pudding, Bread	**-2.0**	1/2	cup	Grain
Pudding, Choc. Pudding Snacks, Jell-O	**-3.5**	4	wt oz	Milk/Dairy
Pudding, Chocolate	**-3.5**	1/2	cup	Milk/Dairy
Pudding, Chocolate, Snack Pack, Hunts	**-4.0**	4	wt oz	Milk/Dairy
Pudding, Fat-Free, Swiss Miss (all flavors)	**-2.5**	1/2	cup	Milk/Dairy
Pudding, Low Cal	**3.0**	1	cup	Milk/Dairy
Pudding, Rice	**-1.0**	1/4	cup	Grain
Pudding, Sustacal	**2.0**	1/2	cup	Milk/Dairy
Pudding, Tapioca	**-0.5**	1/2	cup	Milk/Dairy

Food Name—Alphabetical	Nutripoints	Serving Size		Nutrigroup
Pudding, Tapioca, Healthy Choice Lowfat	**-2.5**	1/2	cup	Milk/Dairy
Pudding, Tapioca, Jello Fat Free	**-3.5**	1/2	cup	Milk/Dairy
Pudding, Vanilla	**-1.5**	1/2	cup	Milk/Dairy
Pudding, Vanilla, Snack Pack, Hunts	**-4.0**	4	wt oz	Milk/Dairy
Pumpkin, Canned	**25.5**	1/2	cup	Vegetable
Pumpkin, Cooked	**17.5**	1/2	cup	Vegetable
Quail, w/o Skin	**6.0**	4	wt oz	Meat/Fish/Poultry
Quiche, Cheese	**-6.0**	1/2	piece	Milk/Dairy
Quiche, Cheese/Bacon	**-4.5**	1/4	piece	Milk/Dairy
Quince	**6.0**	1	whole	Fruit
Quinine Water	**-5.5**	8	fl oz	Sugar
Quinoa, Dry, Arrowhead Mills	**5.5**	1	wt oz	Grain
Rabbit, Domestic, Breaded, Fried	**3.0**	3	wt oz	Meat/Fish/Poultry
Rabbit, Stewed	**2.0**	3	wt oz	Meat/Fish/Poultry
Rabbit, Wild	**3.0**	3	wt oz	Meat/Fish/Poultry
Radishes, Raw	**29.0**	1	cup	Vegetable
Raisins	**4.0**	1/4	cup	Fruit
Raisins, California Golden, Sun-Maid	**3.0**	2	Tbls	Fruit
Raisins, Carob-Covered	**-1.0**	1	wt oz	Fruit
Raisins, Chocolate-Covered	**-1.5**	1	wt oz	Fruit
Raisins, Thompson Seedless, Natural, Sun-Maid	**3.0**	2	Tbls	Fruit
Ramen, Natural Mushroom, Westbrae	**2.0**	1/2	cup	Grain
Ramen, Natural Spinach, Westbrae	**2.0**	1	wt oz	Grain
Ramen, Natural Whole Wheat, Westbrae	**2.0**	1	wt oz	Grain
Raspberries, Fresh	**12.5**	1/2	cup	Fruit
Raspberries, Frozen, Sweetened	**4.5**	1/4	cup	Fruit
Raspberry, Peccavi, Nutripoint Recipe	**-1.0**	1	serving	Fruit
Ratatouille, Frozen Dinner	**1.0**	1	portion	Vegetable
Ravioli	**4.5**	1/2	cup	Grain
Ravioli, Baked Cheese, Fzn, Weight Watchers	**1.0**	1/2	portion	Milk/Dairy
Ravioli, Cheese, Slim, Fzn, Budget Gourmet	**0.5**	1/2	portion	Milk/Dairy
Ravioli, Frozen, Celentano	**0.0**	1/2	portion	Grain
Ravioli, Mini, Frozen, Celentano	**2.0**	1/2	portion	Grain
Red Snapper, Baked	**7.0**	6	wt oz	Meat/Fish/Poultry
Red Snapper, Vera Cruz Style, Nutripoint Recipe	**13.0**	3	wt oz	Meat/Fish/Poultry
Relish, Hot Dog, Vlasic	**-2.5**	2	Tbls	Vegetable
Relish, Sweet, Heinz	**-3.5**	2	Tbls	Vegetable
Rhubarb, Cooked, w/Sugar	**-2.0**	1/4	cup	Vegetable
Rice Cakes, Plain, Lightly Salted, Quaker	**3.0**	3	cakes	Grain
Rice Cakes, Plain, Salt-Free, Quaker	**3.0**	3	cakes	Grain
Rice Cakes, Sesame, Lt. Salted, Quaker	**3.0**	3	cakes	Grain
Rice Milk, Rice Dream Original, 1% Fat	**3.0**	8	fl oz	Grain

Food Name—Alphabetical	Nutripoints	Serving Size		Nutrigroup
Rice, Brown Pilaf, w/Vegetables & Herbs, Pritikin	**3.0**	1/2	cup	Grain
Rice, Brown, Cooked w/o Salt	**4.0**	1/2	cup	Grain
Rice, Brown, Instant, Minute	**3.5**	1/2	cup	Grain
Rice, Brown, Natural Long Grain, Mahatma	**3.5**	1/2	cup	Grain
Rice, Brown, Quick, Vegetable Herb, Arrowhead Mills	**2.5**	1/2	cup	Grain
Rice, Chicken Rice-A-Roni	**0.5**	1/2	cup	Grain
Rice, Converted, Uncle Ben's	**2.5**	1/2	cup	Grain
Rice, Ext Long Grain Enriched, Carolina	**2.0**	1/2	cup	Grain
Rice, Fried, w/Chicken, Frozen, Chun King	**1.5**	1/2	portion	Grain
Rice, Fried, w/Pork, Frozen, Chun King	**1.0**	1/2	serving	Grain
Rice, Long Grain Enriched, Mahatma	**2.0**	1/2	cup	Grain
Rice, Minute Rice	**2.5**	1/2	cup	Grain
Rice, Oriental, Vegetables, Fzn, Budget Gourmet	**0.0**	1/2	portion	Grain
Rice, Pilaf	**2.0**	1/2	cup	Grain
Rice, Rice A Roni	**0.0**	1/2	cup	Grain
Rice, Rice A Roni, Spanish	**1.5**	1/2	cup	Grain
Rice, Spanish	**4.0**	1/2	cup	Grain
Rice, White, Instant, Cooked	**3.0**	2/3	cup	Grain
Rice, White, Regular, Cooked, w/o Salt	**3.0**	1/2	cup	Grain
Rice, White, Regular, w/Added Salt	**3.0**	1/2	cup	Grain
Rice, Whole Grain Brown, Uncle Ben's	**4.5**	2/3	cup	Grain
Rice, Wild & Long Grain, Veg. & Herb, Uncle Ben's	**4.0**	1	serving	Grain
Rice, Wild, Cooked w/o Salt	**5.5**	1/2	cup	Grain
Rice, Wild, Sherry, Frozen, Green Giant	**4.5**	1/2	cup	Grain
Rigatoni, Baked, w/Meat Sauce/Cheese, Fzn, Stouffer's	**0.5**	1/2	portion	Grain
Roll, Cracked Wheat	**3.0**	1	roll	Grain
Roll, Diet	**2.5**	1	roll	Grain
Roll, Dinner, Wheat Loaf, Pipin' Hot	**1.5**	2	rolls	Grain
Roll, Dinner, White Loaf, Pipin' Hot	**1.5**	2	rolls	Grain
Roll, Frankfurter, Side-Sliced, Pepperidge Farm	**1.5**	1	roll	Grain
Roll, Frankfurter, Wonder	**2.0**	1	roll	Grain
Roll, French or Vienna	**2.5**	1	roll	Grain
Roll, French, Brown 'n Serve, Pepperidge Farm	**2.5**	1/2	roll	Grain
Roll, Hard	**2.0**	1	roll	Grain
Roll, Rye	**3.5**	1	roll	Grain
Roll, Sourdough	**2.5**	1	roll	Grain
Roll, Sourdough, French Extra, Earth Grains	**2.5**	2	rolls	Grain
Roll, Sweet	**-2.5**	1/2	roll	Grain
Roll, Sweet, Apple, Frozen, Weight Watchers	**-1.5**	1	roll	Grain
Roll, Sweet, Cinnamon Bun, Frosted	**-1.0**	1	roll	Grain

Food Name—Alphabetical	Nutripoints	Serving Size		Nutrigroup
Roll, Sweet, Cinnamon, w/Icing, Pillsbury	**-2.5**	1	roll	Grain
Roll, Sweet, w/Fruit	**1.5**	1	roll	Grain
Roll, Sweet, w/Fruit & Nuts, Frosted	**0.0**	1	roll	Grain
Roll, Sweet, w/Fruit, Frosted	**0.0**	1	roll	Grain
Roll, White	**2.0**	1	roll	Grain
Roll, Whole Wheat	**4.5**	1	roll	Grain
Root Beer	**-6.0**	12	fl oz	Sugar
Rosemary	**0.5**	1	tsp	Condiment
Rotini Cheddar, Garden Gourmet, Green Giant	**4.0**	1/2	cup	Grain
Rotini, Rainbow, Creamette	**3.0**	1	wt oz	Grain
Rum	**-16.5**	2	fl oz	Alcohol
Rum and Carbonated Beverage	**-10.5**	6	fl oz	Alcohol
Rum, Hot Buttered	**-12.5**	3	fl oz	Alcohol
Rutabagas, Cooked	**18.0**	1/2	cup	Vegetable
Rye Cakes, Quaker	**4.5**	3	cups	Grain
Sage	**0.5**	1	tsp	Condiment
Salad, Chef, w/Ham/Cheese, w/o Dressing	**-1.5**	1/2	cup	Vegetable
Salad, Greens, Balsamic Vinegar, Nutripoint Recipe	**42.0**	1	cup	Vegetable
Salad, Mixed Vegetable, Nutripoint Recipe	**17.0**	1/2	cup	Vegetable
Salad, Spinach, Nutripoint Recipe	**65.0**	2	cups	Vegetable
Salad, Spinach, w/Egg/Bacon/Tomato	**4.0**	1/2	cup	Vegetable
Salad, Three Bean	**1.5**	1	cup	Legume/Nut/Seed
Salad, Tossed, No Dressing	**33.0**	1	cup	Vegetable
Salad, Tossed, Nutripoint Recipe	**51.5**	2	cups	Vegetable
Salad, Tossed, w/Tomato	**21.5**	1	cup	Vegetable
Salad, Waldorf	**-2.0**	1/2	cup	Fruit
Salami, Beef	**0.0**	2	wt oz	Meat/Fish/Poultry
Salami, Cooked, Armour	**-4.0**	2	wt oz	Meat/Fish/Poultry
Salami, Cotto Beef, Eckrich	**-4.0**	1	wt oz	Meat/Fish/Poultry
Salami, Cotto, Oscar Mayer	**-2.0**	2	slices	Meat/Fish/Poultry
Salami, Hard (Genoa), Oscar Mayer	**-2.5**	4	slices	Meat/Fish/Poultry
Salami, Meatless, Worthington	**2.5**	3	slices	Legume/Nut/Seed
Salami, Pork	**1.0**	4	slices	Meat/Fish/Poultry
Salami, Slices, Frozen, Loma Linda Foods	**5.5**	2	wt oz	Legume/Nut/Seed
Salami, Turkey Cotto, Louis Rich	**-2.0**	3	slices	Meat/Fish/Poultry
Salisbury Steak, Frozen, Healthy Choice	**1.5**	1	portion	Meat/Fish/Poultry
Salmon Patty, Fried	**1.0**	3	wt oz	Meat/Fish/Poultry
Salmon w/Basil, Frozen, Lean Cuisine	**3.0**	1	serving	Meat/Fish/Poultry
Salmon, Baked w/Butter	**2.0**	3	wt oz	Meat/Fish/Poultry
Salmon, Baked/Broiled	**5.5**	3	wt oz	Meat/Fish/Poultry
Salmon, Canned In Water	**6.5**	1/2	cup	Meat/Fish/Poultry

Food Name—Alphabetical	Nutripoints	Serving Size		Nutrigroup
Salmon, Lettuce Wrapped, w/Herb Sauce, Nutripoint Recipe	**10.5**	4	wt oz	Meat/Fish/Poultry
Salmon, Pink, Bumble Bee	**4.0**	1/2	cup	Meat/Fish/Poultry
Salmon, Pink, Chunk, Skinless/Boneless, Water, Chicken of the Sea	**4.5**	3/4	cup	Meat/Fish/Poultry
Salmon, Red Sockeye, Bumble Bee	**3.0**	1/2	cup	Meat/Fish/Poultry
Salmon, Red, Chunk, Skinless/Boneless, Chicken of the Sea	**3.5**	1/2	cup	Meat/Fish/Poultry
Salmon, Smoked	**3.0**	3	wt oz	Meat/Fish/Poultry
Salmon, Steamed/Poached	**7.5**	3	wt oz	Meat/Fish/Poultry
Salt	**0.0**	1	tsp	Condiment
Salt Pork, Raw	**-4.0**	1	wt oz	Meat/Fish/Poultry
Salt, Iodized, Morton	**0.0**	1	tsp	Condiment
Salt, Lite	**0.0**	1	tsp	Condiment
Sandwich, BLT, White Bread	**1.0**	1/2	serving	Meat/Fish/Poultry
Sandwich, BLT, Whole Wheat Bread	**2.0**	1/2	serving	Meat/Fish/Poultry
Sandwich, Chicken Salad, White Bread	**3.5**	1/2	serving	Meat/Fish/Poultry
Sandwich, Chicken Salad, Whole Wheat Bread	**4.0**	1/2	serving	Meat/Fish/Poultry
Sandwich, Chicken, White Bread	**2.0**	1/2	serving	Meat/Fish/Poultry
Sandwich, Chicken, Whole Wheat Bread	**2.0**	1/2	serving	Meat/Fish/Poultry
Sandwich, Corned Beef, Rye Bread	**1.5**	1/2	serving	Meat/Fish/Poultry
Sandwich, Egg Salad, White Bread	**-3.5**	1/2	serving	Milk/Dairy
Sandwich, Egg Salad, Whole Wheat Bread	**-3.0**	1/2	serving	Milk/Dairy
Sandwich, Grilled Cheese, White	**0.0**	1/2	serving	Milk/Dairy
Sandwich, Ham Salad, White	**-0.5**	1/2	serving	Meat/Fish/Poultry
Sandwich, Ham Salad, Whole Wheat	**0.0**	1/2	serving	Meat/Fish/Poultry
Sandwich, Ham/Cheese, Rye	**0.5**	1/2	serving	Meat/Fish/Poultry
Sandwich, Ham/Cheese, White	**0.0**	1/2	serving	Meat/Fish/Poultry
Sandwich, Ham/Cheese, Whole Wheat	**0.5**	1/2	serving	Meat/Fish/Poultry
Sandwich, Manwich, Original, Hunts	**0.0**	2	Tbls	Condiment
Sandwich, Open Face Pita, Nutripoint Recipe	**5.0**	1/2	serving	Grain
Sandwich, Peanut Butter, White	**1.5**	1/2	serving	Legume/Nut/Seed
Sandwich, Peanut Butter, Whole Wheat	**2.0**	1/2	serving	Legume/Nut/Seed
Sandwich, Peanut Butter/Jelly, White	**0.5**	1/2	serving	Legume/Nut/Seed
Sandwich, Peanut Butter/Jelly, Whole Wheat	**0.5**	1/2	serving	Legume/Nut/Seed
Sandwich, Roast Beef, Hot	**1.0**	1/2	serving	Meat/Fish/Poultry
Sandwich, Sloppy Joe w/Bun	**1.0**	1/2	serving	Meat/Fish/Poultry
Sandwich, Steak, Frozen, Steak-Um	**-3.0**	2	wt oz	Meat/Fish/Poultry
Sandwich, Submarine	**0.0**	1/4	serving	Meat/Fish/Poultry
Sandwich, Tuna Salad, White	**3.0**	1/2	serving	Meat/Fish/Poultry
Sandwich, Tuna Salad, Whole Wheat	**3.5**	1/2	serving	Meat/Fish/Poultry
Sandwich, Turkey, Nutripoint Recipe	**4.0**	1	whole	Meat/Fish/Poultry

Food Name—Alphabetical	Nutripoints	Serving Size		Nutrigroup
Sandwich, Turkey, White Bread	**1.5**	1/2	serving	Meat/Fish/Poultry
Sandwich, Turkey, Whole Wheat Bread	**2.5**	1/2	serving	Meat/Fish/Poultry
Sardines, Canned In Oil	**4.5**	3	pieces	Meat/Fish/Poultry
Sardines, Canned, Mustard Sauce	**1.5**	6	pieces	Meat/Fish/Poultry
Sardines, Canned, Tomato Sauce	**3.5**	6	pieces	Meat/Fish/Poultry
Sauce Mix, Béarnaise, w/Milk-Butter	**-5.5**	1/4	cup	Fat/Oil
Sauce Mix, Curry, w/Milk	**0.0**	1/4	cup	Fat/Oil
Sauce Mix, Mushroom, Prepared w/Milk	**1.0**	1/4	cup	Fat/Oil
Sauce Mix, Stroganoff, Prepared w/Milk/Water	**1.5**	1/4	cup	Fat/Oil
Sauce Mix, Sweet and Sour, Prepared	**0.0**	1/4	cup	Fat/Oil
Sauce Mix, Teriyaki, Prepared	**-2.5**	1/4	cup	Fat/Oil
Sauce, Banana Mint, Nutripoint Recipe	**6.5**	1/4	cup	Milk/Dairy
Sauce, BBQ	**0.0**	1	Tbls	Condiment
Sauce, BBQ, All-Natural Hot & Zesty, Hunts	**-1.5**	1	Tbls	Condiment
Sauce, BBQ, All-Natural Original Flavor, Hunts	**-0.5**	1	Tbls	Condiment
Sauce, BBQ, Hickory Smoke Flavor, Open Pit	**-1.0**	1	Tbls	Condiment
Sauce, BBQ, Kraft	**-2.5**	1	Tbls	Condiment
Sauce, BBQ, Onion Bits, Kraft	**-1.5**	1	Tbls	Condiment
Sauce, BBQ, Original Flavor, Open Pit	**-1.5**	1	Tbls	Condiment
Sauce, Butterscotch	**-4.5**	2	Tbls	Sugar
Sauce, Butterscotch, Smucker's	**-5.0**	2	Tbls	Sugar
Sauce, Cheese	**-5.5**	1/4	cup	Milk/Dairy
Sauce, Chili	**1.0**	1	Tbls	Condiment
Sauce, Chocolate	**-5.0**	2	Tbls	Sugar
Sauce, Chocolate Fudge	**-3.5**	2	Tbls	Sugar
Sauce, Cranberry, Canned, Sweetened	**-3.0**	2	Tbls	Fruit
Sauce, Cranberry, Whole Berry, Ocean Spray	**-4.5**	1/4	cup	Fruit
Sauce, Custard	**-4.0**	1/4	cup	Milk/Dairy
Sauce, Heinz 57	**-1.0**	1	Tbls	Condiment
Sauce, Hollandaise	**-5.0**	1/4	cup	Fat/Oil
Sauce, Juniper Berry, Nutripoint Recipe	**0.0**	2	Tbls	Condiment
Sauce, Picante	**4.0**	1/4	cup	Condiment
Sauce, Soy	**0.0**	1	tsp	Condiment
Sauce, Soy, Kikkoman	**-0.5**	1	tsp	Condiment
Sauce, Spaghetti, Extra Chunky Mushroom/Onion, Prego	**-0.5**	1/4	cup	Vegetable
Sauce, Spaghetti, Extra Thick & Zesty, w/Meat, Ragu	**-0.5**	1/2	cup	Vegetable
Sauce, Spaghetti, Garden Tomato w/Mushroom, Prego	**-0.5**	1/4	cup	Vegetable
Sauce, Spaghetti, Meat Flavor, Prego	**-1.0**	1/4	cup	Vegetable
Sauce, Spaghetti, Meatless, Aunt Millie's	**4.0**	1/2	cup	Vegetable

Food Name—Alphabetical	Nutripoints	Serving Size		Nutrigroup
Sauce, Spaghetti, No Salt Added, Prego	**4.0**	1/2	cup	Vegetable
Sauce, Spaghetti, Plain, Extra Thick & Zesty, Ragu	**0.0**	1/2	cup	Vegetable
Sauce, Spaghetti, Plain, Ragu	**0.0**	1/2	cup	Vegetable
Sauce, Spaghetti, Prego	**0.5**	1/2	cup	Vegetable
Sauce, Spaghetti, Pritikin	**9.5**	1/2	cup	Vegetable
Sauce, Spaghetti, w/Meat, Ragu	**0.0**	1/2	cup	Vegetable
Sauce, Spaghetti, w/Mushrooms, Homestyle, Ragu	**3.0**	1/2	cup	Vegetable
Sauce, Spaghetti, w/Mushrooms, Prego	**0.5**	1/2	cup	Vegetable
Sauce, Spaghetti, w/Pepperoni/Sausage, Aunt Millie's	**3.5**	1/2	cup	Vegetable
Sauce, Steak	**1.5**	1	Tbls	Condiment
Sauce, Sweet and Sour	**-1.5**	1	Tbls	Condiment
Sauce, Tartar	**-3.5**	2	Tbls	Fat/Oil
Sauce, Tartar, Sauce Works, Kraft	**-0.5**	1	Tbls	Fat/Oil
Sauce, Teriyaki	**-0.5**	1	Tbls	Condiment
Sauce, Tomato, Canned	**17.5**	1/2	cup	Vegetable
Sauce, Tomato, Del Monte	**10.5**	1/2	cup	Vegetable
Sauce, Tomato, Hunts	**9.0**	1/2	cup	Vegetable
Sauce, Tomato, Nutripoint Recipe	**19.0**	1/2	cup	Vegetable
Sauce, Tomato, Thick & Zesty, Contadina	**15.5**	1/2	cup	Vegetable
Sauce, Traditional Pizza Quick, Ragu	**-0.5**	3	Tbls	Vegetable
Sauce, White	**-1.0**	1/4	cup	Fat/Oil
Sauce, Worcestershire	**1.0**	1	tsp	Condiment
Sauce, Zabaglione	**-10.5**	1/4	cup	Milk/Dairy
Sauerkraut, Canned	**17.0**	1	cup	Vegetable
Sausage Link, Pork	**-2.5**	2	links	Meat/Fish/Poultry
Sausage Links, Healthy Choice	**1.0**	3	links	Meat/Fish/Poultry
Sausage Links, Veggie, Morningstar Farms	**10.0**	4	links	Legume/Nut/Seed
Sausage Patty	**3.0**	1	patty	Meat/Fish/Poultry
Sausage Patty, Breakfast, Fzn, Morningstar Farms	**10.5**	2	patties	Legume/Nut/Seed
Sausage, Italian	**-0.5**	2	wt oz	Meat/Fish/Poultry
Sausage, Italian, 1 Link	**-1.5**	3	wt oz	Meat/Fish/Poultry
Sausage, Little, Jones	**-3.0**	2	wt oz	Meat/Fish/Poultry
Sausage, Meatless, Prosage Patties, Worthington	**6.0**	2	pieces	Legume/Nut/Seed
Sausage, Polish	**0.0**	2	wt oz	Meat/Fish/Poultry
Sausage, Pork, Jimmy Dean	**-3.5**	2	wt oz	Meat/Fish/Poultry
Sausage, Summer	**-1.0**	2	pieces	Meat/Fish/Poultry
Sausage, Vienna	**-3.5**	3	pieces	Meat/Fish/Poultry
Scallions	**24.0**	10	pieces	Vegetable
Scallop Kabob, Nutripoint Recipe	**16.0**	2	pieces	Meat/Fish/Poultry
Scallops & Shrimp Mariner, Fzn, Budget Gourmet	**0.5**	1/2	portion	Meat/Fish/Poultry
Scallops, Baked/Broiled	**4.0**	6	wt oz	Meat/Fish/Poultry
Scallops, Fried	**1.0**	3	wt oz	Meat/Fish/Poultry
Screwdriver	**-9.5**	8	fl oz	Alcohol

Food Name—Alphabetical	Nutripoints	Serving Size		Nutrigroup
Scrod, Baked, Stuffed, Frozen, Gorton's	**-2.5**	4	wt oz	Meat/Fish/Poultry
Seafood Newberg, Frozen, Budget Gourmet	**-0.5**	1/2	portion	Meat/Fish/Poultry
Seasoning, Poultry	**0.5**	1	tsp	Condiment
Seasoning, Shake 'n Bake for Pork	**-1.0**	1	Tbls	Condiment
Seasoning, Shake 'n Bake Original Chick	**0.0**	1	Tbls	Condiment
Seeds, Flax	**5.0**	2	Tbls	Legume/Nut/Seed
Seeds, Pumpkin & Squash	**2.0**	1/4	cup	Legume/Nut/Seed
Seeds, Pumpkin & Squash, Roasted, Salted	**2.5**	1	wt oz	Legume/Nut/Seed
Seeds, Pumpkin & Squash, Roasted, Unsalted	**2.5**	1	wt oz	Legume/Nut/Seed
Seeds, Sesame	**0.0**	1/4	cup	Legume/Nut/Seed
Seeds, Sunflower, Hulled, Arrowhead Mills	**2.0**	2	Tbls	Legume/Nut/Seed
Seeds, Sunflower, Unsalted	**4.5**	1/4	cup	Legume/Nut/Seed
Sesame Butter (tahini)	**1.5**	1	wt oz	Legume/Nut/Seed
Shallots, Raw	**8.5**	1/4	cup	Vegetable
Shark, Mixed Species, Batter-Dipped & Fried	**0.0**	3	wt oz	Meat/Fish/Poultry
Shark, Mixed Species, Raw	**4.0**	4	wt oz	Meat/Fish/Poultry
Shells & Cheese Dinner, Velveeta	**0.0**	1/2	cup	Grain
Shells, Frozen, Broccoli Stuffed, Celentano	**1.5**	1/4	portion	Milk/Dairy
Shells, Stuffed, 3 Cheese, Frozen, Le Menu	**1.0**	1/2	portion	Milk/Dairy
Shells, Stuffed, Frozen, Celentano	**2.0**	1/2	portion	Milk/Dairy
Sherbet, Orange	**-2.5**	1/2	cup	Fruit
Sherbet, Orange, Borden	**-4.0**	1/2	cup	Milk/Dairy
Shortbread, Lorna Doone	**-2.5**	3	pieces	Grain
Shortcake, Sponge Type w/Fruit	**-1.0**	1/2	piece	Grain
Shortcake, Strawberry, Frozen, Weight Watchers	**-2.0**	1	piece	Grain
Shortening, Crisco	**-3.5**	1	Tbls	Fat/Oil
Shortening, Lard and Veg Oil	**-4.5**	1	Tbls	Fat/Oil
Shortening, Soybean and Cottonseed	**-3.5**	1	Tbls	Fat/Oil
Shortening, Soybean and Palm	**-4.0**	1	Tbls	Fat/Oil
Shrimp Creole, Frozen, Healthy Choice	**0.5**	1	portion	Meat/Fish/Poultry
Shrimp Etouffé (1 pc = 1.5 c)	**2.0**	1	piece	Meat/Fish/Poultry
Shrimp, Fried	**-1.0**	3	pieces	Meat/Fish/Poultry
Shrimp, Fried, Frozen, Mrs. Paul's	**-3.5**	3	wt oz	Meat/Fish/Poultry
Shrimp, Steamed	**0.0**	15	pieces	Meat/Fish/Poultry
Singapore Sling	**-13.5**	6	fl oz	Alcohol
Slow Gin Fizz	**-14.5**	8	fl oz	Alcohol
Smelt, Rainbow, Baked	**4.5**	4	wt oz	Meat/Fish/Poultry
Smoothie, All Flavors, Horizon Organic	**6.0**	12	fl oz	Milk/Dairy
Smoothie, Slim-Fast Optima	**15.0**	10.5	fl oz	Fruit
Snack Bar, Atkins Advantage Bar	**9.5**	1	bar	Legume/Nut/Seed
Snack Bar, Balance Bar 40-30-30	**8.5**	1	bar	Legume/Nut/Seed
Snack Bar, Barbell Energy Bar	**18.5**	1	bar	Milk/Dairy
Snack Bar, Bio-X Bar	**15.0**	1	bar	Milk/Dairy
Snack Bar, Breakthrough, Honey Graham	**13.0**	1	bar	Legume/Nut/Seed
Snack Bar, Clif Bar	**5.5**	1	bar	Legume/Nut/Seed
Snack Bar, Clif Builder's Bar	**5.5**	1/2	bar	Legume/Nut/Seed

Food Name—Alphabetical	Nutripoints	Serving Size		Nutrigroup
Snack Bar, Clif Luna Bar	**28.5**	1	bar	Legume/Nut/Seed
Snack Bar, Clif ZBar	**8.5**	1	bar	Grain
Snack Bar, DrSoy Healthy Snacker Bar	**6.5**	1	bar	Legume/Nut/Seed
Snack Bar, DrSoy Protein Bar	**34.5**	1	bar	Legume/Nut/Seed
Snack Bar, Energia	**23.0**	1	bar	Grain
Snack Bar, Ensure	**4.5**	1	bar	Grain
Snack Bar, FIBAR (all flavors)	**6.0**	1	bar	Grain
Snack Bar, Genisoy	**6.5**	1	bar	Legume/Nut/Seed
Snack Bar, Genisoy Xtreme	**7.0**	1	bar	Legume/Nut/Seed
Snack Bar, GOLEAN Crunchy, Kashi	**3.0**	1	bar	Grain
Snack Bar, GOLEAN, Kashi	**-2.0**	1	bar	Grain
Snack Bar, Marathon, Snickers	**23.5**	1	bar	Milk/Dairy
Snack Bar, Melaleuca Access Activity bar	**-1.0**	1	bar	Milk/Dairy
Snack Bar, Melaleuca Fruit & Fiber Bar	**2.5**	1	bar	Fruit
Snack Bar, MetaForm	**10.0**	1	bar	Milk/Dairy
Snack Bar, MET-Rx Big-100 Meal Replacement	**7.5**	1	bar	Milk/Dairy
Snack Bar, MET-Rx Protein Plus	**6.0**	1	bar	Milk/Dairy
Snack Bar, Nutra Blast	**6.0**	1	bar	Grain
Snack Bar, Nutri-Grain, Kellogg's (all flavors)	**3.5**	1	bar	Grain
Snack Bar, Pounds Off Bar	**29.5**	1	bar	Grain
Snack Bar, Power Bar, All Flavors	**22.5**	1	bar	Grain
Snack Bar, PR Nutrition Bar	**14.0**	1	bar	Legume/Nut/Seed
Snack Bar, Pria Carb Select, Power Bar	**16.5**	1	bar	Legume/Nut/Seed
Snack Bar, Pria, Power Bar	**21.0**	1	bar	Legume/Nut/Seed
Snack Bar, Promax	**5.5**	1/2	bar	Milk/Dairy
Snack Bar, Promax Carb Conscious	**6.0**	1/2	bar	Milk/Dairy
Snack Bar, Protein Plus, Power Bar, All Flavors	**19.5**	1	bar	Milk/Dairy
Snack Bar, Pure Protein	**25.5**	1	bar	Milk/Dairy
Snack Bar, Slim-Fast Optima	**5.0**	1	bar	Legume/Nut/Seed
Snack Bar, SmartZone, Hershey's	**6.5**	1	bar	Milk/Dairy
Snack Bar, SnackWells	**4.5**	1	bar	Fruit
Snack Bar, Think! Bar	**6.5**	1	bar	Fruit
Snack Bar, Tiger's Milk	**9.0**	1	bar	Milk/Dairy
Snack Bar, Tiger's Sports Bar	**25.0**	1	bar	Grain
Snack Bar, VO2 MAX	**9.0**	1	bar	Milk/Dairy
Snack Bar, ZonePerfect	**14.5**	1	bar	Grain
Snack Cake, 97% Fat-Free, Hostess (all flavors)	**-1.5**	1	cake	Grain
Snack Cake, Apple Delight, Little Debbie	**-5.5**	2	pieces	Grain
Snack Cake, Dessert Light, Apple 'n Spice, Pepperidge Farm	**-2.0**	1	piece	Grain
Snack Cake, Ding Dong, Hostess	**-2.0**	1	piece	Grain
Snack Cake, Drake's Devil Dogs	**-2.5**	1	piece	Grain
Snack Cake, Drake's Ring Ding Jr.	**-3.0**	1	piece	Grain
Snack Cake, Lights, Hostess	**-1.0**	1	piece	Grain
Snack Cake, Oatmeal Creme Pie, Little Debbie	**-6.5**	2	pieces	Grain
Snack Cake, Peanut Butter Bar, Little Debbie	**-7.0**	2	pieces	Grain

Food Name—Alphabetical	Nutripoints	Serving Size		Nutrigroup
Snack Cake, Star Crunch, Little Debbie	**-8.5**	2	pieces	Grain
Snack Cake, Suzy Q's	**-3.5**	1/2	piece	Grain
Snails	**4.0**	4	wt oz	Meat/Fish/Poultry
Soft Drink, 7-Up	**-5.5**	12	fl oz	Sugar
Soft Drink, Coke w/Caffeine	**-6.0**	12	fl oz	Sugar
Soft Drink, Cream Soda	**-5.5**	12	fl oz	Sugar
Soft Drink, Diet, w/Caffeine	**-3.0**	12	fl oz	Miscellaneous
Soft Drink, Diet, w/o Caffeine	**0.0**	12	fl oz	Miscellaneous
Soft Drink, Dr. Pepper	**-5.5**	12	fl oz	Sugar
Soft Drink, Ginger Ale	**-5.0**	12	fl oz	Sugar
Soft Drink, Lemon Lime, w/o Caffeine	**-5.5**	12	fl oz	Sugar
Soft Drink, Mountain Dew	**-6.5**	12	fl oz	Sugar
Soft Drink, w/Caffeine	**-7.0**	12	fl oz	Sugar
Soft Drink, w/o Caffeine	**-5.0**	12	fl oz	Sugar
Sole Au Gratin, Frozen, Healthy Choice	**1.5**	1	portion	Meat/Fish/Poultry
Sole Fillet, Fishmarket Fresh, Frozen, Gorton's	**-2.0**	4	wt oz	Meat/Fish/Poultry
Sole Fillet, Light, Mrs. Paul's	**-1.0**	1	serving	Meat/Fish/Poultry
Sole, Baked	**6.0**	6	wt oz	Meat/Fish/Poultry
Sole, Stuffed, Newburg Sauce, Fzn, Weight Watchers	**1.5**	1/2	portion	Meat/Fish/Poultry
Sopaipilla	**-3.0**	1	piece	Grain
Soufflé, Cheese	**-3.0**	1/2	cup	Milk/Dairy
Soufflé, Corn, Frozen, Stouffer's	**0.5**	1/2	portion	Vegetable
Soufflé, Spinach	**-3.0**	1/2	cup	Vegetable
Soup Mix, Chicken Noodle, Dehydrated	**-1.5**	1	serving	Miscellaneous
Soup Mix, Chicken Noodle, w/Chicken Meat, Lipton	**-2.5**	1	cup	Meat/Fish/Poultry
Soup Mix, Chicken Rice, Lipton	**-2.5**	1	cup	Meat/Fish/Poultry
Soup Mix, Country Vegetable, Lipton	**2.0**	1	cup	Vegetable
Soup Mix, Cream of Mushroom, Cup-A-Soup, Lipton	**-2.5**	1	cup	Vegetable
Soup Mix, Green Pea, Cup-A-Soup, Lipton	**0.5**	1/2	cup	Vegetable
Soup Mix, Onion, Dehydrated	**-1.5**	2	Tbls	Miscellaneous
Soup Mix, Onion, Lipton	**-5.5**	1	cup	Vegetable
Soup Mix, Tomato, Cup-A-Soup, Lipton	**-2.5**	1	cup	Vegetable
Soup, Bean	**3.5**	1	cup	Legume/Nut/Seed
Soup, Bean, Black	**5.0**	1	cup	Legume/Nut/Seed
Soup, Bean, Black, Health Valley	**7.5**	1	cup	Legume/Nut/Seed
Soup, Beef	**4.0**	1	cup	Meat/Fish/Poultry
Soup, Beef Lentil, ZonePerfect	**3.0**	1/2	serving	Meat/Fish/Poultry
Soup, Beef Noodle	**1.0**	1	cup	Meat/Fish/Poultry
Soup, Beef, Campbell's	**0.5**	1	cup	Meat/Fish/Poultry
Soup, Blueberry, Chilled, Nutripoint Recipe	**6.0**	3/4	cup	Fruit
Soup, Broccoli, Creamy Organic, Imagine Foods	**5.0**	1	cup	Vegetable
Soup, Cheese	**-1.0**	1/2	cup	Milk/Dairy
Soup, Chicken	**1.5**	1	cup	Meat/Fish/Poultry

Food Name—Alphabetical	Nutripoints	Serving Size		Nutrigroup
Soup, Chicken Broth, Low Sodium, Campbell's	**3.5**	1	cup	Condiment
Soup, Chicken Gumbo	**5.5**	3/4	cup	Meat/Fish/Poultry
Soup, Chicken Gumbo, ZonePerfect	**0.5**	1/2	serving	Meat/Fish/Poultry
Soup, Chicken Noodle	**0.5**	1	cup	Meat/Fish/Poultry
Soup, Chicken Noodle, Campbell's	**-1.5**	1	cup	Meat/Fish/Poultry
Soup, Chicken Rice	**-1.5**	1	cup	Meat/Fish/Poultry
Soup, Chicken Vegetable, Campbell's	**2.0**	1	cup	Meat/Fish/Poultry
Soup, Chicken Vegetable, Couscous, Nile Spice Foods	**2.0**	1	cup	Meat/Fish/Poultry
Soup, Chicken w/Noodles, Low Sodium, Campbell's	**1.5**	1	cup	Meat/Fish/Poultry
Soup, Chicken w/Rice, Healthy Choice	**3.0**	1	cup	Grain
Soup, Chicken, Home Style, Progresso	**5.5**	1 1/2	cups	Meat/Fish/Poultry
Soup, Chicken, w/Ribbon Pasta, Pritikin	**4.5**	1	cup	Meat/Fish/Poultry
Soup, Chowder, Fish	**1.0**	1	cup	Meat/Fish/Poultry
Soup, Chunky 5 Bean Vegetable, Health Valley	**11.0**	1	cup	Vegetable
Soup, Chunky Beef & Potato, Healthy Choice	**1.0**	1	cup	Meat/Fish/Poultry
Soup, Chunky Beef, Campbell's	**4.0**	1	cup	Meat/Fish/Poultry
Soup, Chunky Chicken Noodle, Campbell's	**0.5**	1	cup	Meat/Fish/Poultry
Soup, Chunky Minestrone, Campbell's	**3.5**	1	cup	Vegetable
Soup, Chunky Old Fashioned Bean 'n Ham, Campbell's	**2.0**	1/2	cup	Legume/Nut/Seed
Soup, Chunky Steak 'n Potato, Campbell's	**0.5**	1	cup	Meat/Fish/Poultry
Soup, Chunky Vegetable, Campbell's	**5.0**	1	cup	Vegetable
Soup, Clam Chowder, Manhattan Tomato Base	**0.0**	2	cups	Meat/Fish/Poultry
Soup, Clam Chowder, New England Milk Base	**4.5**	1	cup	Meat/Fish/Poultry
Soup, Cream	**1.5**	1	cup	Milk/Dairy
Soup, Cream of Asparagus	**1.0**	1/2	cup	Vegetable
Soup, Cream of Celery	**-0.5**	1/2	cup	Vegetable
Soup, Cream of Celery, Campbell's	**-3.0**	1	cup	Vegetable
Soup, Cream of Chicken	**0.0**	1	cup	Meat/Fish/Poultry
Soup, Cream of Chicken, 1/3 Less Salt, Campbell's	**-1.5**	1	cup	Meat/Fish/Poultry
Soup, Cream of Chicken, Campbell's	**-2.0**	1	cup	Meat/Fish/Poultry
Soup, Cream of Mushroom	**-1.0**	1/4	cup	Vegetable
Soup, Cream of Mushroom, 1/3 Less Salt, Campbell's	**-2.0**	1	cup	Vegetable
Soup, Cream of Mushroom, Campbell's	**-4.5**	1	cup	Vegetable
Soup, Creamy Natural Broccoli w/Milk, Campbell's	**-1.0**	1/2	cup	Vegetable
Soup, Creamy Natural Broccoli, Campbell's	**-1.0**	1	cup	Vegetable
Soup, Creamy Natural Potato w/Milk, Campbell's	**-2.5**	1/2	cup	Vegetable
Soup, Creamy Natural Potato, Campbell's	**-4.0**	1/2	cup	Vegetable
Soup, French Market, Nutripoint Recipe	**17.0**	1 1/2	cups	Legume/Nut/Seed
Soup, French Onion, Campbell's	**-3.5**	1	cup	Vegetable
Soup, Garden Vegetable, Healthy Choice	**4.5**	1	cup	Vegetable
Soup, Green Pea, Campbell's	**2.5**	8	wt oz	Legume/Nut/Seed
Soup, Healthy Classics, Beef Vegetable, Progresso	**4.5**	1	cup	Meat/Fish/Poultry

Food Name—Alphabetical	Nutripoints	Serving Size		Nutrigroup
Soup, Healthy Classics, Chicken Noodle, Progresso	**6.0**	1	cup	Meat/Fish/Poultry
Soup, Healthy Classics, Garlic & Pasta, Progresso	**4.5**	1	cup	Grain
Soup, Healthy Request, Chicken Noodle, Campbell's	**2.5**	1	cup	Meat/Fish/Poultry
Soup, Healthy Request, Vegetable Beef, Campbell's	**5.5**	1	cup	Meat/Fish/Poultry
Soup, Healthy Request, Vegetable, Campbell's	**7.0**	1	cup	Vegetable
Soup, Hearty Lentil & Vegetable, Wolfgang Puck's	**6.0**	1	cup	Legume/Nut/Seed
Soup, Hot and Sour, Nutripoint Recipe	**4.0**	1	cup	Legume/Nut/Seed
Soup, Lentil	**5.5**	1	cup	Legume/Nut/Seed
Soup, Lentil Curry, Couscous, Nile Spice Foods	**6.5**	1	cup	Legume/Nut/Seed
Soup, Lentil, Health Valley	**8.0**	1/2	cup	Legume/Nut/Seed
Soup, Lentil, Lenticchie, Alessi (dry mix)	**3.0**	1	cup	Legume/Nut/Seed
Soup, Lentil, Nutripoint Recipe	**13.5**	1	cup	Legume/Nut/Seed
Soup, Lentil, w/Ham	**4.5**	1	cup	Legume/Nut/Seed
Soup, Minestrone	**5.0**	1	cup	Vegetable
Soup, Minestrone, Campbell's	**3.5**	1	cup	Vegetable
Soup, Minestrone, Health Valley	**14.0**	1 1/2	cups	Legume/Nut/Seed
Soup, Minestrone, Healthy Choice	**5.0**	1	cup	Legume/Nut/Seed
Soup, Minestrone, Progresso	**4.0**	1	cup	Legume/Nut/Seed
Soup, Mushroom, Beefy, Campbell's	**-3.5**	1	cup	Meat/Fish/Poultry
Soup, Mushroom, Cream Of, Campbell's	**-1.0**	1/4	cup	Vegetable
Soup, New England Clam Chowder w/Milk, Campbell's	**-0.5**	1	cup	Meat/Fish/Poultry
Soup, Old Fashioned Chicken Noodle, Healthy Choice	**1.0**	1	cup	Meat/Fish/Poultry
Soup, Onion	**-1.5**	1	cup	Vegetable
Soup, Oyster Stew, w/Milk, Campbell's	**-1.5**	8	wt oz	Meat/Fish/Poultry
Soup, Pea	**4.0**	1	cup	Legume/Nut/Seed
Soup, Pea, Split Green, Health Valley	**10.0**	1/2	cup	Legume/Nut/Seed
Soup, Pea, Split Green, Progresso	**2.5**	1/2	cup	Legume/Nut/Seed
Soup, Pea, Split Naturals, Hain	**4.0**	1	cup	Legume/Nut/Seed
Soup, Potato	**0.5**	1/2	cup	Vegetable
Soup, Seafood Gumbo	**3.5**	1	cup	Meat/Fish/Poultry
Soup, Spinach, Clear, Nutripoint Recipe	**23.5**	1	cup	Vegetable
Soup, Squash, Creamy Organic, Imagine Foods	**2.0**	1/2	cup	Vegetable
Soup, Tomato	**2.5**	1	cup	Vegetable
Soup, Tomato Minestrone, Couscous, Nile Spice Foods	**2.5**	1/2	cup	Vegetable
Soup, Tomato Rice, Old Fashioned, Campbell's	**-1.5**	1	cup	Vegetable
Soup, Tomato w/ Vegetables, Progresso	**6.5**	1	cup	Vegetable
Soup, Tomato w/Milk, 1/3 Less Salt, Campbell's	**0.0**	1/2	cup	Vegetable
Soup, Tomato w/Milk, Campbell's	**-1.0**	1/2	cup	Vegetable
Soup, Tomato, 1/3 Less Salt, Campbell's	**0.5**	1	cup	Vegetable
Soup, Tomato, Campbell's	**0.5**	1	cup	Vegetable
Soup, Tomato, Health Valley	**11.5**	1/2	cup	Vegetable
Soup, Tomato, Low Sodium, w/Pieces, Campbell's	**1.0**	1/2	cup	Vegetable
Soup, Tomato, No Salt, Health Valley	**12.0**	1/2	cup	Vegetable

Food Name—Alphabetical	Nutripoints	Serving Size		Nutrigroup
Soup, Turkey Vegetable, Campbell's	2.5	1	cup	Meat/Fish/Poultry
Soup, Vegetable	12.0	1	cup	Vegetable
Soup, Vegetable Beef	4.5	1	cup	Vegetable
Soup, Vegetable Parmesan, Couscous, Nile Spice Foods	2.5	1/2	cup	Vegetable
Soup, Vegetable, 1/3 Less Salt, Campbell's	3.0	1	cup	Vegetable
Soup, Vegetable, Campbell's	2.0	1	cup	Vegetable
Soup, Vegetable, Health Valley	12.5	1	cup	Vegetable
Soup, Vegetable, No Salt, Health Valley	13.0	1	cup	Vegetable
Soup, Vegetable, Pritikin	6.5	1	cup	Vegetable
Soup, Vegetarian Vegetable, Campbell's	4.5	8	wt oz	Vegetable
Soup, Wild Rice, Nutripoint Recipe	10.5	1	cup	Grain
Soup, Wonton	-1.0	1	cup	Miscellaneous
Soybean Nuts, Roasted, Salted	5.0	1	wt oz	Legume/Nut/Seed
Soybeans, Cooked	7.0	3/4	cup	Legume/Nut/Seed
Soybeans, Dry, Arrowhead Mills	7.5	1	wt oz	Legume/Nut/Seed
Soybeans, Roasted, Unsalted	3.5	1	wt oz	Legume/Nut/Seed
Soyburger Patty	4.0	3	wt oz	Legume/Nut/Seed
Soyburger, w/Bun	3.0	1/2	serving	Legume/Nut/Seed
Spaghetti Substitute, Spinach, Deboles	2.5	1	wt oz	Grain
Spaghetti, Beef & Mushroom Sauce, Stouffer's	0.5	1/2	serving	Grain
Spaghetti, Cooked (1 C=2 wt oz Dry)	3.0	1/2	cup	Grain
Spaghetti, Creamette, Borden	2.5	1/2	cup	Grain
Spaghetti, Hi-Protein	4.0	1/2	cup	Grain
Spaghetti, Low Cal, Frozen Dinner	2.5	1/2	portion	Grain
Spaghetti, Meat Sauce, Fzn, Weight Watchers	2.5	1/2	portion	Grain
Spaghetti, Ronzoni	3.0	1/2	cup	Grain
Spaghetti, San Giorgio	3.0	1/2	cup	Grain
Spaghetti, w/Meat Sauce	2.0	1/2	cup	Grain
Spaghetti, w/Meat Sauce, Frozen, Stouffer's	0.0	1/2	portion	Grain
Spaghetti, w/Meatball Dinner, Frozen, Morton	3.5	1	portion	Grain
Spaghetti, w/Meatballs	1.5	1/2	cup	Grain
Spaghetti, w/Meatballs/Tomato Sauce, Chef Boyardee	-1.0	7.5	wt oz	Grain
Spaghetti, w/Sauce	4.0	1/2	cup	Grain
Spam	-1.5	2	wt oz	Meat/Fish/Poultry
Spicer's Cheddar Cheese Wheat Snacks	6.0	1	wt oz	Grain
Spinach, Au Gratin, Frozen, Budget Gourmet	3.0	1/2	portion	Vegetable
Spinach, Chopped, Fzn, 365 Organic, Whole Foods	41.5	1 1/2	cup	Vegetable
Spinach, Cut Leaf, In Butter, Frozen, Green Giant	20.0	1/2	cup	Vegetable
Spinach, Early Garden, Canned, Del Monte	35.5	3/4	cup	Vegetable
Spinach, Fresh, Cooked	53.5	1	cup	Vegetable
Spinach, Frozen, Cooked	42.5	3/4	cup	Vegetable
Spinach, Leaf, No Salt Added, Canned, Del Monte	29.5	1	cup	Vegetable
Spinach, Raw, Chopped	75.0	2	cups	Vegetable

Food Name—Alphabetical	Nutripoints	Serving Size		Nutrigroup
Spinach, Whole Leaf, Frozen, Birds Eye	**57.0**	1	cup	Vegetable
Sports Drink, Accelerade Powder Mix	**2.0**	12	fl oz	Sugar
Sports Drink, Accelerade Ready to Drink	**-4.0**	8	fl oz	Sugar
Sports Drink, All Sport	**-2.0**	8	fl oz	Miscellaneous
Sports Drink, AminoVital Ready to Drink	**1.5**	20	fl oz	Sugar
Sports Drink, AminoVital Shake Mix	**5.0**	8	fl oz	Sugar
Sports Drink, Bodyfuel	**4.0**	8	fl oz	Fruit
Sports Drink, Cytomax Energy and Recovery Drink	**3.5**	1	serving	Sugar
Sports Drink, Endurox R4	**0.5**	12	fl oz	Sugar
Sports Drink, Exceed	**1.5**	8	fl oz	Fruit
Sports Drink, Gatorade Endurance Hydration Formula	**-5.5**	8	fl oz	Sugar
Sports Drink, Gatorade Energy Drink	**2.5**	12	fl oz	Sugar
Sports Drink, LowOz	**3.0**	8	fl oz	Fruit
Sports Drink, Lucozade	**-2.0**	500	ml	Sugar
Sports Drink, Motion Potion	**24.5**	16	fl oz	Fruit
Sports Drink, Power Bar Recovery Drink	**-2.0**	8	fl oz	Sugar
Sports Drink, Powerade	**-3.0**	8	fl oz	Sugar
Sports Drink, Recharge	**1.0**	8	fl oz	Fruit
Sports Drink, Zing	**13.5**	8	fl oz	Sugar
Sports Gel, Accelerade Accel Gel	**4.5**	1	serving	Sugar
Sports Powder, AminoVital Fast Charge	**8.5**	1	serving	Sugar
Squash, Acorn, Baked	**11.5**	1/2	cup	Vegetable
Squash, Butternut, Baked	**26.5**	1/2	cup	Vegetable
Squash, Fried, w/Breading	**-1.0**	1/4	cup	Vegetable
Squash, Summer, Cooked	**24.5**	1	cup	Vegetable
Squash, Winter, Baked	**16.0**	1/2	cup	Vegetable
Squash, Winter, Cooked, Frozen, Birds Eye	**23.0**	1/2	cup	Vegetable
Squid, Boiled	**-1.5**	6	wt oz	Meat/Fish/Poultry
Squid, Fried	**0.0**	3	wt oz	Meat/Fish/Poultry
Squid, Raw	**2.0**	6	wt oz	Meat/Fish/Poultry
Squirrel	**3.0**	3	wt oz	Meat/Fish/Poultry
Stinger	**-12.5**	2	fl oz	Alcohol
Strawberries, Fresh	**19.0**	1	cup	Fruit
Strawberries, Frozen, Heavy Syrup, Birds Eye	**5.0**	1/4	cup	Fruit
Strawberries, Frozen, Sweetened	**6.5**	1/2	cup	Fruit
Strawberries, Frozen, Unsweetened	**17.0**	1	cup	Fruit
Strawberries, Halved, Light Syrup, Fzn, Birds Eye	**8.5**	1/2	cup	Fruit
Strawberries, Organic, Fzn, Cascadian Farm	**16.5**	1	cup	Fruit
Stuffing	**-1.5**	1/2	cup	Grain
Stuffing Mix, American New England, Stove Top	**-0.5**	1/2	cup	Grain
Stuffing Mix, Cornbread, w/Butter, Stove Top	**-1.5**	1/2	cup	Grain
Stuffing Mix, Herb Seasoned, Pepperidge Farm	**1.0**	1/2	cup	Grain
Sturgeon, Steamed	**5.5**	4	wt oz	Meat/Fish/Poultry

Food Name—Alphabetical	Nutripoints	Serving Size		Nutrigroup
Subway Barbeque Chicken Sandwich (6")	**5.0**	1	serving	Meat/Fish/Poultry
Subway Cheese Steak Sandwich (6")	**3.5**	1	serving	Meat/Fish/Poultry
Subway Classic Tuna Sandwich (6")	**3.0**	1/2	serving	Meat/Fish/Poultry
Subway Club Sandwich (6")	**3.5**	1	serving	Meat/Fish/Poultry
Subway Cold Cut Combo Sandwich (6")	**1.5**	1/2	serving	Meat/Fish/Poultry
Subway Gardenburger Sandwich (6")	**3.5**	1/2	serving	Grain
Subway Honey Mustard Ham Sandwich (6")	**3.5**	1	serving	Meat/Fish/Poultry
Subway Italian BMT Sandwich (6")	**1.0**	1/2	serving	Meat/Fish/Poultry
Subway Meatball Marinara Sandwich (6")	**2.5**	1/2	serving	Meat/Fish/Poultry
Subway Onion Chicken Teriyaki Sandwich (6")	**3.0**	1	serving	Meat/Fish/Poultry
Subway Oven Roasted Chicken Breast Sandwich (6")	**3.5**	1	serving	Meat/Fish/Poultry
Subway Roast Beef Sandwich (6")	**4.5**	1	serving	Meat/Fish/Poultry
Subway Savory Turkey Breast Sandwich (6")	**5.0**	1	serving	Meat/Fish/Poultry
Subway Seafood Sensation Sandwich (6")	**4.0**	1/2	serving	Meat/Fish/Poultry
Subway Turkey Breast, Ham & Bacon Melt Sandwich (6")	**2.5**	1/2	serving	Meat/Fish/Poultry
Subway Turkey Pastrami Sandwich (6")	**4.5**	1	serving	Meat/Fish/Poultry
Subway Veggie Delight Sandwich (6")	**5.0**	1	serving	Grain
Subway Veggie-Max Sandwich (6")	**3.0**	1/2	serving	Legume/Nut/Seed
Succotash, Cooked	**7.5**	1/2	cup	Vegetable
Succotash, Frozen, Cooked	**7.0**	1/2	cup	Vegetable
Sugar, Brown	**-5.0**	2	Tbls	Sugar
Sugar, Cinnamon	**-5.5**	2	Tbls	Sugar
Sugar, Maple	**-5.5**	3	Tbls	Sugar
Sugar, Powdered	**-4.5**	3	Tbls	Sugar
Sugar, Raw	**-5.0**	2	Tbls	Sugar
Sugar, White	**-6.0**	2	Tbls	Sugar
Sugar, White Confectioner's	**-5.5**	4	Tbls	Sugar
Sushi/Raw Fish	**2.5**	6	wt oz	Meat/Fish/Poultry
Sustacal	**8.0**	4	fl oz	Milk/Dairy
Sweet Potato/Yam, Baked	**12.0**	1/2	piece	Vegetable
Sweet Potato/Yam, Canned	**8.0**	1/2	piece	Vegetable
Sweet Potatoes, Candied	**4.0**	1/2	piece	Vegetable
Sweetbreads (organ meats)	**-52.0**	3	wt oz	Meat/Fish/Poultry
Swiss Chard, Cooked	**42.0**	1	cup	Vegetable
Swordfish Fillet, Breaded, Fried	**1.0**	3	wt oz	Meat/Fish/Poultry
Swordfish, Baked	**6.5**	3	wt oz	Meat/Fish/Poultry
Syrup, Butter Blends	**-6.0**	2	tsp	Sugar
Syrup, Butterlite, Aunt Jemima	**-6.0**	1	fl oz	Sugar
Syrup, Cane	**-5.0**	2	tsp	Sugar
Syrup, Corn	**-5.0**	2	Tbls	Sugar
Syrup, Lite, Aunt Jemima	**-4.5**	1	fl oz	Sugar
Syrup, Maple	**-5.0**	2	Tbls	Sugar
Syrup, Maple Low Cal	**-4.0**	2	Tbls	Sugar
Syrup, Original, Aunt Jemima	**-5.5**	1	fl oz	Sugar

Food Name—Alphabetical	Nutripoints	Serving Size		Nutrigroup
Syrup, Sorghum	**-3.5**	2	tsp	Sugar
Taco Bell Bean Burrito w/Green Sauce	**4.0**	1/2	serving	Legume/Nut/Seed
Taco Bell Bean Burrito w/Red Sauce	**4.0**	1/2	serving	Legume/Nut/Seed
Taco Bell Bean Burrito, Fresco Style	**3.5**	1	serving	Legume/Nut/Seed
Taco Bell Bean/Cheese Taco, Fresco Style	**1.5**	1	serving	Legume/Nut/Seed
Taco Bell Beef Burrito w/Green Sauce	**1.5**	1/2	serving	Legume/Nut/Seed
Taco Bell Beef Burrito w/Red Sauce	**1.0**	1/2	serving	Legume/Nut/Seed
Taco Bell Beef Enchirito w/Green Sauce	**0.0**	1/2	serving	Meat/Fish/Poultry
Taco Bell Beef Enchirito w/Red Sauce	**0.0**	1/2	serving	Meat/Fish/Poultry
Taco Bell Beef Enchirito, Fresco Style	**4.0**	1	serving	Meat/Fish/Poultry
Taco Bell Beef Gordita Baja, Fresco Style	**3.0**	1	serving	Meat/Fish/Poultry
Taco Bell Burrito Supreme w/Green Sauce	**2.0**	1/2	serving	Legume/Nut/Seed
Taco Bell Burrito Supreme w/Red Sauce	**2.0**	1/2	serving	Legume/Nut/Seed
Taco Bell Chicken Burrito Supreme, Fresco Style	**3.0**	1	serving	Meat/Fish/Poultry
Taco Bell Chicken Enchirito, Fresco Style	**2.5**	1	serving	Meat/Fish/Poultry
Taco Bell Chicken Fajita	**0.5**	1	serving	Meat/Fish/Poultry
Taco Bell Chicken Gordita Baja, Fresco Style	**3.5**	1	serving	Meat/Fish/Poultry
Taco Bell Cinnamon Crispas	**-2.0**	1/2	piece	Grain
Taco Bell Double Beef Burrito Supreme w/Green Sauce	**1.0**	1/2	serving	Meat/Fish/Poultry
Taco Bell Double Beef Burrito Supreme w/Red Sauce	**1.0**	1/2	serving	Meat/Fish/Poultry
Taco Bell Fiesta Chicken Burrito Supreme, Fresco Style	**2.5**	1	serving	Meat/Fish/Poultry
Taco Bell Grilled Steak Soft Taco, Fresco Style	**2.5**	1	serving	Meat/Fish/Poultry
Taco Bell Guacamole	**1.0**	1	Tbls	Fruit
Taco Bell Jalapeno Peppers	**-1.5**	2	Tbls	Condiment
Taco Bell Mexican Pizza	**-0.5**	1/4	piece	Grain
Taco Bell Meximelt	**-1.0**	1/2	serving	Grain
Taco Bell Nachos	**-0.5**	1/2	serving	Grain
Taco Bell Nachos Bellgrande	**0.0**	1/4	serving	Grain
Taco Bell Pico de Gallo	**1.0**	2	Tbls	Condiment
Taco Bell Pintos & Cheese, Green Sauce	**2.5**	1	serving	Legume/Nut/Seed
Taco Bell Pintos & Cheese, Red Sauce	**2.5**	1	serving	Legume/Nut/Seed
Taco Bell Ranch Dressing	**-4.0**	1	Tbls	Fat/Oil
Taco Bell Salsa	**2.0**	1	Tbls	Condiment
Taco Bell Soft Beef Taco, Fresco Style	**1.5**	1	taco	Meat/Fish/Poultry
Taco Bell Soft Chicken Taco, Fresco Style	**2.5**	1	serving	Meat/Fish/Poultry
Taco Bell Soft Taco	**0.0**	1	taco	Meat/Fish/Poultry
Taco Bell Sour Cream	**-3.5**	2	Tbls	Fat/Oil
Taco Bell Steak Burrito Supreme, Fresco Style	**3.0**	1	serving	Meat/Fish/Poultry
Taco Bell Steak Fajita	**1.0**	1	serving	Meat/Fish/Poultry
Taco Bell Steak Gordita Baja, Fresco Style	**3.5**	1	serving	Meat/Fish/Poultry
Taco Bell Super Combo Taco	**-0.5**	1	taco	Meat/Fish/Poultry
Taco Bell Supreme Soft Taco	**-0.5**	1	taco	Meat/Fish/Poultry
Taco Bell Taco	**-1.0**	1	taco	Meat/Fish/Poultry

Food Name—Alphabetical	Nutripoints	Serving Size		Nutrigroup
Taco Bell Taco Bellgrande	**-1.5**	1/2	taco	Meat/Fish/Poultry
Taco Bell Taco Hot Sauce	**0.0**	1	tsp	Condiment
Taco Bell Taco Light	**-1.5**	1/2	taco	Meat/Fish/Poultry
Taco Bell Taco Salad w/o Shell	**0.0**	1/4	serving	Vegetable
Taco Bell Taco Salad w/Salsa w/o Shell	**0.5**	1/4	serving	Vegetable
Taco Bell Taco Salad w/Salsa w/Shell	**0.0**	1/8	serving	Vegetable
Taco Bell Taco Sauce	**0.0**	1	tsp	Condiment
Taco Bell Tostada Green Sauce	**1.5**	1/4	serving	Vegetable
Taco Bell Tostada Red Sauce	**1.5**	1/4	serving	Vegetable
Taco Bell Tostada, Fresco Style	**3.5**	1	serving	Legume/Nut/Seed
Taco Salad	**1.5**	1/4	cup	Vegetable
Taco, Bean/Cheese	**0.5**	1/2	taco	Legume/Nut/Seed
Taco, Beef/Cheese	**2.5**	1	taco	Meat/Fish/Poultry
Taco, Chicken	**2.0**	1/2	taco	Meat/Fish/Poultry
Tamale	**-1.5**	1/2	piece	Grain
Tamales, In Chili Sauce, Old El Paso	**-0.5**	1	piece	Grain
Tangerine	**13.0**	1	whole	Fruit
Tarragon	**0.5**	1	tsp	Condiment
Tarts, Fat-Free, Health Valley (all flavors)	**2.0**	1	tart	Grain
Tea Mix, Iced, Lemon, Sugar-Free, Lipton	**-2.5**	8	fl oz	Miscellaneous
Tea Mix, Iced, Lipton	**-7.5**	8	fl oz	Sugar
Tea, American Black	**-3.0**	1	cup	Miscellaneous
Tea, Arizona Herbal w/Honey	**-2.0**	8	fl oz	Miscellaneous
Tea, Decaffeinated	**0.0**	1	cup	Miscellaneous
Tea, Herb	**0.5**	6	fl oz	Miscellaneous
Tequila Sunrise	**-10.0**	6	fl oz	Alcohol
Thins, Juice Plus+® Fiber Snack	**2.0**	2	tablets	Fruit
Thyme	**0.5**	1	tsp	Condiment
Tofu	**5.0**	1/2	cup	Legume/Nut/Seed
Tofu Burger, Frozen, Island Spring Oriental	**0.0**	1	burger	Legume/Nut/Seed
Tom Collins	**-14.0**	8	fl oz	Alcohol
Tomato Paste, Canned	**20.0**	1/4	cup	Vegetable
Tomato Paste, Contadina	**12.5**	1/4	cup	Vegetable
Tomato, Fresh	**30.0**	1	whole	Vegetable
Tomatoes, Canned	**23.0**	1/2	cup	Vegetable
Tomatoes, Peeled, Del Monte	**14.0**	1	cup	Vegetable
Tomatoes, Stewed, Hunts	**7.0**	1/2	cup	Vegetable
Tonic Water, Sweetened	**-5.5**	12	fl oz	Sugar
Topping, Blueberry, Hot, Nutripoint Recipe	**2.5**	1/2	cup	Fruit
Topping, Extra Creamy, Cool Whip, Birds Eye	**-6.0**	1/4	cup	Milk/Dairy
Topping, Lite, Cool Whip	**-3.0**	1/2	cup	Milk/Dairy
Topping, Marshmallow Cream	**-5.5**	2	Tbls	Sugar
Topping, Non-Dairy, Cool Whip, Birds Eye	**-4.5**	1/4	cup	Milk/Dairy
Topping, Peach, Hot, Nutripoint Recipe	**7.0**	1/2	cup	Fruit
Topping, Red Raspberry, Hot, Nutripoint Recipe	**9.0**	1/2	cup	Fruit
Topping, Strawberry, Smucker's	**-3.5**	1	Tbls	Fruit

Food Name—Alphabetical	Nutripoints	Serving Size		Nutrigroup
Topping, Whipped, La Creme	**-5.5**	1/4	cup	Milk/Dairy
Tortellini, Cheese, w/Tomato Sauce, Fzn Stouffer's	**0.0**	1/2	portion	Milk/Dairy
Tortellini, Veal w/Tomato Sauce, Fzn, Stouffer's	**1.5**	1/2	portion	Meat/Fish/Poultry
Tortellini, Veal, Alfredo, Frozen, Stouffer's	**-1.0**	1/2	portion	Meat/Fish/Poultry
Tortilla Chips	**0.5**	15	chips	Grain
Tortilla Chips, Doritos	**-0.5**	18	chips	Grain
Tortilla Chips, Doritos, Light, Lowfat, Nacho Cheese	**0.5**	11	chips	Vegetable
Tortilla Chips, Light Nacho Cheese, Doritos	**1.0**	15	chips	Grain
Tortilla Chips, Nacho Cheese, Doritos	**-0.5**	15	chips	Grain
Tortilla, Corn	**4.0**	2	pieces	Grain
Tortilla, Flour	**2.0**	1	piece	Grain
Tortilla, Whole Wheat	**4.5**	1	piece	Grain
Tostada	**1.0**	1/4	piece	Vegetable
Trail Mix	**2.0**	1/4	cup	Legume/Nut/Seed
Treet	**-4.5**	2	wt oz	Meat/Fish/Poultry
Trout, Baked	**5.0**	3	wt oz	Meat/Fish/Poultry
Tuna Helper, Prepared	**2.5**	1/2	cup	Meat/Fish/Poultry
Tuna Noodle Casserole	**3.5**	1	cup	Meat/Fish/Poultry
Tuna Noodle Casserole, Frozen, Stouffer's	**0.0**	1/2	portion	Meat/Fish/Poultry
Tuna Salad	**3.0**	1/2	cup	Meat/Fish/Poultry
Tuna Salad, Nutripoint Recipe	**5.0**	1/2	cup	Meat/Fish/Poultry
Tuna, Albacore Solid White, Oil, Chicken of the Sea	**4.0**	1/2	cup	Meat/Fish/Poultry
Tuna, Canned In Oil	**2.0**	1/2	cup	Meat/Fish/Poultry
Tuna, Canned In Water	**7.5**	3/4	cup	Meat/Fish/Poultry
Tuna, Chunk Light, In Oil, Star-Kist	**1.5**	1/2	cup	Meat/Fish/Poultry
Tuna, Chunk Light, Oil, Chicken of the Sea	**3.5**	1/2	cup	Meat/Fish/Poultry
Tuna, Chunk Light, Water, Chicken of the Sea	**6.5**	3/4	cup	Meat/Fish/Poultry
Tuna, Chunk Light, Water, Low Sodium, Chicken of the Sea	**8.0**	1/2	cup	Meat/Fish/Poultry
Tuna, Diet Albacore, Chunk White, Water, Low Sodium, Chicken/Sea	**5.0**	1/2	cup	Meat/Fish/Poultry
Tuna, Fresh, Broiled	**6.5**	3	wt oz	Meat/Fish/Poultry
Tuna, Light Chunk, In Water, Bumble Bee	**7.0**	1/2	cup	Meat/Fish/Poultry
Tuna, Lite Chunk Light, Water & Oil, Chicken of the Sea	**6.0**	1/2	cup	Meat/Fish/Poultry
Tuna, Solid White, In Water, Star-Kist	**5.5**	1/2	cup	Meat/Fish/Poultry
Tuna, Solid White, Water, Chicken of the Sea	**5.5**	1/2	cup	Meat/Fish/Poultry
Tuna, Tonno, Solid Light, Oil, Chicken of the Sea	**4.0**	1/2	cup	Meat/Fish/Poultry
Tuna, White Solid, In Water, Bumble Bee	**6.5**	1/2	cup	Meat/Fish/Poultry
Tuno, Meatless Tuna, Worthington	**4.0**	1/2	cup	Legume/Nut/Seed
Turkey A La King, w/Rice, Fzn, Budget Gourmet	**-0.5**	1/2	portion	Meat/Fish/Poultry
Turkey Breast Slices, Louis Rich	**3.5**	3	slices	Meat/Fish/Poultry
Turkey Breast, Frozen, Healthy Choice	**2.0**	1	portion	Meat/Fish/Poultry
Turkey Breast, Grilled, Fzn, Healthy Choice	**1.0**	1	serving	Meat/Fish/Poultry

Food Name—Alphabetical	Nutripoints	Serving Size		Nutrigroup
Turkey Breast, Roasted, No Sodium Added, Mr. Turkey	**1.0**	4	wt oz	Meat/Fish/Poultry
Turkey Breast, Sliced, Frozen, Budget Gourmet	**0.5**	1/2	portion	Meat/Fish/Poultry
Turkey Breast, Sliced, Mr. Turkey	**1.0**	3	wt oz	Meat/Fish/Poultry
Turkey Breast, Sliced, Mushroom Sauce, Fzn, Stouffer's	**1.0**	1	portion	Meat/Fish/Poultry
Turkey Breast, Stuffed, Frozen, Weight Watchers	**-1.0**	1/2	portion	Meat/Fish/Poultry
Turkey Dinner, Frozen, Morton	**4.0**	1	portion	Meat/Fish/Poultry
Turkey Ham, Louis Rich	**1.0**	4	slices	Meat/Fish/Poultry
Turkey Pie, Frozen, Stouffer's	**-1.0**	1/2	pie	Meat/Fish/Poultry
Turkey Pot Pie	**0.5**	1/2	pie	Meat/Fish/Poultry
Turkey Pot Pie, Swanson	**-1.0**	1/2	pie	Meat/Fish/Poultry
Turkey Roll, Light Meat	**3.0**	3	wt oz	Meat/Fish/Poultry
Turkey Roll, Light/Dark Meat	**1.0**	4	wt oz	Meat/Fish/Poultry
Turkey Roll, White, Cooked, Mr. Turkey	**-0.5**	4	wt oz	Meat/Fish/Poultry
Turkey Sausage, Lean Italian, Jennie-O, Turkey Store	**1.0**	4	wt oz	Meat/Fish/Poultry
Turkey Slices, Veggie, Yves	**7.0**	4	slices	Legume/Nut/Seed
Turkey, Breast Slices, Turkey Store	**6.5**	4	wt oz	Meat/Fish/Poultry
Turkey, Breast Tenderloins, Turkey Store	**6.5**	4	wt oz	Meat/Fish/Poultry
Turkey, Burger Patties, Turkey Store	**2.5**	3.5	wt oz	Meat/Fish/Poultry
Turkey, Dark Meat and Skin, Baked	**1.0**	3 1/2	wt oz	Meat/Fish/Poultry
Turkey, Dark Meat, Baked w/o Skin	**3.0**	3	wt oz	Meat/Fish/Poultry
Turkey, Divan, Frozen, Le Menu	**0.5**	1	portion	Meat/Fish/Poultry
Turkey, Frozen Dinner	**3.5**	1/2	portion	Meat/Fish/Poultry
Turkey, Glazed, Slim, Frozen, Budget Gourmet	**0.5**	1	portion	Meat/Fish/Poultry
Turkey, Ground Breast Meat, Turkey Store	**6.5**	4	wt oz	Meat/Fish/Poultry
Turkey, Light Meat and Skin, Baked	**2.5**	3 1/2	wt oz	Meat/Fish/Poultry
Turkey, Light Meat Baked w/o Skin	**4.0**	3	wt oz	Meat/Fish/Poultry
Turkey, Light/Dark Meat, w/o Skin, Baked	**3.5**	3	wt oz	Meat/Fish/Poultry
Turkey, Luncheon Loaf, Louis Rich	**-1.0**	4	slices	Meat/Fish/Poultry
Turkey, Pie, Frozen, Morton	**-0.5**	1/2	pie	Meat/Fish/Poultry
Turkey, Slices, Frozen, Loma Linda Foods	**6.5**	2	wt oz	Legume/Nut/Seed
Turkey, w/Dressing & Potatoes, Fzn, Swanson	**-0.5**	1	portion	Meat/Fish/Poultry
Turkey, w/Dressing, Frozen, Morton	**4.0**	1	portion	Meat/Fish/Poultry
Turkey, White & Dark, Canned, Premium Chunk, Swanson	**0.0**	4	wt oz	Meat/Fish/Poultry
Turkey, White, Canned, Premium Chunk, Swanson	**3.5**	4	wt oz	Meat/Fish/Poultry
Turmeric	**0.5**	1	tsp	Condiment
Turnip Greens, Allen's	**44.5**	3	wt oz	Vegetable
Turnip Greens, Chopped, Cooked	**79.0**	1	cup	Vegetable
Turnip Greens, Seasoned, Nutripoint Recipe	**67.0**	1	cup	Vegetable
Turnips, Cooked	**19.5**	1	cup	Vegetable
Turnips, Raw	**18.0**	1/2	cup	Vegetable
Turnover, Blueberry, Frozen, Pepperidge Farm	**-2.0**	1/2	piece	Grain
Turnover, Fruit	**-1.5**	1	piece	Grain
Twinkies, Hostess	**-3.0**	1	piece	Grain

Food Name—Alphabetical	Nutripoints	Serving Size		Nutrigroup
Vanilla Extract	**0.0**	1	tsp	Condiment
Veal Chop, Medium Fat, Fried	**-0.5**	3	wt oz	Meat/Fish/Poultry
Veal Cutlet, Medium Fat, Braised	**1.0**	3	wt oz	Meat/Fish/Poultry
Veal Cutlet/Steak, Lean, Braised	**3.5**	3	wt oz	Meat/Fish/Poultry
Veal Marsala, Frozen, Le Menu	**-0.5**	1	portion	Meat/Fish/Poultry
Veal Parmigiana	**-1.5**	1/2	serving	Meat/Fish/Poultry
Veal Parmigiana Patty, Frozen, Weight Watchers	**1.0**	1	portion	Meat/Fish/Poultry
Veal Parmigiana, Frozen, Budget Gourmet	**0.0**	1/2	portion	Meat/Fish/Poultry
Veal Parmigiana, Frozen, Morton	**2.0**	1	portion	Meat/Fish/Poultry
Veal Patty, Fried	**1.0**	2	wt oz	Meat/Fish/Poultry
Veal Primavera, Frozen, Stouffer's	**-0.5**	1	portion	Meat/Fish/Poultry
Veal Roast, Lean, Braised	**2.0**	3	wt oz	Meat/Fish/Poultry
Veal Roast, Medium Fat, Braised	**0.5**	3	wt oz	Meat/Fish/Poultry
Vegeburger, Loma Linda Foods	**8.5**	4	wt oz	Legume/Nut/Seed
Vegetable Medley, Nutripoint Recipe	**48.5**	1	cup	Vegetable
Vegetable Melange, Peas, Carrots, Cauliflower, Corn, Trader Joe's	**1.0**	2/3	cup	Vegetable
Vegetable Stir Fry, Nutripoint Recipe	**13.5**	1/2	cup	Vegetable
Vegetables, Custom Cuisine w/Dijon, Fzn, Birds Eye	**18.0**	1/2	cup	Vegetable
Vegetables, Italian Style, Frozen, Birds Eye	**3.0**	1/2	cup	Vegetable
Vegetables, Japanese Style, Frozen, Birds Eye	**2.5**	1/2	cup	Vegetable
Vegetables, Mixed, Canned	**22.0**	1/2	cup	Vegetable
Vegetables, Mixed, Frozen, Birds Eye	**18.0**	1/2	cup	Vegetable
Vegetables, Mixed, Frozen, Cooked	**18.0**	1/2	cup	Vegetable
Vegetables, Pasta Primavera Style, Fzn, Birds Eye	**7.0**	1/2	cup	Vegetable
Vegetables, San Francisco Style, Fzn, Birds Eye	**0.5**	1/2	cup	Vegetable
Vegetables, Spring, Cheese Sauce, Frozen, Budget Gourmet	**4.5**	1/2	portion	Vegetable
Vegetarian Stew	**12.5**	1	cup	Vegetable
Veggie Burger, 365 Organic, Whole Foods	**2.5**	1	serving	Legume/Nut/Seed
Vegi-Patties, Frozen, Lifestream	**1.5**	1	patty	Legume/Nut/Seed
Venison, Baked	**8.5**	4	wt oz	Meat/Fish/Poultry
Venison, w/Juniper Berry Sauce, Nutripoint Recipe	**6.5**	6	wt oz	Meat/Fish/Poultry
ViaViente Nutritional Drink	**22.0**	8	fl oz	Fruit
Vinegar	**0.0**	1	Tbls	Condiment
Vitamin Water, Essential Orange-Orange, Glaceau	**6.0**	8	fl oz	Fruit
Vitamin Water, Formula 50 Grape, Glaceau	**5.5**	8	fl oz	Fruit
Vitamin Water, Stress-B Lemon-Lime, Glaceau	**12.5**	8	fl oz	Fruit
Vodka	**-16.5**	2	fl oz	Alcohol
Waffles	**4.0**	1	waffle	Grain
Waffles, Blueberry, Aunt Jemima	**2.0**	2	waffles	Grain
Waffles, Buttermilk, Jumbo, Downyflake	**0.0**	2	waffles	Grain
Waffles, Common Sense Oat Bran, Eggo	**3.5**	1 1/2	waffles	Grain
Waffles, Homestyle, Frozen, Eggo	**1.0**	1 1/2	waffles	Grain
Waffles, Honey Oat, Heart to Heart, Kashi	**15.5**	2	waffles	Grain

Food Name—Alphabetical	Nutripoints	Serving Size		Nutrigroup
Waffles, Nutri-Grain, Frozen, Eggo	**1.5**	1 1/2	waffles	Grain
Waffles, Organic Gorilla Banana, Nature's Path	**1.0**	2	waffles	Grain
Waffles, Original, Aunt Jemima	**1.0**	2	waffles	Grain
Waffles, Whole Grain Wheat/Oat Bran, Aunt Jemima	**10.5**	2	waffles	Grain
Walnuts, Baking, Diamond	**-0.5**	1	wt oz	Legume/Nut/Seed
Walnuts, Black	**0.5**	12	nuts	Legume/Nut/Seed
Walnuts, English or Persian	**0.0**	12	nuts	Legume/Nut/Seed
Water Chestnuts, Canned	**5.5**	1	cup	Vegetable
Watercress	**52.5**	20	pieces	Vegetable
Watermelon	**10.5**	1	cup	Fruit
Wendy's Apple Danish	**-1.0**	1/2	piece	Grain
Wendy's Bacon Swiss Hamburger	**-0.5**	1/4	burger	Meat/Fish/Poultry
Wendy's Breakfast Sandwich	**-2.5**	1/2	serving	Milk/Dairy
Wendy's Buttermilk Biscuit	**-1.5**	1/2	serving	Grain
Wendy's Butterscotch Pudding	**-2.5**	1/4	cup	Milk/Dairy
Wendy's Caesar Side Salad	**0.5**	1/3	serving	Vegetable
Wendy's California Coleslaw	**1.0**	1/4	cup	Vegetable
Wendy's Cheddar Chips	**-1.5**	1	wt oz	Grain
Wendy's Cheese Danish	**-1.5**	1/2	piece	Grain
Wendy's Chef Salad (take Out)	**6.0**	1/4	serving	Vegetable
Wendy's Chicken BLT Salad	**-1.5**	1/3	serving	Meat/Fish/Poultry
Wendy's Chicken Club Sandwich	**0.5**	1/2	serving	Meat/Fish/Poultry
Wendy's Chicken Fried Steak	**-2.0**	1/3	serving	Meat/Fish/Poultry
Wendy's Chicken Sandwich	**2.0**	1/2	serving	Meat/Fish/Poultry
Wendy's Chicken Strips Sandwich	**-1.5**	1/2	serving	Meat/Fish/Poultry
Wendy's Chocolate Chip Cookie	**-3.0**	1/2	cookie	Grain
Wendy's Chocolate Pudding	**-2.0**	1/4	cup	Milk/Dairy
Wendy's Cinnamon w/Raisin Danish	**-1.5**	1/2	piece	Grain
Wendy's Classic Hamburger	**0.0**	1/3	burger	Meat/Fish/Poultry
Wendy's Classic Hamburger w/Cheese	**-0.5**	1/3	piece	Meat/Fish/Poultry
Wendy's Creamy Peppercorn Dressing	**-6.0**	1	Tbls	Fat/Oil
Wendy's Crispy Chicken Nuggets (animal Oil)	**-2.0**	4	pieces	Meat/Fish/Poultry
Wendy's Crispy Chicken Nuggets (vegetable Oil)	**-1.5**	4	pieces	Meat/Fish/Poultry
Wendy's Crushed Red Peppers	**13.5**	1	Tbls	Vegetable
Wendy's Deluxe Three Bean Salad	**2.0**	1/4	cup	Vegetable
Wendy's Fish Sandwich	**0.0**	1/2	serving	Meat/Fish/Poultry
Wendy's French Toast	**-2.0**	1	piece	Grain
Wendy's Fresh Fruit Bowl	**8.5**	1/2	serving	Fruit
Wendy's Frosty Dairy Dessert	**-3.5**	1/2	serving	Milk/Dairy
Wendy's Garden Salad (take Out)	**16.5**	1/2	serving	Vegetable
Wendy's Homestyle Chicken Fillet	**0.5**	1/2	serving	Meat/Fish/Poultry
Wendy's Homestyle Chicken Strips Salad	**0.5**	1/3	serving	Meat/Fish/Poultry
Wendy's Hot Stuffed Potato	**4.5**	1/4	potato	Vegetable
Wendy's Hot Stuffed Potato w/Bacon & Cheese	**-0.5**	1/4	potato	Vegetable
Wendy's Hot Stuffed Potato w/Broccoli & Cheese	**1.5**	1/4	potato	Vegetable

Food Name—Alphabetical	Nutripoints	Serving Size		Nutrigroup
Wendy's Hot Stuffed Potato w/Cheese	**-2.0**	1/4	potato	Vegetable
Wendy's Hot Stuffed Potato w/Sour Cream & Chives	**0.0**	1/4	potato	Vegetable
Wendy's Imitation Cheese, Salad Bar	**1.5**	1	wt oz	Milk/Dairy
Wendy's Imitation Parmesan Cheese	**4.5**	1	wt oz	Milk/Dairy
Wendy's Imitation Sour Topping	**-3.5**	2	wt oz	Fat/Oil
Wendy's Jr. Cheeseburger	**1.0**	1/2	burger	Meat/Fish/Poultry
Wendy's Jr. Hamburger	**1.0**	1/2	burger	Meat/Fish/Poultry
Wendy's Mandarin Chicken Salad	**0.5**	1/3	serving	Meat/Fish/Poultry
Wendy's Mediterranean Chicken Salad	**1.0**	1/2	serving	Meat/Fish/Poultry
Wendy's New Beef Chili	**1.5**	1/2	serving	Meat/Fish/Poultry
Wendy's Old Fashioned Corn Relish	**-0.5**	1/4	cup	Vegetable
Wendy's Omelet #1 (eggs, Ham, Cheese)	**-7.0**	1/2	serving	Milk/Dairy
Wendy's Omelet #2 (eggs, Ham, Cheese, Mushroom)	**-10.0**	1/2	serving	Milk/Dairy
Wendy's Omelet #3 (eggs, Ham, Cheese, Onion)	**-10.0**	1/2	serving	Milk/Dairy
Wendy's Omelet #4 (eggs, Mushroom, Green Pepper, Onion)	**-11.5**	1	serving	Milk/Dairy
Wendy's Pasta Deli Salad	**1.5**	1	cup	Grain
Wendy's Philly Swiss Hamburger	**0.0**	1/2	burger	Meat/Fish/Poultry
Wendy's Picante Sauce	**3.0**	2	wt oz	Condiment
Wendy's Plain Single Hamburger	**0.5**	1/2	burger	Meat/Fish/Poultry
Wendy's Plain Single Hamburger w/Cheese	**0.0**	1/2	burger	Meat/Fish/Poultry
Wendy's Potato Chili Cheese	**-1.0**	1	wt oz	Milk/Dairy
Wendy's Red Bliss Potato Salad	**-1.5**	1/4	cup	Vegetable
Wendy's Sausage Gravy	**-3.0**	3	wt oz	Fat/Oil
Wendy's Sausage Patty	**-3.0**	1	patty	Meat/Fish/Poultry
Wendy's Side Salad	**29.0**	1	serving	Vegetable
Wendy's Single Cheese Hamburger w/Everything	**0.5**	1/2	burger	Meat/Fish/Poultry
Wendy's Single Hamburger w/Everything	**0.5**	1/2	burger	Meat/Fish/Poultry
Wendy's Sliced Pepperoni	**0.0**	1	wt oz	Meat/Fish/Poultry
Wendy's Small Cheeseburger	**1.0**	1/2	burger	Meat/Fish/Poultry
Wendy's Small Hamburger	**1.0**	1/2	burger	Meat/Fish/Poultry
Wendy's Spicy Chicken Fillet	**0.0**	1/3	serving	Meat/Fish/Poultry
Wendy's Spring Mix Salad	**0.5**	1/4	serving	Vegetable
Wendy's Taco Beef Salad	**2.0**	1	cup	Meat/Fish/Poultry
Wendy's Taco Chips	**0.0**	1	wt oz	Grain
Wendy's Taco Supreme Salad	**0.0**	1/3	serving	Legume/Nut/Seed
Wendy's Ultimate Chicken Grill Sandwich	**2.5**	1/2	serving	Meat/Fish/Poultry
Western Dinner, Frozen, Morton	**0.0**	1	portion	Meat/Fish/Poultry
Wheat Cakes, Quaker	**4.5**	3	cups	Grain
Wheat Germ	**10.5**	1/4	cup	Grain
Wheat Germ, Kretschmer	**12.0**	1/4	cup	Grain
Wheat Germ, Kretschmer, Honey Crunch	**8.0**	1	wt oz	Grain
Wheat, Whole Grain, Dry, Arrowhead Mills	**4.5**	2	wt oz	Grain
Whiskey	**-16.5**	2	fl oz	Alcohol
Whiskey Sour	**-19.0**	3	fl oz	Alcohol

Food Name—Alphabetical	Nutripoints	Serving Size		Nutrigroup
White Russian	**-13.0**	2	fl oz	Alcohol
Whiting, Broiled, Baked	**2.0**	4	wt oz	Meat/Fish/Poultry
Wine Cooler	**-9.0**	8	fl oz	Alcohol
Wine Spritzer	**-14.5**	6	fl oz	Alcohol
Wine, Chinese	**-14.5**	6	fl oz	Alcohol
Wine, Light	**-14.0**	6	fl oz	Alcohol
Wine, Sweet	**-13.0**	4	fl oz	Alcohol
Wine, Table	**-14.0**	6	fl oz	Alcohol
Yeast, Active Dry, Fleischmann's	**0.5**	0.25	wt oz	Miscellaneous
Yeast, Brewers	**3.5**	1	Tbls	Miscellaneous
Yeast, Dry Active	**4.5**	1	packet	Miscellaneous
Yellowtail, Raw	**-0.5**	4	wt oz	Meat/Fish/Poultry
Yogurt Drink, Frusion Smoothie, Dannon	**-0.5**	6	fl oz	Milk/Dairy
Yogurt Drink, Lowfat, Dan'Up, All Flavors, Dannon	**0.5**	1	cup	Milk/Dairy
Yogurt Drink, Nouriche Light, All Flavors, Yoplait	**10.5**	11	fl oz	Milk/Dairy
Yogurt Drink, Nouriche, All Flavors, Yoplait	**6.0**	6	fl oz	Milk/Dairy
Yogurt, Banana Custard Style, Yoplait	**-1.0**	4	wt oz	Milk/Dairy
Yogurt, Blended Lowfat, All Flavors, Horizon Organic	**1.0**	3/4	cup	Milk/Dairy
Yogurt, Blended Multipack, Columbo	**1.5**	1	cup	Milk/Dairy
Yogurt, Colombo Classic w/Fruit on Bottom	**0.0**	1	cup	Milk/Dairy
Yogurt, Creamy Fruit Blends, Dannon	**0.0**	6	wt oz	Milk/Dairy
Yogurt, Custard Style, All Flavors, Yoplait	**-0.5**	6	wt oz	Milk/Dairy
Yogurt, Fat Free, All Flavors, Horizon Organic	**2.0**	3/4	cup	Milk/Dairy
Yogurt, Fat-Free Light, Columbo	**4.0**	1	cup	Milk/Dairy
Yogurt, Frozen	**1.5**	4	wt oz	Milk/Dairy
Yogurt, Frozen, 90% Fat Free, Peanut Butter Cup, Colombo	**-1.5**	3	fl oz	Milk/Dairy
Yogurt, Frozen, 92% Fat Free, Mocha Swiss Almond, Colombo	**-1.5**	3	fl oz	Milk/Dairy
Yogurt, Frozen, 94% Fat Free, Bavarian Chocolate Crunch, Colombo	**-1.0**	3	fl oz	Milk/Dairy
Yogurt, Frozen, 94% Fat Free, Caramel Pecan Chunk, Colombo	**-0.5**	3	fl oz	Milk/Dairy
Yogurt, Frozen, 96% Fat Free, Vanilla Dream, Colombo	**0.0**	4	fl oz	Milk/Dairy
Yogurt, Frozen, 97% Fat Free, Strawberry Passion, Colombo	**0.0**	4	fl oz	Milk/Dairy
Yogurt, Frozen, Almond Amaretto, Brice's	**-0.5**	1/2	cup	Milk/Dairy
Yogurt, Frozen, Lowfat, Chocolate, Tuscan Pop	**-2.0**	1	piece	Milk/Dairy
Yogurt, Frozen, Lowfat, Peach, Blue Bell	**1.0**	1/2	cup	Milk/Dairy
Yogurt, Frozen, Lowfat, Raspberry, Blue Bell	**0.0**	1/2	cup	Milk/Dairy
Yogurt, Frozen, TCBY	**9.0**	5	wt oz	Milk/Dairy
Yogurt, Fruit	**2.0**	6	wt oz	Milk/Dairy
Yogurt, Fruit on the Bottom, Dannon	**0.5**	6	wt oz	Milk/Dairy
Yogurt, Go-GURT!, All Flavors, Yoplait	**-0.5**	2.25	wt oz	Milk/Dairy
Yogurt, Grande!, All Flavors, Yoplait	**0.0**	4	wt oz	Milk/Dairy

Food Name—Alphabetical	Nutripoints	Serving Size		Nutrigroup
Yogurt, Light 'N Fit Carb Control, Dannon	**3.0**	8	wt oz	Milk/Dairy
Yogurt, Light 'N Fit Creamy, Dannon	**5.0**	6	wt oz	Milk/Dairy
Yogurt, Light 'N Fit Smoothie Carb Control, Dannon	**3.0**	8	wt oz	Milk/Dairy
Yogurt, Light 'N Fit Smoothie, Dannon	**5.5**	8	wt oz	Milk/Dairy
Yogurt, Light 'N Fit, Dannon	**4.5**	8	wt oz	Milk/Dairy
Yogurt, Light, All Flavors, Yoplait	**5.5**	6	wt oz	Milk/Dairy
Yogurt, Lowfat, Boysenberry, Yoplait	**-0.5**	4	wt oz	Milk/Dairy
Yogurt, Lowfat, Cherry Vanilla, Borden	**-0.5**	4	wt oz	Milk/Dairy
Yogurt, Lowfat, Fruit On Bottom, All Flavors, Dannon	**1.0**	4	wt oz	Milk/Dairy
Yogurt, Lowfat, Nuts/Raisins/Fruit, Dannon	**0.5**	4	wt oz	Milk/Dairy
Yogurt, Lowfat, Nuts/Raisins/Vanilla, Dannon	**0.0**	4	wt oz	Milk/Dairy
Yogurt, Lowfat, Peach, Borden	**-0.5**	4	wt oz	Milk/Dairy
Yogurt, Lowfat, Plain	**7.0**	8	wt oz	Milk/Dairy
Yogurt, Lowfat, Plain, Dannon	**5.5**	8	wt oz	Milk/Dairy
Yogurt, Lowfat, Strawberry, Borden	**-0.5**	4	wt oz	Milk/Dairy
Yogurt, Lowfat, Strawberry, Yoplait	**-0.5**	4	wt oz	Milk/Dairy
Yogurt, Lowfat, Swiss Style Plain, Lite-Line, Borden	**1.5**	1	cup	Milk/Dairy
Yogurt, Natural Flavors Vanilla, Dannon	**2.5**	6	wt oz	Milk/Dairy
Yogurt, Nonfat, Plain, Dannon	**9.0**	1	cup	Milk/Dairy
Yogurt, Original, All Flavors, Yoplait	**0.5**	6	wt oz	Milk/Dairy
Yogurt, Pineapple All Natural, Breyer's	**-2.0**	4	wt oz	Milk/Dairy
Yogurt, Soft Frozen Peach, Yoplait	**-2.0**	1/2	cup	Milk/Dairy
Yogurt, Strawberry All Natural, Breyer's	**-2.0**	4	wt oz	Milk/Dairy
Yogurt, Trix, Yoplait	**0.0**	4	wt oz	Milk/Dairy
Yogurt, Ultra Low-Carb, All Flavors, Yoplait	**3.5**	6	wt oz	Milk/Dairy
Yogurt, Whips, All Flavors, Yoplait	**0.0**	4	wt oz	Milk/Dairy
Yogurt, Whole Milk, Plain	**2.5**	8	wt oz	Milk/Dairy
Yogurt, YoBaby Drinkable, Stonyfield Farm Organic	**2.0**	6	fl oz	Milk/Dairy
Yogurt, Yumsters, Yoplait	**0.0**	4	wt oz	Milk/Dairy
Zucchini, Cooked	**15.0**	1	cup	Vegetable
Zucchini, Raw	**16.0**	1	cup	Vegetable

POSTSCRIPT

"If your lifestyle does not control your body, eventually your body will control your lifestyle. The choice is yours."

Ern Baxter
Author of *I Almost Died*

WE ALL PAY LIP SERVICE TO THE VALUE OF GOOD HEALTH HABITS. We hear retired people say things such as, "As long as you've got your health ... ," and we agree, even if we're years from thinking that anything could go wrong with our health. But as the years go by, and we begin to see how things *can* go wrong—how friends and family members can be stricken by chronic illness—we begin to appreciate the idea that good health is a very valuable commodity. Unfortunately, for many people, it can be too late.

Ern Baxter had a heart attack in middle age that frightened him more than he ever thought he could be frightened. Suddenly, he faced the possibility of his life ending much sooner than he'd thought. After a sea change in his attitudes about health and fitness, he rehabilitated himself to the point where he feels better than he had ever felt before his brush with death. I've quoted above from his book because I think his comment crystallizes everything you need to know about respecting your body and doing your best to keep it in optimum condition.

Good nutrition is a major component of a healthy life. I think that Nutripoints will help you achieve the best level of nutrition you've ever experienced. I would like to point out that to achieve an optimum sense of well-being, you must make both exercise and stress control part of your regimen. I strongly suggest that you investigate these areas and adopt some form of exercise, as well as techniques for stress control, so that you can enjoy the maximum benefits of Nutripoints.

Some excellent books on exercise include Dr. Kenneth Cooper's *Aerobics Program for Total Well-Being* (Bantam, 1985) and Casey Meyer's *Walking: A Complete Guide to the Exercise* (Random House, 1992).

For a good introduction to stress management I recommend Dr. Robert Eliot's *Is it Worth Dying For?* (Bantam, 1989); Drs. Kreigel and Kriegel's *The C Zone: Peak Performance Under Pressure* (Ballantine, 1985); Dr. Herbert Bensen's *Beyond the Relaxation Response* (Berkeley, 1985); and Alan Lakein's *How to Get Control of Your Time and Your Life* (Signet, 1996).

As a final note, I'd like to say that I don't think nutrition, exercise, and stress control are the most important things in life. I think eating should be pleasurable. I think exercise should be fun. I think time spent with loved ones and devotion to spiritual goals are at the core of a happy life. But I've seen that optimum health can affect life for the better, and I know that good health is achievable. So I want to convince you that it's a gift you can give yourself. It can enhance every other aspect of your life. I hope that *Nutripoints* will make your ultimate life goals easier to achieve.

REFERENCES

Association of Vitamin Chemists, The. *Methods of Vitamin Assay.* New York: Interscience Publishers, 1966.

Bland, Dr. Jeffrey. *Nutraerobics.* San Francisco: Harper & Row, 1983.

Brody, Jane. *Jane Brody's Nutrition Book.* New York: Norton, 1981.

Carper, Jean. *Jean Carper's Total Nutrition Guide.* New York: Bantam, 1987.

Colbert, Don, MD. *Toxic Relief.* Siloam, 2003.

Connor, Sonja L., and William Connor. *The New American Diet.* New York: Simon & Schuster, 1986.

Cybersoft, Inc. *The NutriBase Nutrition Facts Desk Reference,* 2nd Edition. New York: Avery, 2001.

Hendler, Sheldon Saul, MD. *The Complete Guide to Anti-Aging Nutrients.* New York: Simon & Schuster, 1984.

Katch, Frank I., and William D. McArdle. *Nutrition, Weight Control, and Exercise.* Boston: Houghton Mifflin, 1988.

Last, John M., MD, ed. *Maxcy-Rosenau: Public Health and Preventive Medicine,* 11th ed. New York: Appleton-Century-Crofts, 1980.

Mayer, Jean. *A Diet for Living.* New York: David McKay, 1975.

McArdle, William D., Frank I. Katch, and Victor L. Katch. *Exercise Physiology: Energy, Nutrition, And Human Performance,* 5th Edition. Lippincott Williams & Wilkins, 2004.

National Cancer Institute. *Cancer Facts 3.19:* "Artificial Sweeteners", 2003.

National Research Council. *Diet and Health: Implications for Reducing Chronic Disease.* Washington, DC: National Academy Press, 1989.

National Research Council. *Recommended Dietary Allowances,* 10th revised ed. Washington, DC: National Academy of Sciences, 1992.

Ornish, Dean, MD. *Dr. Dean Ornish's Program for Reversing Heart Disease,* revised ed. Ballantine, 2004.

Paige, David M., MD, ed. *Manual of Clinical Nutrition.* Pleasantville, NJ: Nutrition Publications, 1983.

Pennington, Jean A. T., Ph.D., R.D., and Judith Spungen-Douglass, M.S.,R.D. *Bowes and Church's Food Values of Portions Commonly Used,* 18th ed. Lippincott Williams & Wilkins, 2004.

Saltman, Paul, Joel Gurin, and Ira Mothner. *California Nutrition Book.* Boston: Little Brown, 1987.

Schmid, Dr. Ronald F. *Traditional Foods Are Your Best Medicine.* New York: Ballantine, 1987.

Stunkard, Albert J., MD, ed. *Obesity.* Philadelphia: W. B. Saunders, 1980.

United States Department of Agriculture, Agricultural Research Service. *USDA National Nutrient Database for Standard Reference.* Release 18, 2005.

United States Department of Agriculture. *Composition of Foods.* Agriculture Handbooks 8-1 through 8-17 and 8-21, Washington, DC: USDA, 1978-1989.

United States Department of Agriculture. *Nutritive Value of Foods.* Home and Garden Bulletin No. 72, Washington, DC: U.S. Government Printing Office, 2002.

United States Department of Health and Human Services, Public Health Service, Centers for Disease Control. *Foodborne* Disease *Surveillance.* Annual Summary, 1982. Atlanta: U.S. Department of Health and Human Services, issued September 1985.

Walford, Roy L., MD. *Beyond the 120-Year Diet: How to Double Your Vital Years,* revised edition. Four Walls Eight Windows, 2004.

Weiner, Michael A. *The Way of the Skeptical Nutritionist.* New York: Macmillan, 1981.

Whalen, Dr. Elizabeth, and Dr. Frederic J. Stare. *The 100% Natural, Purely Organic, Cholesterol-Free, Megavitamin, Low-Carbohydrate Nutrition Hoax.* New York: Atheneum, 1983.

Worthington, Virginia, Sc.D. "Nutritional Quality of Organic Versus Conventional Fruits, Vegetables, and Grains." *The Journal of Alternative and Complementary Medicine,* Vol. 7:2, 2001, pp.161-173.

INDEX

D

E

F

M

N

O

P

Q

R

S

T

U

V

W

X

Y

Z

ABOUT THE AUTHOR

Roy E. Vartabedian, Dr.P.H., M.P.H., F.A.P.C.A. is a clinical preventive care specialist in private practice in Southern California, and President of Vartabedian & Associates/Designs for Wellness. A frequent lecturer and popular guest speaker, Dr. Vartabedian has appeared on the *Today Show, Live With Regis & Kathy Lee, Everyday With Joan Lunden* and a variety of other national and regional TV and radio programs. His breakthrough Nutripoint method has also been the subject of numerous articles in leading newspapers and magazines across the country such as *Ladies Home Journal, The New York Daily News* and *The Dallas Morning News.*

Previously, he held the position of Executive Director of the Cooper Clinic Residential Wellness Programs in Dallas for 6 years. He received his Doctor of Public Health degree (clinical preventive care) and Master of Public Health degree (nutrition, health education) from Loma Linda University, Loma Linda, California. Prior to his work in Dallas he taught Preventive Medicine at the Florida Hospital Family Practice Residency in Orlando for 4 years.

Dr. Vartabedian is available for public speaking engagements to your group. He also works as a consultant in the development of nutrition, wellness, and preventive medicine programs.

To contact Dr. Vartabedian, write to:

Vartabedian & Associates
P.O. Box 1671
Carlsbad, CA 92018
760 804-5999

Order Form

Please send the following *Nutripoint* Products immediately to:

Name: ______________________________

Address: ______________________________

City, State, Zip: ______________________________

Phone: ______________________

	Quantity	Price	Total
***Nutripoint* Program**	____	$65.00	____
Sales Tax (for California Deliveries)	____	5.04	____
Shipping/Handling	____	9.95	____
Planning & Tracking Software for *Nutripoints* (for use with Nutripoint Program)	____	$75.00	____
Sales Tax (for California Deliveries)	____	5.81	____
Shipping/Handling	____	3.95	____

TOTAL ____________

Send order form along with check, money order, or credit card # to:

Vartabedian & Associates or Phone: 1-888-796-5229
P.O. Box 1671 Fax: (760) 804-5996
Carlsbad, CA 92018-1671 **www.Nutripoints.com**

Card #: ______________________ Exp Date: __________

✓ one: ❑ MC ❑ VISA ❑ AMEX ❑ Discover

Signature: ______________________________

Thank you for your order. Please allow 1-2 weeks for delivery.
Volume discounts available. Please call for details.